Trigger Point Dry Needling

Content Strategist: Poppy Garraway/Serena Castelnovo
Content Development Specialist: Veronika Watkins
Senior Project Manager: Kamatchi Madhavan
Designer: Bridget Hoette

Trigger Point Dry Needling

An Evidence and Clinical-Based Approach

Second Edition

Edited by

JAN DOMMERHOLT, PT, DPT, MPS
Myopain Seminars, LLC, Bethesda, MD, USA; Bethesda Physiocare, Inc,
Bethesda, MD, USA

CÉSAR FERNÁNDEZ-DE-LAS-PEÑAS, PT, PhD,
Dr. SciMed
Department of Physical Therapy, Occupational Therapy, Physical
Medicine and Rehabilitation of Universidad Rey Juan Carlos, Alcorcón,
Madrid, Spain; Esthesiology Laboratory of Universidad Rey Juan Carlos,
Alcorcón, Madrid, Spain; and, Centre for Sensory-Motor Interaction
(SMI), Department of Health Science and Technology, Aalborg University,
Aalborg, Denmark

ELSEVIER

ELSEVIER

First edition 2013
Second edition 2018

ISBN 978-0-7020-7416-5
e-book 978-0-7020-7518-6

British Library Cataloguing in Publication Data
A catalogue record for this book is available from the British Library

Library of Congress Cataloging in Publication Data
A catalog record for this book is available from the Library of Congress

Notice
Knowledge and best practice in this field are constantly changing. As new research and experience broaden our knowledge, changes in practice, treatment and drug therapy may become necessary or appropriate. Readers are advised to check the most current information provided (i) on procedures featured or (ii) by the manufacturer of each product to be administered, to verify the recommended dose or formula, the method and duration of administration, and contraindications. It is the responsibility of the practitioner, relying on their own experience and knowledge of the patient, to make diagnoses, to determine dosages and the best treatment for each individual patient, and to take all appropriate safety precautions. To the fullest extent of the law, neither the Publisher nor the Editor assumes any liability for any injury and/or damage to persons or property arising out of or related to any use of the material contained in this book.

The Publisher

Printed in India

Last digit is the print number: 9 8 7

Contents

PART 3
OTHER DRY NEEDLING APPROACHES

Preface

Since the publication of the first edition of this book, the utilisation of dry needling in clinical practice has expanded dramatically throughout the world. Whereas initially mostly physiotherapists, chiropractors, and (Australian) myotherapists used dry needling, more recently, other healthcare providers have also started to incorporate dry needling into daily patient management. In many jurisdictions occupational therapists, athletic trainers, acupuncturists, osteopaths, dentists, physicians, and veterinary physicians are using dry needling for a wide variety of patients. Many professional sports teams in the United States and Europe are employing 'dry needlers' in the care of their athletes. Organizations such as the Association of Tennis Professionals and the Women's Tennis Association rely on physiotherapists to provide comprehensive therapy services that include dry needling. In the United States dry needling has even made its way into the emergency rooms with one hospital reporting a decrease of over 50% in opioid prescriptions in the year after the introduction of dry needling for musculoskeletal pain and dysfunction as reported by National Public Radio (All Things Considered, 20 February 2018). Dry needling is a cost effective remedy as part of a multimodal therapy program.

The range of dry needling applications has also expanded. Whereas most clinicians are targeting trigger points, dry needling is increasingly used for the treatment of individuals with tendinopathy, enthesopathy, and spasticity. Although research of dry needling for these conditions is still in its infancy, there is enough evidence to support adding new chapters to this book (Chapters 3 and 4). In addition, we have updated all other chapters with recent, up-to-date research and streamlined the clinical chapters with new colour illustrations. We made an exception for Chapter 13, authored by the late Dr. Peter Baldry (1920–2016). Baldry, who at one time was president of the British Medical Acupuncture Society, had a distinguished medical career that started well before the introduction of penicillin. At a time when most physicians would consider slowing down, Baldry started practicing acupuncture and trigger point dry needling, culminating in the publication of several textbooks and articles about superficial dry needling approach. In memory of Dr. Baldry, we included his original chapter in this volume.

As with the first edition, the ultimate objective of a clinical textbook is to contribute to developing optimal treatment approaches to benefit our patients. Dry needling is effective for reducing acute and chronic pain and improving motor performance, range of motion, and strength. We hope that the research on underlying mechanisms and clinical outcomes will continue in the years ahead.

Jan Dommerholt
Bethesda, MD, USA

César Fernández-de-las-Peñas
Madrid, Spain

Acknowledgements

A book on the current status of dry needling is dependent on the contributions of the authors. We would like to thank José L. Arias-Buría, Peter Baldry, Betty T.M. Beersma, Carel Bron, Cory B. Choma, Li-Wei Chou, Mike Cummings, Ana Isabel-de-la-Llave-Rincón, Michelle Finnegan, Jo L.M. Franssen, Zhonghua Fu, Javier González Iglesias, Steven R. Goodman, Blair Green, Christian Gröbli, Orlando Mayoral-del-Moral, Johnson McEvoy, Ricardo Ortega-Santiago, María Palacios-Ceña, Jaime Salom Moreno, Bárbara Torres-Chica, and María Torres-Lacomba for taking the time to share their experiences and insights.

We would also like to acknowledge the team at Elsevier, especially Serena Castelnovo and Poppy Garraway Smith (Content Strategist), Kamatchi Madhavan (Senior Project Manager), and Veronika Watkins (Content Development Specialist). We appreciate their patience, persistence, professionalism, and encouragement throughout the entire process of producing this second edition of the book.

DEDICATION

Jan Dommerholt would like to dedicate this book to Mona Mendelson, and Taliah and Aram Dommerholt.

César Fernández-de-las-Peñas would like to dedicate this book to his daughters, Marta, Sofia, and Estela Fernández-Alonso, and his second son, Miguel Angel, for his love from heaven.

Contributors

José L. Arias-Buría, PT, MSc, PhD
Department of Physical Therapy, Occupational Therapy, Physical Medicine and Rehabilitation of Universidad Rey Juan Carlos, Alcorcón, Madrid, Spain
Cátedra de Investigación y Docencia en Fisioterapia: Terapia Manual y Punción Seca, Universidad Rey Juan Carlos, Alcorcón, Madrid, Spain

Peter Baldry, MB, FRCP (deceased)
Formerly Consultant Physician, Ashford Hospital, North West London, UK
(Past President of British Medical Acupuncture Society and Acupuncture Association of Chartered Physiotherapists)

Betty T.M. Beersma, MPT
Practice for Musculoskeletal Disorders of the Neck, Shoulder, and Upper Extremity, Groningen, the Netherlands

Carel Bron, MPT, PhD
Practice for Musculoskeletal Disorders of the Neck, Shoulder, and Upper Extremity, Groningen, the Netherlands

Cory B. Choma, BscPT, Bsc (Chem.), CGIMS, Clinical Specialist (Pain Science)
Gunn IMS instructor for University of British Columbia
CSA Physiotherapy, Associate Clinic Owner
Director of Chronic Pain Department
Honorary Fellow of iSTOP, Edmonton, Alberta, Canada

Li-Wei Chou, MD, PhD
Director, Department of Physical Therapy and Graduate Institute of Rehabilitation Science, China Medical University, Taichung, Taiwan
Professor, Graduate Institute of Acupuncture Science, China Medical University, Taichung, Taiwan
Attending Physician, Department of Physical Medicine and Rehabilitation, China Medical University Hospital, Taichung, Taiwan
Chairman, Department of Physical Medicine and Rehabilitation, Asia University Hospital, Taichung, Taiwan

Dr Mike Cummings, MB ChB, DipMedAc
Medical Director, British Medical Acupuncture Society

Ana Isabel de-la-Llave-Rincón, PT, MSc, PhD
Department of Physical Therapy, Occupational Therapy, Rehabilitation and Physical Medicine, Universidad Rey Juan Carlos, Alcorcón, Madrid, Spain
Cátedra de Investigación y Docencia en Fisioterapia: Terapia Manual y Punción Seca, Universidad Rey Juan Carlos, Alcorcón, Madrid, Spain

Jan Dommerholt, PT, DPT, MPS
Myopain Seminars, LLC, Bethesda, MD, USA
Bethesda Physiocare, Inc, Bethesda, MD, USA

César Fernández-de-las-Peñas, PT, PhD, Dr. SciMed
Department of Physical Therapy, Occupational Therapy, Physical Medicine and Rehabilitation of Universidad Rey Juan Carlos, Alcorcón, Madrid, Spain
Centre for Sensory-Motor Interaction (SMI), Department of Health Science and Technology, Aalborg University, Aalborg, Denmark
Cátedra de Investigación y Docencia en Fisioterapia: Terapia Manual y Punción Seca, Universidad Rey Juan Carlos, Alcorcón, Madrid, Spain

Michelle Finnegan, PT, DPT, OCS, MTC, CMTPT, CCTT, FAAOMPT
Bethesda Physiocare, Bethesda, MD, USA
Myopain Seminars, Bethesda, MD, USA

Jo L.M. Franssen, PT
Myofasciale Pijn Seminars, Groningen, the Netherlands

Zhonghua Fu, MD, PhD
Professor, FSN Institute, Nanjing University of Chinese Medicine, Nanjing, China
Visiting Professor, Guangzhou University of Chinese Medicine, Guangzhou, China
Distinguished Expert, Beijing University of Chinese Medicine, Beijing, China

Steven R. Goodman, MS, MD
LearnIMS Continuing Education, Spokane, Washington
Gunn-IMS Instructor, Honorary Fellow, International Advisory Board, Institute for the Study and Treatment of Pain, Vancouver, BC, Canada
Clinical Assistant Professor, Department of Rehabilitation Medicine, University of Washington, Seattle, Washington, USA

Blair H. Green, PT, DPT, OCS, PHC, CMTPT
Catalyst Physical Therapy, Atlanta, GA, USA
Myopain Seminars, Bethesda, MD, USA

Christian Gröbli, PT
David G Simons Academy, DGSA®, Winterthur, Switzerland

Javier González Iglesias, PT, DO, PhD
Candás Fisioterapia Integral, Asturias, Spain

Johnson McEvoy, PT, DPT, MSc, MISCP
United Physiotherapy Clinic, Limerick, Ireland

Orlando Mayoral del Moral, PT, PhD
Physical Therapy Unit, Hospital Provincial de Toledo, Spain
Clínica de fisioterapia Orlando Mayoral, Madrid, Spain
Seminarios Travell y Simons®, Toledo, Spain

Jaime Salom Moreno, PT, PhD
Department of Physical Therapy, Occupational Therapy, Physical Medicine and Rehabilitation of Universidad Rey Juan Carlos, Alcorcón, Madrid, Spain

Cátedra de Investigación y Docencia en Fisioterapia: Terapia Manual y Punción Seca, Universidad Rey Juan Carlos, Alcorcón, Madrid, Spain

Ricardo Ortega-Santiago, PT, MSc, PhD
Department of Physical Therapy, Occupational Therapy, Rehabilitation and Physical Medicine, Universidad Rey Juan Carlos, Alcorcón, Madrid, Spain
Cátedra de Investigación y Docencia en Fisioterapia: Terapia Manual y Punción Seca, Universidad Rey Juan Carlos, Alcorcón, Madrid, Spain

María Palacios-Ceña, PT, MSc, PhD
Department of Physical Therapy, Occupational Therapy, Rehabilitation and Physical Medicine, Universidad Rey Juan Carlos, Alcorcón, Spain
Cátedra de Investigación y Docencia en Fisioterapia: Terapia Manual y Punción Seca, Universidad Rey Juan Carlos, Alcorcón, Madrid, Spain

Bárbara Torres-Chica, PT, PhD
Department of Physical Therapy, Universidad Nebrija, Madrid, Spain

María Torres-Lacomba, PT, PhD
Head of the Physiotherapy in Women's Health Research Group
Physical Therapy Department, Physical Therapy College, University of Alcalá, Alcalá de Henares, Madrid, Spain

CHAPTER 1

Basic Concepts of Myofascial Trigger Points

CÉSAR FERNÁNDEZ-DE-LAS-PEÑAS • JAN DOMMERHOLT

MYOFASCIAL TRIGGER POINT OVERVIEW

Myofascial trigger points (TrPs) are one of the most overlooked and ignored causes of acute and chronic pain (Hendler & Kozikowski, 1993). At the same time, TrPs constitute one of the most common musculoskeletal pain conditions (Hidalgo-Lozano et al., 2010; Bron et al., 2011a). There is overwhelming evidence that muscle pain is commonly a primary dysfunction (Mense, 2010a) and not necessarily secondary to other diagnoses. Muscles feature many types of nociceptors, which can be activated by a variety of mechanical and chemical means (Mense, 2009). As a primary problem, TrPs may occur in absence of other medical issues; however, TrPs can also be associated with underlying medical conditions (e.g., systemic diseases) or certain metabolic, parasitical, and nutritional disorders. As a comorbid condition, TrPs can be associated with other conditions such as osteoarthritis of the shoulder, hip, or knee (Bajaj et al., 2001) as well as with injuries such as whiplash (Freeman et al., 2009). Pain elicited by muscle TrPs constitutes a separate and independent cause of acute and especially chronic pain that may compound the symptoms of other conditions and persist long after the original initiating condition has been resolved. TrPs are also associated with visceral conditions and dysfunctions, including endometriosis, interstitial cystitis, irritable bowel syndrome, dysmenorrhea, and prostatitis (Weiss, 2001; Anderson, 2002; Doggweiler-Wiygul, 2004; Jarrell, 2004). The presence of abdominal TrPs was 90% predictive of endometriosis (Jarrell, 2004).

Throughout history TrPs have been referred to by different names (Simons, 1975). The current TrP terminology has evolved during the past several decades (Simons et al., 1999; Dommerholt et al., 2006; Dommerholt & Shah, 2010). Although different definitions of TrPs are used among different disciplines, the most commonly accepted definition maintains that 'a TrP is a hyperirritable spot in a taut band of a skeletal muscle that is painful on compression, stretch, overload, or contraction of the tissue, which usually responds with a referred pain that is perceived distant from the spot' (Simons et al., 1999).

From a clinical viewpoint, we can distinguish active and latent TrPs. The local and referred pain from active TrPs reproduces the symptoms reported by patients and is recognised by patients as their usual or familiar pain (Simons et al., 1999). Both active and latent TrPs cause allodynia at the TrP and secondary hyperalgesia after applied pressure. Allodynia is pain due to a stimulus that does not normally provoke pain. In latent muscle TrPs the local and referred pain do not reproduce any symptoms familiar or usual to the patient (Simons et al., 1999). Active and latent TrPs have similar physical findings. The difference is that latent TrPs do not reproduce any spontaneous symptoms other than referred pain. In patients with lateral epicondylalgia, active TrPs commonly reproduce the symptoms within the affected arm (Fernández-Carnero et al., 2007); however, patients may also present with latent TrPs on the nonaffected side without experiencing any symptoms on that side (Fernández-Carnero et al., 2008). In a recent Delphi study with 60 experts from 12 countries, 80% of the participants agreed that referred pain from TrPs can include different sensory sensations, including pain, a dull ache, tingling, or burning pain. Eighty-four percent of the experts agreed that the reproduction of symptoms experienced by patients and the recognition of pain are the main clinical differences between active and latent TrPs (Fernández-de-las-Peñas & Dommerholt, 2018).

Although latent TrPs are not spontaneously painful, they provide nociceptive input into the dorsal horn (Ge et al., 2008, 2009; Li et al., 2009; Zhang et al., 2009; Wang et al., 2010; Xu et al., 2010; Zhang et al., 2009; Ge & Arendt-Nielsen, 2011). The underlying mechanism is not clear at this point in time and requires more research. Certain regions within a muscle may only be connected via ineffective synapses to dorsal horn neurons and referred pain may occur when these ineffective synapses are sensitised (Mense, 2010b). Latent TrPs can easily turn into active TrPs, which is at least partially dependent on the degree of sensitisation and increased synaptic efficacy in the dorsal horn. For example, the pain pressure threshold of latent TrPs in the forearm muscles decreased significantly after only 20 minutes of continuous piano playing (Chen et al., 2000). Active TrPs induce larger referred pain areas and higher pain intensities than latent TrPs (Hong et al., 1997). Active TrPs and their overlying cutaneous and subcutaneous tissues are usually more sensitive to pressure and electrical stimulation than latent TrPs (Vecchiet et al., 1990, 1994).

Both active and latent TrPs can provoke motor dysfunctions, for example, muscle weakness, inhibition, increased motor irritability, spasm, muscle imbalance, and altered motor recruitment (Lucas et al., 2004, 2010) in either the affected muscle or in functionally related muscles (Simons et al., 1999). Lucas and colleagues (2010) demonstrated that latent TrPs were associated with impaired motor activation pattern, confirmed more recently by Bohlooli and colleagues (2016). Elimination of these latent TrPs induces normalisation of the impaired motor activation pattern (Lucas et al., 2010). In another study, restrictions in ankle range of motion were corrected after manual release of latent TrPs in the soleus muscle (Grieve et al., 2011). Manual treatment of latent TrPs in the upper trapezius muscle significantly decreased TrP sensitivity, increased flexibility of muscle fibres, and improved range of motion (Ganesh et al., 2016; Kojidi et al., 2016).

NEUROPHYSIOLOGICAL BASIS OF MUSCLE REFERRED PAIN

Referred pain is a phenomenon described for more than a century and has been used extensively as a diagnostic tool in the clinical setting. Typically pain from deep structures such as muscles, joints, ligaments, tendons, and viscera is described as deep, diffuse, and difficult to locate accurately in contrast to superficial types of pain such as pain originating in the skin (Mense, 1994). Pain located at the source of pain is termed *local pain* or *primary pain*, whereas pain felt in a different region away from the source of pain is termed *referred pain* or *secondary hyperalgesia* (Ballantyne et al., 2010). Referred pain can be perceived in any region of the body, but

the size of the referred pain area is variable and can be influenced by pain-induced changes in central somatosensory maps (Kellgren, 1938; Gandevia & Phegan, 1999). Referred pain is a very common phenomenon in clinical practice; most patients with chronic pain present with what is commonly described as 'a summation of referred pain from several different structures'. Understanding at least the basic neurophysiological mechanisms of muscle referred pain is required to make a proper diagnosis of myofascial pain and to manage patients with TrPs.

Clinical Characteristics of Muscle Referred Pain

Clinical characteristics of muscle referred pain (Arendt-Nielsen & Ge, 2009; Fernández-de-las-Peñas et al., 2011) include the following:

1. The duration of referred pain can last for as short as a few seconds or as long as a few hours, days, or weeks, or occasionally indefinitely.
2. Muscle referred pain is described as deep, diffuse, burning, tightening, or pressing pain, which is completely different from neuropathic or cutaneous pain.
3. Referred pain from muscle tissues may have a similar topographical distribution as referred pain from joints.
4. The referred pain can spread cranial/caudal or ventral/dorsal.
5. The intensity of muscle referred pain and the size of the referred pain area are positively correlated to the degree of irritability of the central nervous system or sensitisation.
6. Referred pain frequently follows the distribution of sclerotomes but not of dermatomes.
7. Muscle referred pain may be accompanied by other symptoms such as numbness, coldness, stiffness, weakness, fatigue, or musculoskeletal motor dysfunction. Perhaps the term 'referred sensation' more accurately describes the phenomenon as nonpainful sensations such as burning and tingling are also associated with TrPs.

Mechanisms and Neurophysiological Models of Referred Pain

The exact neuropathways mediating referred pain are not completely understood, but there are enough data to support that 'muscle referred pain is a process of central sensitisation, which is mediated by a peripheral activity and sensitisation, and which can be facilitated by sympathetic activity and dysfunctional descending inhibition' (Ge et al., 2006; Arendt-Nielsen & Ge,

2009). Increased autonomic activity is likely due to activation of adrenergic receptors at the motor endplate (Gerwin et al., 2004). Stimulation of these adrenergic receptors triggered an increased release of ACh in mice (Bowman et al., 1988). Nociceptive stimuli of latent TrPs can lead to autonomic changes such as vasoconstriction (Kimura et al., 2009). The local or systemic administration of the alpha-adrenergic antagonist phentolamine to TrPs caused an immediate reduction in electrical activity, suggesting that TrPs indeed have an autonomic component (Hubbard & Berkoff, 1993; Lewis et al., 1994; McNulty et al., 1994; Banks et al., 1998). Such increased autonomic activity may facilitate an increased concentration of intracellular ionised calcium and be responsible again for a vicious cycle maintaining TrPs (Gerwin et al., 2004; Gerwin, 2008). Muscle spindle afferents may also contribute to the formation of TrP taut bands via afferent signals to extrafusal motor units through H-reflex pathways (Ge et al., 2009) but are not considered to be the primary cause of TrP formation.

Several neuroanatomical and neurophysiological theories regarding the appearance of referred pain have been suggested. All models agree that nociceptive dorsal horn or brainstem neurons receive convergent inputs from different tissues. Consequently, higher brain centres cannot identify the input source properly. Most recent models have included newer theories in which sensitisation of dorsal horn and brainstem neurons also plays a relevant and central role. Following is a brief summary the most common theories.

Convergent-projection theory

Ruch (1961) proposed that afferent fibres from different tissues such as skin, viscera, muscles, and joints converge onto common spinal neurons, which can lead to a misinterpretation of the source of nociceptive activity from the spinal cord. The source of pain of one tissue can be misinterpreted as originating from other structures. The convergent-projection theory would explain the segmental nature of muscle referred pain and the increased referred pain intensity when local pain is intensified. This theory does not explain, however, the delay in the development of referred pain after the onset of local pain (Graven-Nielsen et al., 1997a).

Convergence-facilitation theory

The somatosensory sensitivity changes reported in referred pain areas can in part be explained by sensitisation mechanisms in the dorsal horn and brainstem neurons, whereas the delay in appearance of referred pain can be explained because the creation of central sensitisation needs time (Graven-Nielsen et al., 1997a).

Axon-reflex theory

Bifurcation of afferents from different tissues was suggested as an explanation of referred pain (Sinclair et al., 1948). Although bifurcation of nociceptive afferents from different tissues exits, it is generally agreed that these pathways are unlikely to occur (McMahon, 1994). The axon-reflex theory cannot explain the delay in the appearance of the referred pain, the different thresholds required for eliciting local pain versus referred pain, or the somatosensory sensitivity changes within the referred pain areas.

Thalamic-convergence theory

Theobald (1949) suggested that referred pain appears as a summation of input from the injured area and from the referred pain area within neurons in the brain but not in the spinal cord. Several decades later, Apkarian and colleagues (1995) described several pathways converging on different subcortical and cortical neurons. There is evidence of pain reduction after anaesthetisation of the referred pain area, which suggests that peripheral processes contribute to referred pain, although central processes are assumed to be the most predominant.

Central hyperexcitability theory

Recordings from dorsal horn neurons in animal models have revealed that new receptive fields at a distance from the original receptive field emerged within minutes after noxious stimuli (Hoheisel et al., 1993): that is, after nociceptive input, dorsal horn neurons that were previously responsive to only one area within a muscle began to respond to nociception from areas that previously did not trigger a response. The appearance of new receptive fields could indicate that latent convergent afferents on the dorsal horn neuron are opened by noxious stimuli from muscle tissues (Mense, 1994) and that this facilitation of latent convergence connections induces the referred pain. More recently, similar patterns have been identified for nociceptive input from fascial structures (Taguchi et al., 2008). In fact, several studies showed that mechanical hyperalgesia was larger in fascia than in muscle (Schilder et al., 2014; Weinkauf et al., 2015).

The central hyperexcitability theory is consistent with most of the characteristics of muscle and fascia referred pain. There is a dependency on the stimulus and a delay in appearance of referred pain compared with local pain. The development of referred pain in healthy subjects is generally distal and not proximal to the site of induced pain, (Arendt-Nielsen et al., 2000), although several clinical studies have demonstrated proximal and distal referred pain in patients with chronic pain (Graven-Nielsen, 2006). The differences between healthy individuals and persons with persistent pain may indicate that preexisting pain may induce a state of hyperexcitability in the spinal cord or brainstem, resulting in proximal and distal referred pain.

NEUROPHYSIOLOGICAL ASPECTS OF MYOFASCIAL TRIGGER POINTS
The Nature of Trigger Points
Taut bands

TrPs are located within discrete bands of contractured muscle fibres, which are commonly referred to as *taut bands* in the TrP literature. Taut bands can be palpated with a flat or pincer palpation and feel like tense strings within the belly of the muscle. It is important to clarify that contractures are not the same as muscle spasms. Muscle spasms require electrogenic activity, meaning that the α-motor neuron and the neuromuscular endplate are active. A muscle spasm is a pathological involuntary electrogenic contraction (Simons & Mense, 1998). In contrast, a taut band signifies a *contracture* arising endogenously within a certain number of muscle fibres independent of electromyogenic activity, which does not involve the entire muscle (Simons & Mense, 1998).

In 1997 Gerwin and Duranleau first described the visualisation of taut bands using sonography, but until recently it was not yet possible to visualise the actual TrP (Lewis & Tehan, 1999), mostly due to technological limitations (Park & Kwon, 2011). With the advancement of technology, more recent studies have found that TrP taut bands can be visualised using sonographic and magnetic resonance elastography (MRE) (Chen et al., 2007, Chen, Basford, & An et al., 2008, 2016; Sikdar et al., 2009; Bubnov, 2010; Rha et al., 2011; Maher et al., 2013; Müller et al., 2015). Chen and colleagues (2007) demonstrated that the stiffness of the taut bands in patients with TrPs is higher than that of the surrounding muscle tissue in the same subject and in people without TrPs. Sikdar and colleagues (2009) showed that vibration amplitudes assessed with spectral Doppler were 27% lower on average within the TrP region compared with surrounding tissue. They also found reduced vibration amplitude within the hypoechoeic region identified as a TrP. In summary, TrP taut bands are detectable and quantifiable, providing potentially useful tools for TrP diagnosis and future studies. Research to determine the correlation of clinician-identified myofascial taut bands with their presence and characteristics on MRE imaging showed that the agreement between physicians and MRE raters was relatively poor. The presence of taut bands as localised areas of increased muscle stiffness was confirmed once again, meaning they can be assessed quantitatively (Chen et al., 2016).

Although TrPs and taut bands can now be visualised, the mechanism for the formation of muscle taut band is still not fully understood (Gerwin, 2008). The current thinking is that the development of the taut band and subsequent pain are related to local muscle overload or overuse when the muscle cannot respond adequately, particularly after unusual or excessive eccentric or concentric loading (Gerwin et al., 2004; Gerwin, 2008; Mense & Gerwin, 2010).

Muscle failure and TrP formation are also common with submaximal muscle contractions as seen, for example, in the upper trapezius muscles of computer operators (Treaster et al., 2006; Hoyle et al., 2011) or in the forearm muscles of pianists (Chen et al., 2000). The failure of the muscle to respond to a particular acute or recurrent overload may be the result of a local energy crisis. Muscle activation in response to a demand is always dispersed throughout the muscle among fibres that are the first to be contracted and the last to relax. These fibres are the most vulnerable to muscle overload. Unusual or excessive eccentric loading may cause local muscle injury. In submaximal contractions, the Cinderella hypothesis and Henneman's size principle apply (Kadefors et al., 1999; Chen et al., 2000; Hägg, 2003; Zennaro et al., 2003; Treaster et al., 2006; Hoyle et al., 2011). Smaller motor units are recruited first and derecruited last without any substitution of motor units. This would lead to local biochemical changes without muscle breakdown, especially in those parts of the muscle that are not substituted and therefore most heavily worked (Gerwin, 2008).

The motor endplate. Under normal physiological conditions, nerve impulses from a α-motor neuron reach the motor nerve terminal orthodromically and open voltage-gated sodium (Na^+) channels, which trigger a Na^+ influx that depolarises the terminal membrane. Next, voltage-gated P-type calcium (Ca^{2+}) channels are opened, causing an influx of Ca^{2+} and a quantal, but graded, release of approximately 100 acetylcholine-containing synaptic vesicles (ACh), adenosine triphosphate (ATP), serotonin (5HT), glutamate, and calcitonin gene-related peptide (CGRP), among other molecules from the nerve terminal into the synaptic cleft (Wessler, 1996; Malomouzh et al., 2007). The release of ACh is highly regulated; normally, inhibitory neuronal receptors, including muscarinic, alpha 2- and beta-adrenoceptors, nitric oxide (NO) receptors, and purinergic P2Y receptors, among others, prevent an excessive release of acetylcholine release (Wessler, 1996). Under normal circumstances, these inhibitory mechanisms prevent the development of persistent contractures as seen in myofascial pain.

Of importance is that ACh release can be quantal and nonquantal. After exocytosis, ACh crosses the synaptic cleft and binds to acetylcholine receptors (AChR) on the motor endplate. In less than a millisecond, ACh is partially diffused and partially hydrolyzed by the enzyme acetylcholinesterase (AChE) into acetate and choline. Choline is reabsorbed into the nerve terminal where, by combining choline and acetyl coenzyme A from the mitochondria, it is synthesised into ACh via acetyltransferase. ACh release is modulated by the concentration of AChE. There are two sources of AChE in the synaptic cleft. A soluble form of AChE prevents ACh from reaching the receptors. The second source is the AChE that is found within the synaptic clefts; this AChE removes ACh from the receptors binding sites. Inhibition of AChE will cause an accumulation of ACh in the synaptic cleft, which may stimulate motor nerve endings and tonically activate nAChRs. Inhibition of AChE may also cause an increase of intracellular levels of Ca^{2+}, which likely contributes to the formation of taut bands. AChE is inhibited in an acidic environment and by calcitonin gene-related peptide. The nAChRs are temporarily inhibited after stimulation by ACh (Magleby & Pallotta, 1981). As a side note, ATP also plays a key role in the synthesis of AChE and nAChR through P2Y1 nucleotide receptors (Choi et al., 2003).

The nonquantal release does not involve activation via the α-motor neuron. Nonquantal release contributes to maintaining the functional properties of skeletal muscles and to various neurotrophic functions of the motor endplate itself. It may also contribute to the formation of abnormal contractures or taut bands seen in myofascial pain conditions. TrPs are often viewed as loci of multiple localised sarcomere contractions, but this has not yet been fully confirmed. Biopsy studies of TrPs in fresh cadavers showed fully contracted sarcomeres with an absence of the I-band and an excess of the A-band (Reitinger et al., 1996; Windisch et al., 1999), but one cannot assume that no changes occurred after the time of death and before the onset of rigor mortis.

Presynaptic ATP inhibits the release of quantal ACh through purinergic P2Y receptors, which implies that a decrease in ATP would lead to an increased release of ACh, which may be involved in the TrP pathophysiology. This process is also redox dependent and, as such, oxidative stress may further facilitate the presynaptic inhibition.

Of interest is that the nonquantal release of ACh is also significantly reduced by ATP, but not by adenosine. Blocking ATP with the purinergic receptor antagonist suramin ceases the effect of ATP and immediately increases the nonquantal secretion of ACh. Suramin also inhibits the activity of NO synthase, and a lack of NO increases the nonquantal release of ACh as well. Malomouzh and colleagues (2011) established that the inhibitory effect of ATP on the nonquantal release of ACh occurs through the phospholipase C via metabotropic P2Y purinergic receptors.

Adenosine is a neurotransmitter that synchronises the release of quantal release of ACh. It is a product of the breakdown of adenosine 5′ triphosphate and acts at the inhibitory adenosine A1 and facilitatory A2a receptors. Activation of A1 receptors reduces the number of ACh molecules released in each quantum. Increasing intracellular Ca^{2+} in the nerve terminal activates the exocytotic process that is mediated by A2a receptors. The A2a receptors also contribute to the facilitatory effect of CGRP on the release of ACh. In addition, modulation of a quantal ACh release occurs through secondary messenger systems involving protein kinase A and C (PKA and PKC).

The potential role of CGRP in myofascial pain and other pain conditions such as migraines cannot be underestimated. CGRP is found in higher concentrations in the immediate environment of active TrP (Shah et al., 2008). It is a potent microvascular vasodilator involved in wound healing, prevention of ischemia, and several autonomic and immune functions (Smillie & Brain, 2011). CGRP and its receptors are widely expressed in the central and peripheral nervous system. For example, CGRP type I is produced in the cell body of motor neurons in the ventral horn of the spinal cord and is excreted via an axoplasmatic transport mechanism. CGRP is also released from the trigeminal ganglion and from trigeminal nerves within the dura and, as such, contributes to peripheral sensitisation (Durham & Vause, 2010). It stimulates the phosphorylation of ACh receptors, which prolongs their sensitivity to ACh (Hodges-Savola & Fernandez, 1995). In addition, CGRP promotes the release of ACh and inhibits AChE.

Interestingly, myofascial tension, as seen with TrPs, may also stimulate an excessive release of ACh, which suggests the presence of a self-sustaining vicious cycle (Chen & Grinnell, 1997; Grinnel et al., 2003). Experimental research of rodents demonstrated that excessive ACh in the synaptic cleft leads to morphological changes resembling TrP contractures (Mense et al., 2003). Consuming excessive amounts of coffee in combination with alcohol triggers a similar response pattern, which has been attributed to the ability of caffeine to release Ca^{2+} from the sarcoplasmic reticulum (Oba et al., 1997a, 1997b; Shabala et al., 2008).

Many human, rabbit, and equine studies of TrPs have confirmed the presence of spontaneous electrical activity of continuous low amplitude referred to as endplate noise (EPN) and intermittent large amplitude spikes referred to as endplate spikes (EPS) (Bron and Dommerholt, 2012). The prevalence of EPN and EPS is correlated with the degree of irritability and pain (Kuan et al., 2007b). Of interest is a recent study of dry needling at myofascial trigger spots in model rats, which showed increased levels of ACh and nAChr at TrP locations, but not in controls without TrPs or in non-TrP sites (Liu et al., 2017). Dry needling caused a significant decrease in ACh, nAChRs, EPN, and EPS. EPN and EPS are hypothesised to be the result of an excess release of ACh at the motor endplate. Failure of the motor endplate is likely an intrinsic dysfunction of the endplate itself, as the degree of endplate noise does not change when the motor nerve is transected (Hong and Yu, 1998).

Local twitch response

Manual strumming or needling of a TrP usually result in a so-called local twitch response (LTR), which is a sudden contraction of muscle fibres in a taut band (Hong & Simons, 1998). LTRs can be observed visually, can be recorded electromyographically, or can be visualised with diagnostic ultrasound (Gerwin & Duranleau, 1997; Rha et al., 2011). The number of LTRs may be related to the irritability of the muscle TrP (Hong et al., 1997), although some muscles such as the triceps brachii commonly feature many LTRs. The irritability appears to be correlated with the degree of sensitisation of muscle nociceptors by bradykinin, serotonin, and prostaglandin, among others. Hong and Torigoe (1994) reported that LTRs could be elicited in an animal model by needling of hypersensitive trigger spots, which are the equivalent of TrPs in humans. LTRs were observed in only a few of the control sites. In addition, LTRs could not be elicited after transection of the innervating nerve. LTRs are spinal cord reflexes elicited by stimulating the sensitive site in the TrP region (Hong et al., 1995). Audette and colleagues (2004) reported that dry needling of active TrPs in the trapezius

and levator scapulae muscles elicited bilateral LTRs in 61.5% of the muscles, whereas dry needling of latent TrPs resulted only in unilateral LTRs.

Eliciting LTRs has been advocated for effective TrP dry needling (Hong, 1994). After LTR, Shah and colleagues (2005) observed an immediate drop in concentrations of several neurotransmitters, including CGRP and substance P, and several cytokines and interleukins in the extracellular fluid of the local TrP milieu. The concentrations did not quite reach the levels of normal muscle tissue. The reductions were observed during approximately 10 minutes before they appeared to slowly rise again. Due to the short observation times, it is not known whether the concentrations stabilised or increased again over time. Recently several authors have questioned whether eliciting LTRs is necessary or even desirable (Koppenhaver et al., 2017; Perreault et al., 2017), which will be addressed in more detail in Chapter 2.

Muscle pain

Muscle pain follows noxious stimuli, which activate specific peripheral nociceptors. If nociceptive impulses exceed the threshold of various nociceptors, they are transmitted through second order neurons in the dorsal horn, through the spinal cord, and to primary and secondary somatosensory areas in the brain, including the amygdala, anterior cingulated gyrus, and the primary sensory cortex. Locally, activation of receptors leads to the release of neuropeptides, which also causes vasodilatation and increase the permeability of the microvasculature (Snijdelaar et al., 2000; Ambalavanar et al., 2006). When neuropeptides are released in sufficient quantity, they trigger the release of histamine from mast cells, BK from kallidin, 5-HT from platelets, and PGs from endothelial cells (Massaad et al., 2004); this release leads to a vicious cycle as these chemicals also activate peripheral nociceptive receptors and potentiate dorsal horn neuron sensitisation. As such, muscle nociceptors play an active role in muscle pain and in the maintenance of normal tissue homoeostasis by assessing the peripheral biochemical milieu and by mediating the vascular supply to peripheral tissue.

The responsiveness of receptors is indeed a dynamic process and can change depending on the concentrations of the sensitising agents. As an example, under normal circumstances the BK receptor, knows as a B2 receptor, triggers only a temporary increase of intracellular calcium and does not play a significant role in sensitisation. When the BK concentration increases, a B1 receptor is synthesised that facilitates a long-lasting increase of intracellular calcium and stimulates the release of tumour necross factor and other interleukins, which in turn lead to increased concentrations of BK and peripheral sensitisation (Calixto et al., 2000; Marceau et al., 2002). There are many interactions between these chemicals making muscle pain a very complicated phenomenon. Babenko and colleagues (1999) found that the combination of BK and 5-HT induced higher sensitisation of nociceptors than each substance in isolation.

Referred pain occurs at the dorsal horn level and is the result of activation of otherwise quiescent axonal connections between affective nerve fibres dorsal horn neurons, which are activated by mechanisms of central sensitisation (Mense & Gerwin, 2010). Referred pain is not unique to myofascial TrPs, but, nevertheless, it is highly characteristic of myofascial pain syndrome. Usually referred pain happens within seconds after mechanical stimulation of active TrPs, suggesting that the induction of neuroplastic changes related to referred pain is a rapid process. Kuan and colleagues (2007a) demonstrated that TrPs are more effective in inducing neuroplastic changes in the dorsal horn neurons than non-TrPs regions.

The multiple contractures found in muscles of patients with myofascial pain can compress regional arteries, resulting in ischemia and hypoxia. Recent Doppler ultrasound studies confirmed a higher outflow resistance or vascular restriction at active TrPs and an increased vascular bed outside the immediate environment of TrPs, which is consistent with the measurement of decreased oxygen saturation levels within TrPs and increased levels outside the core of TrPs (Brückle et al., 1990; Ballyns et al., 2011). Hypoxia may trigger an immediate increased release of ACh at the motor endplate (Bukharaeva et al., 2005). Hypoxia also leads to a decrease of the local pH, which will activate transient receptor potential vanilloid (TRPV) receptors and acid sensing ion channels (ASIC), among many others, via hydrogen ions or protons. Because these channels are nociceptive, they initiate pain, hyperalgesia, and central sensitisation without inflammation or any damage or trauma to the muscle (Sluka et al., 2001, 2002, 2003, 2009; Deval et al., 2010). Research at the US National Institutes of Health has confirmed that the pH in the direct vicinity of active TrPs is well below 5 (Shah et al, 2005), which is sufficient to activate muscle nociceptors (Sahlin et al., 1976; Gautam et al., 2010). Different kinds of ASICs play specific roles (Walder et al., 2010), and it is not known which specific ASICs are activated in myofascial pain. It is likely that multiple types of ASICs are involved in the sensory aspects of TrPs (Dommerholt, 2011) such as the ASIC1a,

which processes noxious stimuli, and the ASIC3, which is involved in inflammatory pain (Shah et al., 2005; Deval et al., 2010). A low pH down-regulates AChE at the neuromuscular junction and can trigger the release of several neurotransmitters and inflammatory mediators such as CGRP, substance P, BK, interleukins, ATP, 5-HT, PG, potassium, and protons; this would result in a decrease in the mechanical threshold and activation of peripheral nociceptive receptors. A sensitised muscle nociceptor has a lowered stimulation threshold into the innocuous range and will respond to harmless stimuli such as light pressure and muscle movement. When nociceptive input to the spinal cord is intense or occurs repeatedly, peripheral and central sensitisation mechanisms occur and spread of nociception at the spinal cord level results in referred pain (Hoheisel et al., 1993).

Sensitisation Mechanisms of Trigger Points
Trigger point as a focus of peripheral sensitisation
As stated, muscle pain is associated with the activation of muscle nociceptors by a variety of endogenous substances, including several neuropeptides and inflammatory mediators, among others. In experimental research different substances are commonly used to elicit local and referred muscle pain (Babenko et al., 1999; Arendt-Nielsen et al., 2000; Arendt-Nielsen & Svensson, 2001; Graven-Nielsen, 2006). In fact, induced referred pain areas obtained in these experimental studies have confirmed the empirical referred pain patterns described by Travell and Simons (Travell & Rinzler, 1952; Simons et al., 1999).

Peripheral sensitisation is described as a reduction in the pain threshold and an increase in responsiveness of the peripheral nociceptors. Scientific evidence has shown that pressure sensitivity is higher at TrPs than at control points (Hong et al., 1996), suggesting an increased nociceptive sensitivity at TrPs and peripheral sensitisation. The concentrations of BK, CGRP, substance P, tumour necrosis factor α (TNF-α), interleukins 1β, IL-6, and IL-8, 5-HT, and norepinephrine were significantly higher near active TrPs than near latent TrP or non-TrP points and in remote pain-free distant areas (Shah et al., 2005, 2008). These chemical mediators may partly be released from peripheral sensitised nociceptors that drive the pain, but also be released from the sustained muscle fibre contraction within the taut band (Gerwin, 2008). Interestingly, the concentrations of these biochemical substances in a pain-free area of the gastrocnemius muscle were also higher in individuals with active TrPs in the upper trapezius muscle compared with those with latent TrPs or non-TrPs (Shah et al., 2008). These studies confirm not only the presence of nociceptive pain hypersensitivity in active TrP, but also establish that TrPs are a focus of peripheral sensitisation. Substances associated with muscle pain and fatigue are apparently not limited to local areas of TrPs or a single anatomical locus. Li and colleagues (2009) reported nociceptive (hyperalgesia) and nonnociceptive (allodynia) hypersensitivity at TrPs, suggesting that TrPs sensitise both nociceptive and nonnociceptive nerve endings. Nevertheless, painful stimulation induced higher pain response than nonnoxious stimulation at TrPs (Li et al., 2009). Hsieh and colleagues (2012) confirmed that the concentrations of multiple chemicals, including β-endorphin, substance P, TNF-α, cyclooxygenase-2 (COX-2), hypoxia-inducible factor-1α (HIF-1α), inducible isoform of nitric oxide synthases (iNOS), and vascular endothelial growth factor (VEGF) were significantly higher. Of interest is that dry needling reduced these concentrations, but this was dosage dependent (Hsieh et al., 2012).

Wang and colleagues (2010) reported that ischemic compression, which mainly blocked large-diameter myelinated muscle afferents, induced increased pressure pain and referred pain thresholds at the TrP, but not at non-TrP regions. After decompression, the pressure sensitivity returned to precompression levels. In other words, nonnociceptive large-diameter myelinated muscle afferents may be involved in the pathophysiology of TrP pain and hyperalgesia (Wang et al., 2010). As nonnociceptive afferents are involved in proprioception, excitation of the large-diameter myelinated afferents by TrPs may explain the presence of altered proprioception in some patients with chronic musculoskeletal pain. Meng and colleagues (2015) confirmed that myelinated afferents influence endplate noise and mechanical hyperalgesia in a rat model.

Trigger point nociception induces central sensitisation

Central sensitisation is an increase in the excitability of neurons within the central nervous system, characterised by allodynia and hyperalgesia. Hyperalgesia is an increased response to a stimulus that is normally painful. Allodynia and hyperalgesia are observed in patients with TrPs. In fact, emerging research suggests a physiological link between the clinical manifestations of TrPs, such as hyperalgesia and consistent referred pain, and the phenomenon of central sensitisation, although the causal relationships and mechanisms are still unclear. Additionally, Arendt-Nielsen and colleagues (2008) demonstrated that experimentally induced muscle pain

is able to impair diffuse noxious inhibitory control mechanisms, supporting an important role of muscle tissues in chronic pain.

Mense (1994) suggested that the presence of multiple TrPs in the same or different muscles or the presence of active TrPs for prolonged periods of time may sensitise spinal cord neurons and supraspinal structures by means of a continued peripheral nociceptive afferent barrage into the central nervous system. Both spatial and temporal summations are important in this pattern. Although the relationship between active TrPs and central sensitisation has been observed clinically for many years, neurophysiological studies have been conducted only during the last decade. Kuan and colleagues (2007a) reported that spinal cord connections of TrPs were more effective in inducing neuroplastic changes in the dorsal horn neurons than non-TrPs. In addition, motor neurons related to TrPs had smaller diameters than neurons of normal tissue. It appears that TrP may be connected to a greater number of small sensory or nociceptive neurons than non-TrP tissues (Kuan et al., 2007a). Mechanical stimulation of latent TrPs can induce central sensitisation in healthy subjects, suggesting that stimulation of latent TrPs can increase pressure hypersensitivity in extrasegmental tissues (Xu et al., 2010). Central sensitisation also increased the TrP pressure sensitivity in segmentally related muscles (Srbely et al., 2010a). Further, Fernández-Carnero and colleagues (2010) reported that central sensitisation related to TrPs in the infraspinatus increased the amplitude of electromyographical (EMG) activity of TrPs in the extensor carpi radialis brevis.

Current evidence suggests that TrPs induce central sensitisation, but sensitisation mechanisms can also promote TrP activity (Fernández-de-las-Peñas & Dommerholt, 2014). It is, however, more likely that TrPs induce central sensitisation, as latent TrPs are present in healthy individuals without evidence of central sensitisation. Finally, active TrP pain is, at least partially, processed at supraspinal levels. Recent imaging data suggest that TrP hyperalgesia is processed in various brain areas as enhanced somatosensory activity involving the primary and secondary somatosensory cortex, inferior parietal, and mid-insula and limbic activity, involving the anterior insula. Suppressed right dorsal hippocampal activity is present in patients with TrPs in the upper trapezius muscle compared with healthy controls (Niddam et al., 2008; Niddam, 2009). Abnormal hippocampal hypoactivity suggests that dysfunctional stress responses play an important role in the generation and maintenance of hyperalgesia from TrPs (Niddam et al., 2008). Current data suggest that a TrP is more painful than normal tissue because of specific physiological changes as well as peripheral and central sensitisation, and not because of anatomical issues.

Muscle referred pain is a process of reversible central sensitisation

A sensitised central nervous system may modulate referred muscle pain. Infusions with the N-methyl-D-aspartate (NMDA) antagonist ketamine in individuals with fibromyalgia reduced their referred pain areas (Graven-Nielsen et al., 2000). As noted previously, the appearance of new receptive fields is characteristic of muscle and fascia referred pain (Mense, 1994; Taguchi et al., 2008; Schilder et al., 2014). Because referred pain area is correlated with the intensity and duration of muscle pain (Graven-Nielsen et al., 1997b), muscle referred pain appears to be a central sensitisation phenomenon maintained by peripheral sensitisation input for example from active TrPs.

Central sensitisation is a reversible process in patients with myofascial pain, although older animal studies suggest that central sensitisation would be an irreversible process (Sluka et al., 2001). Several clinical studies have demonstrated that sensitisation mechanisms related to TrPs may be reversible with proper management. TrP injections into neck muscles produced a rapid relief of palpable scalp or facial tenderness, which would constitute mechanical hyperalgesia and allodynia, and associated symptoms in migraine (Mellick & Mellick, 2003). Anaesthetic injections of active TrPs significantly decreased mechanical hyperalgesia, allodynia, and referred pain in patients suffering from migraine headaches (Giamberardino et al., 2007), fibromyalgia (Affaitati et al., 2011), and whiplash (Freeman et al., 2009). In addition, dry needling of primary TrPs inhibited the activity in satellite TrPs situated in their zone of referred pain (Hsieh et al., 2007). Dry needling of active TrPs has been shown to temporarily increase the mechanical pain threshold in local pain syndromes (Srbely et al., 2010b), suggesting a segmental antinociceptive effect of TrP therapy.

The cause of the rapid decrease in local and referred pains with manual TrP therapy observed in clinical practice is not completely understood but may be, at least partially, the result of the mechanical input from the needle, which would cause local stretching of muscle fibres, elongation of fibroblasts, and microdamage to tissues (Domingo et al., 2013). The resolution of referred pain is related to the decrease in nociceptive input to the dorsal horn of the spinal cord, and interruption of the spread of pain through convergence

and central sensitisation. Nevertheless, the reversal in referred pain is surprisingly fast and suggests that long-standing central sensitisation can be reversed instantaneously with proper treatment. This effect may be related to the up-regulation of the endocannabinoid or endorphin system as a result of myofascial manipulation and other soft tissue therapies (McPartland, 2008). Empirically, dry needling and TrP injections have a much quicker result than strict manual TrP release techniques, presumably due to increased specificity of the stimulus (Dommerholt & Gerwin, 2010). In spite of methodological limitations of many studies, there is ample evidence that manual techniques are effective (Hains et al., 2010a, 2010b; Hains & Hains, 2010; Bron et al., 2011b; Rickards, 2011) without any indication that one particular manual technique would be superior to another (Fernández-de-las-Peñas et al., 2005; Gemmell et al., 2008).

Accumulated evidence indicates that referred pain is a reversible process of central nervous system neuroplasticity (Arendt-Nielsen et al., 2000), which is maintained by increased peripheral nociceptive input from active TrPs. It is conceivable that the degree of central sensitisation may influence whether a patient will eventually be diagnosed with myofascial pain, fibromyalgia, or neuropathic pain. Multiple factors can influence the degree of sensitisation including descending inhibitory mechanisms, sympathetic activity, or neuropathic activation. In clinical practice it is commonly seen that patients with less central sensitisation require a fewer number of treatments.

Sympathetic facilitation of local and referred muscle pain

There is a growing interest in the association between TrPs and the sympathetic nervous system. Rabbit (Chen et al., 1998) and human studies (McNulty et al., 1994; Chung et al., 2004) showed that an increased sympathetic efferent discharge increased the frequency and the amplitude of EMG activity of muscle TrPs, whereas sympathetic blockers decreased the frequency and amplitude of EMG activity. Others reported that sympathetic blockers decreased TrP and tender point pain sensitivity (Bengtsson & Bengtsson, 1988; Martinez-Lavin, 2004), which is consistent with the observed increased concentrations of norepinephrine at active TrPs (Shah et al., 2005).

Ge and colleagues (2006) reported that sympathetic facilitation induced a decrease in the pressure pain thresholds and pressure threshold for eliciting referred pain and an increase in local and referred pain intensities, suggesting a sympathetic-sensory interaction at

TrPs. Zhang and colleagues (2009) found an attenuated skin blood flow response after painful stimulation of latent TrPs compared with non-TrPs, which may be secondary to increased sympathetic vasoconstriction activity at latent TrPs.

TrP sensitivity appears to be maintained by sympathetic hyperactivity, although, once again, the mechanisms of this interaction are not completely understood. Increased sympathetic activity at TrPs may enhance the release of norepinephrine and ATP, among others (Gerwin et al., 2004). Another possible mechanism suggests that the increased level of muscle sympathetic nerve activity may lead to a delayed resolution of inflammatory substances and change the local chemical milieu at TrPs (Macefield & Wallin, 1995). As was discussed previously, Gerwin and colleagues (2004) suggested that the presence of α and β adrenergic receptors at the endplate could provide a possible mechanism for autonomic interaction (Maekawa et al., 2002), although this has not been confirmed in humans.

Pathophysiology of Trigger Points: The Integrated Hypothesis

The activation of a TrP may result from a variety of factors such as repetitive muscle overuse, acute or sustained overload, psychological stress, or other key or primary TrPs. Particular attention has been paid to injured or overloaded muscle fibres after eccentric and intense concentric contractions in the pathogenesis of TrPs (Gerwin et al., 2004). Hong (1996) hypothesised that each TrP contains a sensitive locus, described as a site from which a LTR can be elicited when the TrP is mechanically stimulated, and an active locus, described as an area from which spontaneous electrical activity (SEA) is recorded. In this model, the sensitive locus contains nociceptors and constitutes the sensory component, whereas the active locus consists of dysfunctional motor endplates, which would be the motor component (Simons et al., 1995; Simons, 1996; Hong & Simons, 1998). To date, the presence of these loci has not been confirmed.

Muscle trauma, repetitive low-intensity muscle overload, or intense muscle contractions may create a vicious cycle of events, wherein damage to the sarcoplasmic reticulum or the cell membrane leads to an increase of the calcium concentration, a shortening of the actin and myosin filaments, a shortage of ATP, and an impaired calcium pump (Simons et al., 1999; Gerwin et al., 2004). This vicious cycle leads to the development of the so-called 'energy crisis hypothesis' (Simons & Travell, 1981), which over time evolved into the *integrated trigger point hypothesis*, based

on subsequent scientific research (Simons, 2004). The integrated hypothesis is the most accepted theoretical concept, although other models have been proposed (Dommerholt & Franssen, 2011). The integrated hypothesis is a work in progress and continues to be modified and updated as new scientific evidence emerges (Gerwin et al., 2004; McPartland & Simons, 2006; Jafri, 2014).

The integrated hypothesis proposes that abnormal depolarisation of the postjunctional membrane of motor endplates causes a localised hypoxic energy crisis associated with sensory and autonomic reflex arcs that are sustained by complex sensitisation mechanisms (McPartland & Simons, 2006). The first EMG study of TrPs, conducted by Hubbard and Berkoff (1993), reported the presence of spontaneous EMG activity in a TrP of the upper trapezius muscle. The authors described two components of this spontaneous EMG activity: a low amplitude constant background activity of 50 μV and an intermittent higher amplitude spikelike of 100 to 700 μV. Others confirmed the constant background activity of 10 to 50 μV and, occasionally, 80 μV in animal TrPs (Simons et al., 1995; Chen et al., 1998; Macgregor et al., 2006) and in human TrPs (Simons, 2001; Couppé et al., 2001; Simons et al., 2002).

The origin of this SEA is still controversial; however, clear evidence supports that SEA originates from motor endplate potentials (EPP). Simons concluded that the SEA is the same as endplate noise (EPN) (Simons, 2001; Simons et al., 2002). EPN is more prevalent in active TrPs than in latent TrPs (Mense & Gerwin, 2010). EPN seems to reflect a local depolarisation of the muscle fibres induced by a significantly increased and abnormal spontaneous release of ACh (Ge et al., 2011). Kuan and colleagues (2002), in an animal model, showed that SEA can be decreased by botulinum toxin, which inhibits the release of ACh, CGRP, and other chemicals at the neuromuscular junction. Additionally, analysis of the motor behaviours of a TrP shows that the intramuscular EMG activity at TrPs exhibits similar motor behaviours to the surface EMG activity over a TrP, which supports that the origin of the electrical activity is derived from extrafusal motor endplates and not from intrafusal muscle spindles (Ge et al., 2011).

An interesting study found higher pain intensities and pain features similar to TrPs when noxious stimuli were applied to motor endplate areas compared with silent muscle sites (Qerama et al, 2004). Kuan and colleagues (2007b) reported a high correlation between the irritability, pain intensity, and pressure pain thresholds and the prevalence of EPN loci in a TrP region of the upper trapezius muscle. Lower pressure pain thresholds were associated with greater SEA. From a clinical perspective, several studies showed that treatment of TrPs can eliminate or significantly reduce EPN (Kuan et al., 2002; Gerwin et al., 2004; Qerama et al., 2006; Chen, Hong et al., 2008; Chou et al., 2009). Findings from these studies support that TrPs are associated with dysfunctional motor endplates (Simons et al., 2002). It should be noted that motor endplates are distributed throughout the entire muscle and not just in the muscle belly as frequently is assumed (Edström & Kugelberg, 1968). In studies of cats and rats, motor endplates were identified in 75% of the soleus muscle (Bodine-Fowler et al., 1990; Monti et al., 2001). In the anterior tibialis muscle of a cat, motor endplates were located in 56% to 62% of the muscle (Monti et al., 2001).

Regarding the motor component of the TrPs, the intramuscular and surface EMG activity recorded from a TrP showed that the SEA is similar to a muscle cramp potential and that the increase in local muscle pain intensity is positively associated with the duration and amplitude of muscle cramps (Ge et al., 2008). Localised muscle cramps may induce intramuscular hypoxia, increased concentrations of algogenic mediators, direct mechanical stimulation of nociceptors, and, subsequently, the experience of pain (Simons & Mense, 1998). Therefore it seems that TrP pain and tenderness are closely associated with sustained focal ischemia and muscle cramps within muscle taut bands (Ge et al., 2011).

Although current evidence supports that dysfunctional motor endplates are clearly associated with TrPs, recent evidence suggests that muscle spindles may also be involved in this complex process. Ge and colleagues (2009) found that intramuscular TrP electrical stimulation can evoke H-reflexes and that greater H-reflex amplitudes and lower H-reflex thresholds exist at TrPs compared with non-TrPs. The lower reflex threshold and higher reflex amplitude at TrPs could be related to a greater density or excitability of muscle spindle afferents (Ge et al., 2009). Nevertheless, the mechanisms underlying increased sensitivity of muscle spindle afferents at TrPs are still unclear. The increased chemical mediators in the TrPs (Shah et al., 2005) may contribute to an increased static fusimotor drive to muscle spindles or to increased muscle spindle sensitivity (Thunberg et al., 2002).

Recently Jafri (2015) expanded the integrated hypothesis by incorporating the role of reactive oxygen species (ROS). The integrated hypothesis postulated that when Ca^{2+} is not removed from the cytosol, the actin-myosin crossbridge would remain. Removing Ca^2 by reuptake into the sarcoplasmic reticulum is an energy demanding process that occurs via the Na^+/K^--

ATPase (sarcoendoplasmic reticulum ATPase [SERCA]) system. In Jafri's point of view, the role of Ca^{2+} has been undervalued. He summarised that increased muscle activity, as seen in muscle overload, generates ROS, especially superoxide. Normally, ROS are converted by superoxide dismutase (SOD), which converts superoxide to hydrogen peroxide (H_2O_2). Eventually H_2O_2 is broken down to oxygen and water by glutathione peroxidase or catalase. Under stressful or pathological conditions, the enzyme xanthine oxidase and phospholipase A2 dependent processes have been shown to also produce ROS. During repetitive contractions, nicotinamide adenine dinucleotide phosphate oxidase 2 (NOX2), located within the sarcoplasmic reticulum, the sarcolemma, and the transverse tubules, is the major source of superoxide ROS. Jafri hypothesised that mechanical stress can trigger an excessive release of Ca^{2+} in muscles through so-called X-ROS signaling. Mechanical deformation of the microtubule network can activate NOX2, which would produce ROS. The ROS oxidises ryanodine receptors leading to increases in Ca^{2+} release from the sarcoplasmic reticulum. The Ca^{2+} mobilisation resulting from mechanical stretch through this pathway is referred to as X-ROS signaling. In skeletal muscles, X-ROS sensitises Ca^{2+}—permeable sarcolemmal transient receptor potential or TRP channels, which may be a source of nociceptive input and inflammatory pain. Activating the transient receptor potential vanilloid 1 (TRPV1) leads to a quick increase in intracellular Ca^{2+} concentrations. Jafri suggested that myofascial pain is likely due to a combined activation of several ligand-gated ion channels, including the TRPV1 receptor, other acid sensing ion channels (ASIC3), BK and purinergic receptors, among others.

Gerwin (2017) postulated that dysfunctional ATP-sensitive sodium channels (K_{ATP} receptor channel) may provide further answers to the pathophysiology of TrPs. When ATP concentrations are at normal levels, the K_{ATP} receptor channel is closed. When ATP levels drop, for example with hypoxia, the K_{ATP} receptor channel opens and inhibits the influx of Ca^{2+} from the sarcoplasmic reticulum and the endoplasmic reticulum into the cytosol and prevents the formation of ROS. Dysfunctional K_{ATP} receptor channels may trigger focal regions of supercontracted muscle fibres, which suggest that excessive ACh concentrations may not be the only mechanism leading to intense sarcomere contractures.

Other Hypothetical Models

Although the integrated trigger point hypothesis is the most prominent and most accepted model, other hypothetical TrP models have been developed. Recently

Hocking (2010) postulated the *central modulation hypothesis* and suggested that plateau potentials are critical in the understanding of the aetiology of TrPs. According to Hocking, cell membranes may continue to trigger action potentials without synaptic excitation as a result of plateau potentials (Hocking, 2010). In other words, a sustained α-motoneuron plateau depolarisation would lead to the formation of TrPs. Hocking identified two underlying central nervous system mechanisms. So-called *antecedent* TrPs are thought to be the result of central sensitisation of C-fibre nociceptive withdrawal reflexes, visceromotor reflexes, or nociceptive jaw-opening reflexes; they occur in withdrawal reflex agonist muscles. *Consequent* TrPs would be due to compensatory reticulospinal or reticulotrigeminal motor facilitation; they occur in withdrawal reflex antagonist muscles. A critical difference with the integrated TrP hypothesis is that, in the central modulation model, myofascial pain is not a disorder of the motor endplate, but a nociception-induced central nervous system disorder leading to centrally maintained α-motoneuron plateau depolarisations (Hocking, 2010). There are several aspects of the integrated TrtP hypothesis that are also part of the central modulation hypothesis such as the presence of the energy crisis and low-amplitude motor endplate potentials. When Hocking presented his hypothesis initially, he also suggested several research projects to test the hypothesis. Further research is indeed needed to test this interesting hypothesis.

Srbely (2010) developed the *neurogenic hypothesis,* which is based primarily on his and his associates' research (Srbely & Dickey, 2007; Srbely et al., 2008, 2010a, 2010b). According to the neurogenic hypothesis, TrPs are neurogenic manifestations of primary pathologies in the same neurological segment. Srbely (2010) suggests that central sensitisation is the underlying cause of myofascial pain syndrome. The notion that the inactivation of TrPs can reverse central sensitisation is interpreted as evidence of the neurogenic hypothesis. Other than Srbely's own studies, there is no other research to confirm or dispute the neurogenic hypothesis.

Partanen and colleagues (2010) developed the *neurophysiologic hypothesis,* which maintains that the SEA is not recorded from motor endplates but from intrafusal muscle spindle fibres. According to this hypothesis, taut bands are caused by inflammation of muscle spindles and sensitisation of group III and IV afferents, which in turn leads to activation of the gamma and beta efferent systems (Partanen, 1999; Partanen et al., 2010). As was mentioned already, muscle spindles may be involved in the TrP aetiology (Ge et al., 2009), but there is no convincing evidence that endplate noise would originate in intrafusal fibres (Wiederholt, 1970). There is no research to date to confirm or dispute the neurophysiological hypothesis.

Gunn (1997a, 1997b) developed the *radiculopathy hypothesis,* which is discussed in detail in Chapter 15. Quintner and colleagues (2015) suggested *neuritis* as a possible cause without providing any experimental support.

REFERENCES

Affaitati, G., Costantini, R., Fabrizio, A., Lapenna, D., Tafuri, E., & Giamberardino, M. A. (2011). Effects of treatment of peripheral pain generators in fibromyalgia patients. *European Journal of Pain, 15,* 61–69.

Ambalavanar, R., Dessem, D., Moutanni, A., et al. (2006). Muscle inflammation induces a rapid increase in calcitonin gene-related peptide (CGRP) mRNA that temporally relates to CGRP immunoreactivity and nociceptive behavior. *Neuroscience, 143,* 875–884.

Anderson, R. U. (2002). Management of chronic prostatitis-chronic pelvic pain syndrome. *The Urologic Clinics of North America, 29,* 235–239.

Apkarian, A. V., Brüggemann, J., Shi, T., & Airapetiam, L. (1995). A thalamic model for true and referred visceral pain. In G. F. Gebhart (Ed.), *Visceral pain, progress in pain research and management* (pp. 217–259). Seattle: IASP Press.

Arendt-Nielsen, L., Laursen, R. J., & Drewes, A. M. (2000). Referred pain as an indicator for neural plasticity. *Progress in Brain Research, 129,* 343–356.

Arendt-Nielsen, L., & Svensson, P. (2001). Referred muscle pain: basic and clinical findings. *The Clinical Journal of Pain, 17,* 11–19.

Arendt-Nielsen, L., Sluka, K. A., & Nie, H. L. (2008). Experimental muscle pain impairs descending inhibition. *Pain, 140,* 465–471.

Arendt-Nielsen, L., & Ge, H. Y. (2009). Patho-physiology of referred muscle pain. In C. Fernández-de-las-Peñas, L. Arendt-Nielsen, & R. D. Gerwin (Eds.), *Tension type and cervicogenic headache: patho-physiology, diagnosis and treatment* (pp. 51–59). Boston: Jones & Bartlett Publishers.

Audette, J. F., Wang, F., & Smith, H. (2004). Bilateral activation of motor unit potentials with unilateral needle stimulation of active myofascial trigger points. *American Journal of Physical Medicine & Rehabilitation, 83,* 368–374.

Babenko, V., Graven-Nielsen, T., Svensson, P., Drewes, A. M., Jensen, T. S., & Arendt-Nielsen, L. (1999). Experimental human muscle pain and muscular hyperalgesia induced by combinations of serotonin and bradykinin. *Pain, 82,* 1–8.

Ballantyne, J. C., Rathmell, J. P., & Fishman, S. M. (Eds.), (2010). *Bonica's management of pain.* Lippincott Williams & Williams: Baltimore.

Ballyns, J. J., Shah, J. P., Hammond, J., Gebreab, T., Gerber, L. H., & Sikdar, S. (2011). Objective sonographic measures for characterizing myofascial trigger points associated with cervical pain. *Journal of Ultrasound in Medicine, 30*(10), 1331–1340.

Banks, S. L., Jacobs, D. W., Gevirtz, R., & Hubbard, D. R. (1998). Effects of autogenic relaxation training on electromyographic activity in active myofascial trigger points. *Journal of Musculoskeletal Pain, 6*(4), 23–32.

Bajaj, P., Bajaj, P., Graven-Nielsen, T., & Arendt-Nielsen, L. (2001). Trigger points in patients with lower limb osteoarthritis. *Journal of Musculoskeletal Pain, 9*(3), 17–33.

Bengtsson, A., & Bengtsson, M. (1988). Regional sympathetic blockade in primary fibromyalgia. *Pain, 33*, 161–167.

Bodine-Fowler, S., Garfinkel, A., Roy, R. R., & Edgerton, V. R. (1990). Spatial distribution of muscle fibers within the territory of a motor unit. *Muscle & Nerve, 13*, 1133–1145.

Bohlooli, N., Ahmadi, A., Maroufi, N., Sarrafzadeh, J., & Jaberzadeh, S. (2016). Differential activation of scapular muscles, during arm elevation, with and without trigger points. *Journal of Bodywork and Movement Therapies, 20*, 26–34.

Bowman, W. C., Marshall, I. G., Gibb, A. J., & Harborne, A. J. (1988). Feedback control of transmitter release at the neuromuscular junction. *Trends in Pharmacological Sciences, 9*, 16–20.

Bron, C., & Dommerholt, J. (2012). Etiology of myofascial trigger points. *Current Pain and Headache Reports, 16*(5), 439–444.

Bron, C., Dommerholt, J., Stegenga, B., Wensing, M., & Oostendorp, R. A. (2011a). High prevalence of shoulder girdle muscles with myofascial trigger points in patients with shoulder pain. *BMC Musculoskeletal Disorders, 12*, 139.

Bron, C., de Gast, A., Dommerholt, J., Stegenga, B., Wensing, M., & Oostendorp, R. A. B. (2011b). Treatment of myofascial trigger points in patients with chronic shoulder pain; a randomized controlled trial. *BMC Medicine, 9*, 8.

Brückle, W., Sückfull, M., Fleckenstein, W., Weiss, C., & Müller, W. (1990). Gewebe-Po2-Messung in der verspannten Rückenmuskulatur (m. erector spinae). *Zeitschrift für Rheumatologie, 49*, 208–216.

Bubnov, R. V. (2010). The use of trigger point "dry" needling under ultrasound guidance for the treatment of myofascial pain (technological innovation and literature review). *Likars'ka Sprava, 5-6*, 56–64.

Bukharaeva, E. A., Salakhutdinov, R. I., Vyskocil, F., & Nikolsky, E. E. (2005). Spontaneous quantal and non-quantal release of acetylcholine at mouse endplate during onset of hypoxia. *Physiological Research, 54*, 251–255.

Calixto, J. B., Cabrini, D. A., Ferreira, J., & Campos, M. M. (2000). Kinins in pain and inflammation. *Pain, 87*, 1–5.

Chen, B. M., & Grinnell, A. D. (1997). Kinetics, Ca²⁺ dependence, and biophysical properties of integrin-mediated mechanical modulation of transmitter release from frog motor nerve terminals. *The Journal of Neuroscience, 17*, 904–916.

Chen, J. T., Chen, S. M., Kuan, T. S., Chung, K. C., & Hong, C. Z. (1998). Phentolamine effect on the spontaneous electrical activity of active loci in a myofascial trigger spot of rabbit skeletal muscle. *Archives of Physical Medicine and Rehabilitation, 79*, 790–794.

Chen, S. M., Chen, J. T., Kuan, T. S., Hong, J., & Hong, C. Z. (2000). Decrease in pressure pain thresholds of latent myofascial trigger points in the middle finger extensors immediately after continuous piano practice. *Journal of Musculoskeletal Pain, 8*, 83–92.

Chen, Q., Bensamoun, S., Basford, J. R., Thompson, J. M., & An, K. N. (2007). Identification and quantification of myofascial taut bands with magnetic resonance elastography. *Archives of Physical Medicine and Rehabilitation, 88*, 1658–1661.

Chen, Q., Basford, J. R., & An, K. (2008). Ability of magnetic resonance elastography to assess taut bands. *Clinical Biomechanics, 23*, 623–629.

Chen, K. H., Hong, C. Z., Kuo, F. C., Hsu, H. C., & Hsieh, Y. L. (2008). Electrophysiologic effects of a therapeutic laser on myofascial trigger spots of rabbit skeletal muscles. *American Journal of Physical Medicine & Rehabilitation, 87*, 1006–1014.

Chen, Q., Wang, H. J., Gay, R. E., Thompson, J. M., Manduca, A., An, K. N., et al. (2016). Quantification of Myofascial Taut Bands. *Archives of Physical Medicine and Rehabilitation, 97*(1), 67–73.

Choi, R. C., Siow, N. L., Cheng, A. W., Ling, K. K., Tung, E. K., Simon, J., Barnard, E. A., & Tsim, K. W. (2003). ATP acts via P2Y1 receptors to stimulate acetylcholinesterase and acetylcholine receptor expression: transduction and transcription control. *The Journal of Neuroscience, 23*(11), 4445–4456.

Chou, L. W., Hsieh, Y. L., Kao, M. J., & Hong, C. Z. (2009). Remote influences of acupuncture on the pain intensity and the amplitude changes of endplate noise in the myofascial trigger point of the upper trapezius muscle. *Archives of Physical Medicine and Rehabilitation, 90*, 905–912.

Chung, J. W., Ohrbach, R., & WDJr, McCall. (2004). Effect of increased sympathetic activity on electrical activity from myofascial painful areas. *American Journal of Physical Medicine & Rehabilitation, 83*, 842–850.

Couppé, C., Midttun, A., Hilden, J., Jørgensen, U., Oxholm, P., & Fuglsang-Frederiksen, A. (2001). Spontaneous needle electromyographic activity in myofascial trigger points in the infraspinatus muscle: a blinded assessment. *Journal of Musculoskeletal Pain, 9*(3), 7–17.

Deval, E., Gasull, X., Noel, J., et al. (2010). Acid-sensing ion channels (ASICs): pharmacology and implication in pain. *Pharmacology & Therapeutics, 128*, 549–558.

Doggweiler-Wygul, R. (2004). Urologic myofascial pain syndromes. *Current Pain and Headache Reports, 8*, 445–451.

Domingo, A., Mayoral, O., Monterde, S., & Santafe, M. M. (2013). Neuromuscular damage and repair after dry needling in mice. *Evidence-based Complementary and Alternative Medicine, 2013*, 260806.

Dommerholt, J., Bron, C., & Franssen, J. L. M. (2006). Myofascial trigger points: an evidence informed review. *The Journal of Manual & Manipulative Therapy*, 14, 203–221.

Dommerholt, J., & Gerwin, R. D. (2010). Neurophysiological effects of trigger point needling therapies. In C. Fernández-de-las-Peñas, L. Arendt-Nielsen, & R. D. Gerwin (Eds.), *Tension type and cervicogenic headache: pathophysiology, diagnosis and treatment* (pp. 247–259). Boston: Jones & Bartlett.

Dommerholt, J., & Shah, J. (2010). Myofascial pain syndrome. In J. C. Ballantyne, J. P. Rathmell, & S. M. Fishman (Eds.), *Bonica's management of pain* (pp. 450–471). Baltimore: Lippincott Williams & Williams.

Dommerholt, J., & Franssen, J. (2011). Wetenschappelijke evidentie van myofasciale trigger points. In P. K. Jonckheere, J. Demanet, J. Pattyn, & J. Dommerholt (Eds.), *Trigger points praktisch werkboek myofasciale therapie. Deel 1: bovenste lidmaat*. Brugge: Acu-Qi.

Dommerholt, J. (2011). Dry needling - peripheral and central considerations. *The Journal of Manual & Manipulative Therapy*, 19, 223–237.

Durham, P. L., & Vause, C. V. (2010). Calcitonin gene-related peptide (CGRP) receptor antagonists in the treatment of migraine. *CNS Drugs*, 24, 539–548.

Edström, L., & Kugelberg, E. (1968). Histochemical composition, distribution of fibres and fatiguability of single motor units. Anterior tibial muscle of the rat. *Journal of Neurology, Neurosurgery, and Psychiatry*, 31, 424–433.

Fernández-Carnero, J., Fernández-de-las-Peñas, C., de-la-Llave-Rincón, A. I., et al. (2007). Prevalence of and referred pain from myofascial trigger points in the forearm muscles in patients with lateral epicondylalgia. *The Clinical Journal of Pain*, 23, 353–360.

Fernández-Carnero, J., Fernández-de-las-Peñas, C., De-la-Llave-Rincón, A. I., Ge, H. Y., & Arendt-Nielsen, L. (2008). Bilateral myofascial trigger points in the forearm muscles in chronic unilateral lateral epicondylalgia: a blinded controlled study. *The Clinical Journal of Pain*, 24, 802–807.

Fernandez-Carnero, J., Ge, H. Y., Kimura, Y., Fernandez-de-las-Penas, C., & Arendt-Nielsen, L. (2010). Increased spontaneous electrical activity at a latent myofascial trigger point after nociceptive stimulation of another latent trigger point. *The Clinical Journal of Pain*, 26, 138–143.

Fernández-de-las-Peñas, C., & Dommerholt, J. (2014). Myofascial trigger points: peripheral or central phenomenon? *Current Rheumatology Reports*, 16(1), 395.

Fernández-de-las-Peñas, C., & Dommerholt, J. (2018). International consensus on diagnostic criteria and clinical considerations of myofascial trigger points: a Delphi study. *Pain Medicine*, 19, 142–150.

Fernández-de-las-Peñas, C., Sorbeck Campo, M., Fernández-Carnero, J., & Miangolarra-Page, J. C. (2005). Manual therapies in myofascial trigger point treatment: a systematic review. *Journal of Bodywork and Movement Therapies*, 9, 27–34.

Fernández-de-las-Peñas, C., Ge, H. Y., & Dommerholt, J. (2011). Manual treatment of myofascial trigger points. In C. Fernández-de-las-Peñas, J. Cleland, & P. Huijbregts (Eds.), *Neck and arm pain syndromes: evidence-informed*

screening, diagnosis and conservative management (pp. 451–461). London: Churchill Livingstone-Elsevier.

Freeman, M. D., Nystrom, A., & Centeno, C. (2009). Chronic whiplash and central sensitization; an evaluation of the role of a myofascial trigger points in pain modulation. *Journal of Brachial Plexus and Peripheral Nerve Injury*, 4, 2.

Gandevia, S. C., & Phegan, C. (1999). Perceptual distortions of the human body image produced by local anaesthesia, pain and cutaneous stimulation. *The Journal of Physiology*, 15, 609–616.

Ganesh, G. S., Singh, H., Mushtaq, S., Mohanty, P., & Pattnaik, M. (2016). Effect of cervical mobilization and ischemic compression therapy on contralateral cervical side flexion and pressure pain threshold in latent upper trapezius trigger points. *Journal of Bodywork and Movement Therapies*, 20, 477–483.

Gautam, M., Benson, C. J., & Sluka, K. A. (2010). Increased response of muscle sensory neurons to decreases in pH after muscle inflammation. *Neuroscience*, 170, 893–900.

Ge, H. Y., Fernández-de-las-Penas, C., & Arendt-Nielsen, L. (2006). Sympathetic facilitation of hyperalgesia evoked from myofascial tender and trigger points in patients with unilateral shoulder pain. *Clinical Neurophysiology*, 117, 1545–1550.

Ge, H. Y., Zhang, Y., Boudreau, S., Yue, S. W., & Arendt-Nielsen, L. (2008). Induction of muscle cramps by nociceptive stimulation of latent myofascial trigger points. *Experimental Brain Research*, 187, 623–629.

Ge, H. Y., Serrao, M., Andersen, O. K., Graven-Nielsen, T., & Arendt-Nielsen, L. (2009). Increased H-reflex response induced by intramuscular electrical stimulation of latent myofascial trigger points. *Acupuncture in Medicine*, 27, 150–154.

Ge, H. Y., Fernández-de-las-Peñas, C., & Yue, S. W. (2011). Myofascial trigger points: spontaneous electrical activity and its consequences for pain induction and propagation. *Chinese Medicine*, 6, 13.

Ge, H. Y., & Arendt-Nielsen, L. (2011). Latent myofascial trigger points. *Current Pain and Headache Reports*, 15, 386–392.

Gemmell, H., Miller, P., & Nordstrom, H. (2008). Immediate effect of ischaemic compression and trigger point pressure release on neck pain and upper trapezius trigger points: a randomized controlled trial. *Clinical Chiropractic*, 11, 30–36.

Gerwin, R. D., & Duranleau, D. (1997). Ultrasound identification of the myofascial trigger point. *Muscle & Nerve*, 20, 767–768.

Gerwin, R. D., Dommerholt, J., & Shah, J. (2004). An expansion of Simons' integrated hypothesis of trigger point formation. *Current Pain and Headache Reports*, 8, 468–475.

Gerwin, R. D. (2008). The taut band and other mysteries of the trigger point: an examination of the mechanisms relevant to the development and maintenance of the trigger point. *Journal of Musculoskeletal Pain*, 16, 115–121.

Gerwin, R. D. (2017). New concepts in the initiation of the myofascial trigger point. *Presentation at Myopain 2017 Bangalore, India*. October 2017.

Giamberardino, M. A., Tafuri, E., Savini, A., et al. (2007). Contribution of myofascial trigger points to migraine symptoms. *The Journal of Pain*, 8, 869–878.

Graven-Nielsen, T., Arendt-Nielsen, L., Svensson, P., & Jensen, T. S. (1997a). Quantification of local and referred muscle pain in humans after sequential intra-muscular injections of hypertonic saline. *Pain*, 69, 111–117.

Graven-Nielsen, T., McArdle, A., Phoenix, J., et al. (1997b). In vivo model of muscle pain: quantification of intramuscular chemical, electrical, and pressure changes associated with saline-induced muscle pain in humans. *Pain*, 69, 137–143.

Graven-Nielsen, T., Aspegren-Kendall, S., Henriksson, K. G., et al. (2000). Ketamine attenuates experimental referred muscle pain and temporal summation in fibromyalgia patients. *Pain*, 85, 483–491.

Graven-Nielsen, T. (2006). Fundamentals of muscle pain, referred pain, and deep tissue hyperalgesia. *Scandinavian Journal of Rheumatology*, 122(Suppl), 1–43.

Grieve, R., Clark, J., Pearson, E., Bullock, S., Boyer, C., & Jarrett, A. (2011). The immediate effect of soleus trigger point pressure release on restricted ankle joint dorsiflexion: a pilot randomised controlled trial. *Journal of Bodywork and Movement Therapies*, 15, 42–49.

Grinnell, A. D., Chen, B. M., Kashani, A., Lin, J., Suzuki, K., & Kidokoro, Y. (2003). The role of integrins in the modulation of neurotransmitter release from motor nerve terminals by stretch and hypertonicity. *Journal of Neurocytology*, 32, 489–503.

Gunn, C. C. (1997a). *The Gunn approach to the treatment of chronic pain* (2nd ed.). New York: Churchill Livingstone.

Gunn, C. C. (1997b). Radiculopathic pain: diagnosis, treatment of segmental irritation or sensitization. *Journal of Musculoskeletal Pain*, 5(4), 119–134.

Hägg, G. M. (2003). The Cinderella Hypothesis. In H. Johansson, U. Windhorst, M. Djupsjöbacka, & M. Passatore (Eds.), *Chronic work-related myalgia* (pp. 127–132). Gävle: Gävle University Press.

Hains, G., Descarreaux, M., & Hains, F. (2010a). Chronic shoulder pain of myofascial origin: a randomized clinical trial using ischemic compression therapy. *Journal of Manipulative and Physiological Therapeutics*, 33, 362–369.

Hains, G., Descarreaux, M., Lamy, A. M., & Hains, F. (2010b). A randomized controlled (intervention) trial of ischemic compression therapy for chronic carpal tunnel syndrome. *The Journal of the Canadian Chiropractic Association*, 54, 155–163.

Hains, G., & Hains, F. (2010). Patellofemoral pain syndrome managed by ischemic compression to the trigger points located in the peri-patellar and retro-patellar areas: a randomized clinical trial. *Clinical Chiropractic*, 13, 201–209.

Hendler, N. H., & Kozikowski, J. G. (1993). Overlooked physical diagnoses in chronic pain patients involved in litigation. *Psychosomatics*, 34, 494–501.

Hidalgo-Lozano, A., Fernández-de-las-Peñas, C., Alonso-Blanco, C., Ge, H.-Y., Arendt-Nielsen, L., & Arroyo-Morales, M. (2010). Muscle trigger points and pressure pain hyperalgesia in the shoulder muscles in patients with unilateral shoulder impingement: a blinded, controlled study. *Experimental Brain Research*, 202, 915–925.

Hocking, M. J. L. (2010). Trigger points and central modulation - a new hypothesis. *Journal of Musculoskeletal Pain*, 18(2), 186–203.

Hodges-Savola, C. A., & Fernandez, H. L. (1995). A role for calcitonin gene-related peptide in the regulation of rat skeletal muscle G4 acetylcholinesterase. *Neuroscience Letters*, 190, 117–120.

Hong, C. Z. (1994). Consideration and recommendation of myofascial trigger point injection. *Journal of Musculoskeletal Pain*, 2, 29–59.

Hong, C. Z., & Torigoe, Y. (1994). Electro-physiologic characteristics of localized twitch responses in responsive bands of rabbit skeletal muscle fibers. *Journal of Musculoskeletal Pain*, 2, 17–43.

Hong, C. Z., Torigoe, Y., & Yu, J. (1995). The localized twitch responses in responsive bands of rabbit skeletal muscle fibers are related to the reflexes at spinal cord level. *Journal of Musculoskeletal Pain*, 3, 15–33.

Hong, C. Z. (1996). Pathophysiology of myofascial trigger point. *Journal of the Formosan Medical Association*, 95, 93–104.

Hong, C. Z., Chen, Y. N., Twehous, D., & Hong, D. H. (1996). Pressure threshold for referred pain by compression on the trigger point and adjacent areas. *Journal of Musculoskeletal Pain*, 4, 61–79.

Hong, C. Z., Kuan, T. S., Chen, J. T., & Chen, S. M. (1997). Referred pain elicited by palpation and by needling of myofascial trigger points: a comparison. *Archives of Physical Medicine and Rehabilitation*, 78, 957–960.

Hong, C. Z., & Simons, D. (1998). Pathophysiologic and electrophysiologic mechanism of myofascial trigger points. *Archives of Physical Medicine and Rehabilitation*, 79, 863–872.

Hong, C.-Z., & Yu, J. (1998). Spontaneous electrical activity of rabbit trigger spot after transection of spinal cord and peripheral nerve. *Journal of Musculoskeletal Pain*, 6(4), 45–58.

Hoheisel, U., Mense, S., Simons, D. G., & Yu, X. M. (1993). Appearance of new receptive fields in rat dorsal horn neurons following noxious stimulation of skeletal muscle: a model for referral of muscle pain? *Neuroscience Letters*, 153, 9–12.

Hoyle, J. A., Marras, W. S., Sheedy, J. E., & Hart, D. E. (2011). Effects of postural and visual stressors on myofascial trigger point development and motor unit rotation during computer work. *Journal of Electromyography and Kinesiology*, 21, 41–48.

Hsieh, Y. L., Kao, M. J., Kuan, T. S., Chen, S. M., Chen, J. T., & Hong, C. Z. (2007). Dry needling to a key myofascial trigger point may reduce the irritability of satellite MTrPs. *American Journal of Physical Medicine & Rehabilitation*, 86, 397–403.

Hsieh, Y.-L., Yang, S.-A., Yang, C.-C., & Chou, L.-W. (2012). Dry needling at myofascial trigger spots of rabbit skeletal muscles modulates the biochemicals associated with pain, inflammation, and hypoxia. *Evidence-based Complementary and Alternative Medicine*, 2012, 342165.

Hubbard, D. R., & Berkoff, G. M. (1993). Myofascial trigger points show spontaneous needle EMG activity. *Spine, 18,* 1803–1807.

Jafri, M. S. (2014). Mechanisms of Myofascial Pain. *International Scholarly Research Notices, 2014.*

Jarrell, J. (2004). Myofascial dysfunction in the pelvis. *Current Pain and Headache Reports, 8,* 452–456.

Kadefors, R., Forsman, M., Zoega, B., & Herberts, P. (1999). Recruitment of low threshold motor-units in the trapezius muscle in different static arm positions. *Ergonomics, 42,* 359–375.

Kellgren, J. H. (1938). Observation on referred pain arising from muscle. *Clinical Science, 3,* 175–190.

Kimura, Y., Ge, H. Y., Zhang, Y., Kimura, M., Sumikura, H., & Arendt-Nielsen, L. (2009). Evaluation of sympathetic vasoconstrictor response following nociceptive stimulation of latent myofascial trigger points in humans. *Acta Physiologica, 196,* 411–417.

Kojidi, M. M., Okhovatian, F., Rahimi, A., Baghban, A. A., & Azimi, H. (2016). Comparison between the effects of passive and active soft tissue therapies on latent trigger points of the upper trapezius muscle in women: single-blind, randomized clinical trial. *Journal of Chiropractic Medicine, 15*(4), 235–242.

Koppenhaver, S. L., Walker, M. J., Rettig, C., Davis, J., Nelson, C., Su, J., Fernández-de-Las-Peñas, C., & Hebert, J. J. (2017). The association between dry needling-induced twitch response and change in pain and muscle function in patients with low back pain: a quasi-experimental study. *Physiotherapy, 103*(2), 131–137.

Kuan, T. S., Chen, J. T., Chen, S. M., et al. (2002). Effect of botulinum toxin on endplate noise in myofascial trigger spots of rabbit skeletal muscle. *American Journal of Physical Medicine & Rehabilitation, 81,* 512–520.

Kuan, T. S., Hong, C. Z., Chen, J. T., Chen, S. M., & Chien, C. H. (2007a). The spinal cord connections of the myofascial trigger spots. *European Journal of Pain, 11,* 624–634.

Kuan, T. S., Hsieh, Y. L., Chen, S. M., Chen, J. T., Yen, W. C., & Hong, C. Z. (2007b). The myofascial trigger point region: correlation between the degree of irritability and the prevalence of endplate noise. *American Journal of Physical Medicine & Rehabilitation, 86,* 183–189.

Lewis, C., Gevirtz, R., Hubbard, D., & Berkoff, G. (1994). Needle trigger point and surface frontal EMG measurements of psychophysiological responses in tension-type headache patients. *Biofeedback and Self-Regulation, 3,* 274–275.

Lewis, J., & Tehan, P. (1999). A blinded pilot study investigating the use of diagnostic ultrasound for detecting active myofascial trigger points. *Pain, 79,* 39–44.

Li, L. T., Ge, H. Y., Yue, S. W., & Arendt-Nielsen, L. (2009). Nociceptive and non-nociceptive hypersensitivity at latent myofascial trigger points. *The Clinical Journal of Pain, 25,* 132–137.

Liu, Q. G., Liu, L., Huang, Q. M., Nguyen, T. T., Ma, Y. T., & Zhao, J. M. (2017). Decreased spontaneous electrical activity and acetylcholine at myofascial trigger spots after dry needling treatment: a pilot study. *Evidence-based Complementary and Alternative Medicine, 2017,* 3938191.

Lucas, K. R., Polus, B. I., & Rich, P. A. (2004). Latent myofascial trigger points: their effects on muscle activation and movement efficiency. *Journal of Bodywork and Movement Therapies, 8,* 160–166.

Lucas, K. R., Rich, P. A., & Polus, B. I. (2010). Muscle activation patterns in the scapular positioning muscles during loaded scapular plane elevation: the effects of latent myofascial trigger points. *Clinical Biomechanics, 25,* 765–770.

Maher, R. M., Hayes, D. M., & Shinohara, M. (2013). Quantification of dry needling and posture effects on myofascial trigger points using ultrasound shear-wave elastography. *Archives of Physical Medicine and Rehabilitation, 94*(11), 2146–2150.

Malomouzh, A., Mukhtarov, M. R., NikolskyM, E. E., & Vyskočil, F. (2007). Muscarinic M1 acetylcholine receptors regulate the non-quantal release of acetylcholine in the rat neuromuscular junction via NO-dependent mechanism. *Journal of Neurochemistry, 102*(6), 2110–2117.

Malomouzh, A. I., Nikolsky, E. E., & Vyskočil, F. (2011). Purine P2Y receptors in ATP-mediated regulation of non-quantal acetylcholine release from motor nerve endings of rat diaphragm. *Neuroscience Research, 71*(3), 219–225.

Marceau, F., Sabourin, T., Houle, S., et al. (2002). Kinin receptors: functional aspects. *International Immunopharmacology, 2,* 1729–1739.

Massaad, C. A., Safieh-Garabedian, B., Poole, S., Atweh, S. F., Jabbur, S. J., & Saade, N. E. (2004). Involvement of substance P, CGRP and histamine in the hyperalgesia and cytokine upregulation induced by intraplantar injection of capsaicin in rats. *Journal of Neuroimmunology, 153,* 171–182.

Macefield, V. G., & Wallin, B. G. (1995). Modulation of muscle sympathetic activity during spontaneous and artificial ventilation and apnoea in humans. *Journal of the Autonomic Nervous System, 53,* 137–147.

MacGregor, J., & Graf von Schweinitz, D. (2006). Needle electromyographic activity of myofascial trigger points and control sites in equine cleidobrachialis muscle: an observational study. *Acupuncture in Medicine, 24,* 61–70.

Maekawa, K., Clark, G. T., & Kuboki, T. (2002). Intramuscular hypoperfusion, adrenergic receptors, and chronic muscle pain. *The Journal of Pain, 3,* 251–260.

Magleby, K. L., & Pallotta, B. S. (1981). A study of desensitization of acetylcholine receptors using nerve-released transmitter in the frog. *The Journal of Physiology, 316,* 225–250.

Martinez-Lavin, M. (2004). Fibromyalgia as a sympathetically maintained pain syndrome. *Current Pain and Headache Reports, 8,* 385–389.

McMahon, S. B. (1994). Mechanisms of cutaneous, deep and visceral pain. In P. D. Wall & R. Melzack (Eds.), *Textbook of pain* (pp. 129–151). Edinburgh: Churchill Livingstone.

McNulty, W. H., Gevirtz, R. N., Hubbard, D. R., & Berkoff, G. M. (1994). Needle electromyographic evaluation of trigger point response to a psychological stressor. *Psychophysiology, 31,* 313–316.

McPartland, J. M., & Simons, D. G. (2006). Myofascial trigger points: translating molecular theory into manual therapy. *The Journal of Manual & Manipulative Therapy, 14*, 232–239.

McPartland, J. (2008). Expression of the endocannabinoid system in fibroblasts and myofascial tissues. *Journal of Bodywork and Movement Therapies, 12*, 169–182.

Mellick, G. A., & Mellick, L. B. (2003). Regional head and face pain relief following lower cervical intramuscular anesthetic injection. *Headache, 43*, 1109–1111.

Meng, F., Ge, H. Y., Wang, Y. H., & Yue, S. W. (2015). Myelinated afferents are involved in pathology of the spontaneous electrical activity and mechanical hyperalgesia of myofascial trigger spots in rats. *Evidence-based Complementary and Alternative Medicine, 2015*, 404971.

Mense, S. (1994). Referral of muscle pain. *APS J, 3*, 1–9.

Mense, S., Simons, D. G., Hoheisel, U., & Quenzer, B. (2003). Lesions of rat skeletal muscle after local block of acetylcholinesterase and neuromuscular stimulation. *Journal of Applied Physiology, 94*, 2494–2501.

Mense, S. (2009). Algesic agents exciting muscle nociceptors. *Experimental Brain Research, 196*, 89–100.

Mense, S. (2010a). Functional anatomy of muscle: muscle, nociceptors and afferent fibers. In S. Mense & R. D. Gerwin (Eds.), *Muscle pain: understanding the mechanisms* (pp. 17–48). Berlin: Springer-Verlag.

Mense, S. (2010b). How do muscle lesions such as latent and active trigger points influence central nociceptive neurons? *J Musculokelet Pain, 18*, 348–353.

Mense, S., & Gerwin, R. D. (2010). *Muscle pain: understanding the mechanisms*. Berlin: Springer-Verlag.

Monti, R. J., Roy, R. R., & Edgerton, V. R. (2001). Role of motor unit structure in defining function. *Muscle & Nerve, 24*, 848–866.

Müller, C. E., Aranha, M. F., & Gavião, M. B. (2015). Two-dimensional ultrasound and ultrasound elastography imaging of trigger points in women with myofascial pain syndrome treated by acupuncture and electroacupuncture: a double-blinded randomized controlled pilot study. *Ultrason Imaging, 37(2)*, 152–167.

Niddam, D. M., Chan, R. C., Lee, S. H., Yeh, T. C., & Hsieh, J. (2008). Central representation of hyperalgesia from myofascial trigger point. *NeuroImage, 39*, 1299–1306.

Niddam, D. M. (2009). Brain manifestation and modulation of pain from myofascial trigger points. *Current Pain and Headache Reports, 13*, 370–375.

Oba, T., Koshita, M., Aoki, T., & Yamaguchi, M. (1997a). BAY K 8644 and ClO4- potentiate caffeine contracture without Ca^{2+} release channel activation. *The American Journal of Physiology, 272*, C41–47.

Oba, T., Koshita, M., & Yamaguchi, M. (1997b). Ethanol enhances caffeine-induced Ca^{2+}-release channel activation in skeletal muscle sarcoplasmic reticulum. *The American Journal of Physiology, 272*, C622–627.

Park, G. Y., & Kwon, D. R. (2011). Application of real-time sonoelastography in musculoskeletal diseases related to physical medicine and rehabilitation. *American Journal of Physical Medicine & Rehabilitation, 90*(11), 875–886.

Partanen, J. (1999). End plate spikes in the human electromyogram: revision of the fusimotor theory. *The Journal of Physiology, 93*, 155–166.

Partanen, J. V., Ojala, T. A., & Arokoski, J. P. A. (2010). Myofascial syndrome and pain: a neurophysiological approach. *Pathophysiology, 17*, 19–28.

Perreault, T., Dunning, J., & Butts, R. (2017). The local twitch response during trigger point dry needling: Is it necessary for successful outcomes? *J Bodyw Mov Ther., 21*(4), 940–947.

Qerama, E., Fuglsang-Frederiksen, A., et al. (2004). Evoked pain in motor endplate region of the brachial biceps muscle: an experimental study. *Muscle & Nerve, 29*, 393–400.

Qerama, E., Fuglsang-Frederiksen, A., Kasch, H., Bach, F. W., & Jensen, T. S. (2006). A double-blind, controlled study of botulinum toxin A in chronic myofascial pain. *Neurology, 67*, 241–245.

Quintner, J. L., Bove, G. M., & Cohen, M. L. (2015). A critical evaluation of the trigger point phenomenon. *Rheumatology (Oxford), 54*(3), 392–399.

Reitinger, A., Radner, H., Tilscher, H., Hanna, M., Windisch, A., & Feigl, W. (1996). Morphologische Untersuchung an Triggerpunkten. *Manuelle Medizin, 34*, 256–262.

Rha, D. W., Shin, J. C., Kim, Y. K., et al. (2011). Detecting local twitch responses of myofascial trigger points in the lower-back muscles using ultrasonography. *Archives of Physical Medicine and Rehabilitation, 92*, 1576–1580.

Rickards, L. (2011). Effectiveness of noninvasive treatments for active myofascial trigger point pain: a systematic review. In J. Dommerholt & P. A. Huijbregts (Eds.), *Myofascial trigger points; pathophysiology and evidence-informed diagnosis and management* (pp. 129–158). Jones & Bartlett: Sudbury.

Ruch, T. C. (1961). Patho-physiology of pain. In T. C. Ruch, H. D. Patton, J. W. Woodbury, & A. L. Towe (Eds.), *Neurophysiology* (pp. 350–368). Philadelphia & London: W.B. Saunders Company.

Sahlin, K., Harris, R. C., Nylind, B., & Hultman, E. (1976). Lactate content and pH in muscle obtained after dynamic exercise. *European Journal of Physiology, 367*, 143–149.

Schilder, A., Hoheisel, U., Magerl, W., Benrath, J., Klein, T., & Treede, R. D. (2014). Sensory findings after stimulation of the thoracolumbar fascia with hypertonic saline suggest its contribution to low back pain. *Pain, 155*(2), 222–231.

Shabala, L., Sanchez-Pastor, E., Trujillo, X., Shabala, S., Muniz, J., & Huerta, M. (2008). Effects of verapamil and gadolinium on caffeine-induced contractures and calcium fluxes in frog slow skeletal muscle fibers. *The Journal of Membrane Biology, 221*, 7–13.

Shah, J. P., Phillips, T. M., Danoff, J. V., & Gerber, L. H. (2005). An in-vivo microanalytical technique for measuring the local biochemical milieu of human skeletal muscle. *Journal of Applied Physiology, 99*, 1977–1984.

Shah, J. P., Danoff, J. V., Desai, M. J., Parikh, S., Nakamura, L. Y., Phillips, T. M., et al. (2008). Biochemicals associated with pain and inflammation are elevated in sites near to and remote from active myofascial trigger points. *Archives of Physical Medicine and Rehabilitation, 89*, 16–23.

Sinclair, D. C., Weddell, G., & Feindel, W. H. (1948). Referred pain and associated phenomena. *Brain, 71*, 184–211.

Sikdar, S., Shah, J. P., Gilliams, E., et al. (2009). Novel applications of ultrasound technology to visualize and characterize myofascial trigger points and surrounding soft tissue. *Archives of Physical Medicine and Rehabilitation, 90*, 1829–1838.

Simons, D. G. (1975). Muscle pain syndromes - part 1. *American Journal of Physical Medicine, 54*, 289–311.

Simons, D. G., & Travell, J. (1981). Myofascial trigger points, a possible explanation. *Pain, 10*(1), 106–109.

Simons, D. G., Hong, C. Z., & Simons, L. S. (1995). Prevalence of spontaneous electrical activity at trigger spots and at control sites in rabbit skeletal muscle. *Journal of Musculoskeletal Pain, 3*, 35–48.

Simons, D. G. (1996). Clinical and etiological update of myofascial pain from trigger points. *Journal of Musculoskeletal Pain, 4*, 93–121.

Simons, D. G., & Mense, S. (1998). Understanding and measurement of muscle tone as related to clinical muscle pain. *Pain, 75*, 1–17.

Simons, D. G., Travell, J. G., & Simons, L. S. (1999). *Myofascial pain and dysfunction: the trigger point manual. (1).* Philadelphia: Lippincott William & Wilkins.

Simons, D. G. (2001). Do endplate noise and spikes arise from normal motor endplates? *American Journal of Physical Medicine & Rehabilitation, 80*, 134–140.

Simons, D. G., Hong, C. Z., & Simons, L. S. (2002). Endplate potentials are common to midfiber myofascial trigger points. *American Journal of Physical Medicine & Rehabilitation, 81*, 212–222.

Simons, D. G. (2004). Review of enigmatic MTrPs as a common cause of enigmatic musculoskeletal pain and dysfunction. *Journal of Electromyography and Kinesiology, 14*, 95–107.

Sluka, K. A., Kalra, A., & Moore, S. A. (2001). Unilateral intramuscular injections of acidic saline produce a bilateral, long-lasting hyperalgesia. *Muscle & Nerve, 24*, 37–46.

Sluka, K. A., Rohlwing, J. J., Bussey, R. A., Eikenberry, S. A., & Wilken, J. M. (2002). Chronic muscle pain induced by repeated acid Injection is reversed by spinally administered mu- and delta-, but not kappa-, opioid receptor agonists. *The Journal of Pharmacology and Experimental Therapeutics, 302*, 1146–1150.

Sluka, K. A., Price, M. P., Breese, N. M., Stucky, C. L., Wemmie, J. A., & Welsh, M. J. (2003). Chronic hyperalgesia induced by repeated acid injections in muscle is abolished by the loss of ASIC3, but not ASIC1. *Pain, 106*, 229–239.

Sluka, K. A., Winter, O. C., & Wemmie, J. A. (2009). Acid-sensing ion channels: a new target for pain and CNS diseases. *Current Opinion in Drug Discovery & Development, 12*, 693–704.

Smillie, S. J., & Brain, S. D. (2011). Calcitonin gene-related peptide (CGRP) and its role in hypertension. *Neuropeptides, 45*, 93–104.

Snijdelaar, D. G., Dirksen, R., Slappendel, R., & Crul, B. J. (2000). Substance P. *European Journal of Pain, 4*, 121–135.

Srbely, J. Z., & Dickey, J. P. (2007). Randomized controlled study of the antinociceptive effect of ultrasound on trigger point sensitivity: novel applications in myofascial therapy? *Clinical Rehabilitation, 21*, 411–417.

Srbely, J. Z., Dickey, J. P., Lowerison, M., Edwards, A. M., Nolet, P. S., & Wong, L. L. (2008). Stimulation of myofascial trigger points with ultrasound induces segmental antinociceptive effects: a randomized controlled study. *Pain, 139*, 260–266.

Srbely, J. Z., Dickey, J. P., Bent, L. R., Lee, D., & Lowerison, M. (2010a). Capsaicin-induced central sensitization evokes segmental increases in trigger point sensitivity in humans. *The Journal of Pain, 11*, 636–643.

Srbely, J. Z., Dickey, J. P., Lee, D., & Lowerison, M. (2010b). Dry needle stimulation of myofascial trigger points evokes segmental anti-nociceptive effects. *Journal of Rehabilitation Medicine, 42*, 463–468.

Srbely, J. Z. (2010). New trends in the treatment and management of myofascial pain syndrome. *Current Pain and Headache Reports, 14*, 346–352.

Taguchi, T., Hoheisel, U., & Mense, S. (2008). Dorsal horn neurons having input from low back structures in rats. *Pain, 138*(1), 119–129.

Theobald, G. W. (1949). The role of the cerebral cortex in the apperception of pain. *Lancet, 257*, 41–47.

Thunberg, J., Ljubisavljevic, M., Djupsjobacka, M., & Johansson, H. (2002). Effects on the fusimotor-muscle spindle system induced by intramuscular injections of hypertonic saline. *Experimental Brain Research, 142*, 319–326.

Travell, J., & Rinzler, S. H. (1952). The myofascial genesis of pain. *Postgraduate Medicine, 11*, 425–434.

Treaster, D., Marras, W. S., Burr, D., Sheedy, J. E., & Hart, D. (2006). Myofascial trigger point development from visual and postural stressors during computer work. *Journal of Electromyography and Kinesiology, 16*, 115–124.

Vecchiet, L., Giamberardino, M. A., & Dragani, L. (1990). Latent myofascial trigger points: changes in muscular and subcutaneous pain thresholds at trigger point and target level. *J. Man and Medicine, 5*, 151–154.

Vecchiet, L., Giamberardino, M. A., & Bigontina, P. (1994). *Comparative sensory evaluation of parietal tissues in painful and nonpainful areas in fibromyalgia and myofascial pain syndrome.* In G. B. Gebhart, D. L. Hammond, & J. S. Jensen (Eds.), *Proceedings of the 7th World Congress on Pain: progress in pain research and management* (pp. 177–185). Seattle: IASP Press.

Walder, R. Y., Rasmussen, L. A., Rainier, J. D., Light, A. R., Wemmie, J. A., & Sluka, K. A. (2010). ASIC1 and ASIC3 play different roles in the development of hyperalgesia after inflammatory muscle injury. *The Journal of Pain, 11*, 210–218.

Wang, Y. H., Ding, X., Zhang, Y., et al. (2010). Ischemic compression block attenuates mechanical hyperalgesia evoked from latent myofascial trigger point. *Experimental Brain Research, 202*, 265–267.

Weinkauf, B., Deising, S., Obreja, O., Hoheisel, U., Mense, S., Schmelz, M., et al. (2015). Comparison of nerve growth factor-induced sensitization pattern in lumbar and tibial muscle and fascia. *Muscle & Nerve, 52*(2), 265–272.

Weiss, J. M. (2001). Pelvic floor myofascial trigger points: manual therapy for interstitial cystitis and the urgency-frequency syndrome. *The Journal of Urology, 166,* 2226–2231.

Wessler, I. (1996). Acetylcholine release at motor endplates and autonomic neuroeffector junctions: a comparison. *Pharmacological Research, 33,* 81–94.

Wiederholt, W. C. (1970). "End-plate noise" in electromyography. *Neurology, 20,* 214–224.

Windisch, A., Reitinger, A., Traxler, H., Radner, H., Neumayer, C., Feigl, W., et al. (1999). Morphology and histochemistry of myogelosis. *Clinical Anatomy, 12*(4), 266–271.

Xu, Y. M., Ge, H. Y., & Arendt-Nielsen, L. (2010). Sustained nociceptive mechanical stimulation of latent myofascial trigger point induces central sensitization in healthy subjects. *The Journal of Pain, 11,* 1348–1355.

Zennaro, D., Laubli, T., Krebs, D., Klipstein, A., & Krueger, H. (2003). Continuous, intermitted and sporadic motor unit activity in the trapezius muscle during prolonged computer work. *Journal of Electromyography and Kinesiology, 13,* 113–124.

Zhang, Y., Ge, H. Y., Yue, S. W., Kimura, Y., & Arendt-Nielsen, L. (2009). Attenuated skin blood flow response to nociceptive stimulation of latent myofascial trigger points. *Archives of Physical Medicine and Rehabilitation, 90,* 325–332.

CHAPTER 2

Proposed Mechanisms and Effects of Trigger Point Dry Needling

JAN DOMMERHOLT • CÉSAR FERNÁNDEZ-DE-LAS-PEÑAS

INTRODUCTION

Many physical therapists and other clinicians have adopted a contemporary pain management approach and incorporate graded exercise, restoration of movement, pain science education, and psychosocial perspectives into the examination, assessment, and therapeutic interventions of patients presenting with pain complaints (Gifford & Butler, 1997; George et al., 2010; Nijs et al., 2010; Hodges & Tucker, 2011). The question emerges whether these approaches by themselves are sufficient to address persistent pain states without eliminating peripheral nociceptive input?

Current pain science research supports that pain is an output by the brain, when there is a perception of bodily danger requiring specific action (Moseley, 2003a). In other words, the 'issues are not just in the peripheral tissues' (Butler, 1991) and considering the meaning of pain in the context of the patient's overall situation is critical (Moseley, 2012a). The effects of trigger point (TrP) dry needling (DN) cannot be considered without this broader biopsychosocial model (Dommerholt, 2011). TrP DN must be approached from a pain science perspective, as it is no longer sufficient to consider TrP therapy strictly as a tool to address local muscle pathology.

As Moseley pointed out, nociceptive mechanisms that contribute to threatening information should be treated, where possible (Moseley, 2003a). Especially in persistent pain conditions, TrPs are a constant source of nociceptive input (Melzack, 2001; Giamberardino et al., 2007; Ge et al., 2011), and it follows that removing such peripheral input is indicated and consistent with the concepts of Melzack's neuromatrix (Melzack, 2001). In Moseley's words, 'trigger points are present in all patients with chronic musculoskeletal pain and are thought to reflect sensitisation of nociceptive processing in the central nervous system' and 'elimination of trigger points is an important component of the management of chronic musculoskeletal pain' (Moseley, 2012b).

In addition to their contribution to nociception, TrPs can contribute to abnormal movement patterns (Lucas et al., 2004, 2010; Bohlooli et al., 2016). TrP-DN immediately improved these abnormal muscle activation patterns (Lucas et al., 2004, 2010). The combination of tissue-based interventions, such as TrP-DN (bottom–up techniques) should be combined with neuroscience pain education (top–down techniques) (Louw et al., 2017). TrP-DN is effective when combined with neuroscience pain education in patients with low back pain (Téllez-García et al., 2015). Once patients realise that the somewhat uncomfortable stimulus of DN actually has the potential to reduce or even eliminate their pain, an endogenous inhibitory conditioned pain modulation system will be activated that inhibits early nociceptive processing (Bjorkedal & Flaten, 2012). Fear of needles did not seem to influence pain tolerance and sympathetic responses (Joseph et al., 2013). Pain after DN, usually referred to as postneedling soreness, is a common finding (Brady et al., 2014) that must be addressed as well. Patients must be reassured that postneedling soreness is normal and more or less irrelevant regarding the overall therapeutic outcome. Studies show that spray and stretch (Martin-Pintado Zugasti et al., 2014), local pressure (Martin-Pintado Zugasti et al., 2015), and low-load exercise (Salom-Moreno et al., 2017) can reduce the soreness.

By creating a therapeutic environment in which the expectation of pain reduction combined with an increased sense of self-efficacy are the focus, usually the pain intensity of the treatment can be dissociated from the magnitude of responses in the pain matrix (Bandura et al., 1987; Legrain et al., 2011a, 2011c; Mueller et al., 2012). Expectancy can significantly influence the anticipation and experience of pain (Wager et al., 2004). The context in which a painful stimulus (i.e., DN) is delivered affects patients' experience and anticipation that this noxious stimulus may trigger (Moseley & Amtz, 2007). Legrain and colleagues (2011b) established that patients should be able to focus and maintain their attention on the processing of pain-unrelated information without being too preoccupied by nociceptive stimuli. When applied to using DN in clinical practice, a top–down approach can facilitate an activation of those executive functions that are involved in the control of selective attention and focus on the important overall goal of achieving pain reduction and return to function. In physical therapy, it is often thought that in the presence of central nervous system sensitization, treatments must be pain free to avoid further wind-up of the sensitized central nervous system (Jull 2012). To cause increased wind-up, input from multiple receptors is required over tens of seconds. A single stimulus, such as a pinch or needle stick, is usually insufficient to induce central sensitization.

Increased activity in the anterior cingulate cortex (ACC) is common in chronic pain conditions and is even present when pain is anticipated (Hsieh et al., 1995; Peyron et al., 2000a, 2000b; Sawamoto et al., 2000; Longo et al., 2012), which supports reducing the anticipation of pain during DN. In addition, several studies have shown that TrPs also can activate the ACC and other limbic structures, but suppress hippocampal activity (Svensson et al., 1997; Niddam et al., 2007, 2008). This suggests that TrPs may be linked to stress-related changes and therefore minimising needling-related stress levels and the patients' anticipation is very important. Of interest in this context is that clinicians may underestimate their patients' ability to understand basic concepts of pain neurophysiology (Moseley, 2003b), which emphasises the need for better pain science education of healthcare professionals (Hoeger Bement & Sluka, 2015).

When treating patients with DN techniques, it is imperative to avoid creating the impression that local muscle pathology would be solely responsible for the persistent pain (Nijs et al., 2010; Puentedura & Louw, 2012). Rather than explaining TrPs as a local pathological or anatomical problem, it makes more sense to focus on the nociceptive nature of TrPs and their role in perpetuating central sensitisation (Fernández de las Peñas & Dommerholt, 2014). In general, input from muscle nociceptors is more effective at inducing neuroplastic changes in wide dynamic range dorsal horn neurons than input from cutaneous nociceptive receptors (Wall & Woolf, 1984), and persistent peripheral nociceptive input increases the sensitivity of the central nervous system.

Unfortunately, the contributions of TrPs and the potentially detrimental effect of poorly worded diagnostic considerations with a predominant anatomical emphasis often are not considered, and individual patients may have gone through many unsuccessful treatment regimens with multiple diagnostic pathways. For example, telling patients they have 'a slipped disc' or degenerative disc disease, or even a tear in the rotator cuff muscles, as the main focus of the discussion can contribute to feelings of iatrogenic hopelessness and reduce their expectations (Jull & Sterling, 2009; Puentedura & Louw, 2012; Louw, 2016). Patients may develop fear avoidance or kinesiophobia, poor coping skills, and an anticipation of pain (Bandura et al., 1987; Vlaeyen & Linton, 2000; Wager et al., 2004; Coppieters et al., 2006). Additionally, patients' altered homeostatic systems may start contributing to the overall pain experience (Puentedura & Louw, 2012) with decreased blood flow to the muscles (Zhang et al., 2009), abnormal cytokine production (Watkins et al., 2001; Milligan & Watkins, 2009), constrained breathing patterns (Chaitow, 2004), and abnormal muscle activation patterns (Moreside et al., 2007), among others. In some patients the anticipation of pain and the pain associated with DN itself may activate threatening inputs, at which point DN would become counterproductive. Fortunately, fear of needles does not seem to have a major effect (Joseph et al., 2013), and for most patients TrP DN is a viable intervention (Dilorenzo et al., 2004; Affaitati et al., 2011).

MECHANISMS AND EFFECTS OF TRIGGER POINT DRY NEEDLING

There are no studies of the effect of DN on the ACC and other limbic structures, but several papers suggest that needling acupuncture and nonacupuncture points does seem to involve the limbic system and the descending inhibitory system (Takeshige et al., 1992a, 1992b; Wu et al., 1999; Hui et al., 2000; Biella et al., 2001; Hsieh et al., 2001; Wu et al., 2002). DN studies of patients with fibromyalgia, which is a diagnosis of central sensitisation (Dommerholt & Stanborough, 2012; Bennet et al., 2014), demonstrate that DN of a few TrPs does not only reduce the nociceptive input from the treated TrPs, but reduces the overall widespread pain and sensitivity (Ge et al., 2009, 2010, 2011; Affaitati et al., 2011). TrP DN often evokes patients' referred pain patterns and their primary pain complaint (Hong et al., 1997). Needling of TrPs in the gluteus minimus or teres minor muscles may initiate pain resembling a L5 or C8 radiculopathy, respectively (Escobar & Ballesteros, 1988; Facco & Ceccherelli, 2005). Needling of TrPs in the sternocleidomastoid or upper trapezius muscles may trigger a patient's migraine or tension-type headache (Calandre et al., 2006). Experimentally induced muscle pain impairs diffuse noxious inhibitory control mechanisms (Arendt-Nielsen et al., 2008), and DN does seem to effect central sensitisation, presumably by altering the nociceptive processing (Kuan et al., 2007a; Mense, 2010; Mense & Masi, 2011). It is known that TrP DN reduces segmental nociceptive input and as such is therapeutically indicated (Srbely et al., 2010).

The exact mechanisms of DN continue to be elusive. Because many studies and case reports have confirmed the clinical efficacy of DN, future research must be directed towards examining the underlying mechanisms (Lewit, 1979; Carlson et al., 1993; Hong, 1994, 1997; Hong & Hsueh, 1996; McMillan et al., 1997; Chen et al., 2001; Cummings, 2003; Mayoral & Torres, 2003; Dilorenzo et al., 2004; Ilbuldu et al., 2004; Itoh et al., 2004, 2007; Lucas et al., 2004; Furlan et al., 2005; Kamanli et al., 2005; Mayoral-del-Moral, 2005; Weiner & Schmader, 2006; Giamberardino et al., 2007; Hsieh et al., 2007, 2012, 2014; Fernandez-Carnero et al., 2010; Lucas et al., 2010; Osborne & Gatt, 2010; Tsai et al., 2010; Srbely et al., 2010; Affaitati et al., 2011; Gonzalez-Perez et al., 2012; Mahmoudzadeh et al., 2016; Gattie et al., 2017). Recent systematic reviews confirm the evidence for DN (Furlan et al., 2005; Cagnie et al., 2015; Liu et al., 2015; Espejo-Antúnez et al., 2017). The quality of myofascial pain treatment studies is also improving (Stoop et al., 2017). TrP-DN was more effective than DN randomly in a muscle (Pecos-Martin et al., 2015). Slowly, bits and pieces of the myofascial pain and DN puzzle are beginning to be explored, even though some studies did not observe any significant advantage to adding DN to the options clinicians may use to treat patients with pain and movement dysfunction (Mason et al., 2016; Espi-Lopez et al., 2017; Perez-Palomares et al., 2017).

Mechanically, deep DN may disrupt contraction knots, stretch contractured sarcomere assemblies, and reduce the overlap between actin and myosin filaments. It may destroy motor endplates and cause distal axon denervation and changes in the endplate cholinesterase and acetylcholine receptors similarly to the normal muscle regeneration process (Gaspersic et al., 2001; Domingo et al., 2013). DN may also change the excitability of spinal motor neurons and improve muscle tone separate from its analgesic effect (Casale et al., 2017).

Of particular interest are local twitch responses (LTR), which are involuntary spinal cord reflexes of muscle fibres in a taut band after DN, injections, or snapping palpation (Dexter & Simons, 1981; Fricton et al., 1985; Hong, 1994; Hong & Torigoe, 1994; Simons & Dexter, 1995; Wang & Audette, 2000; Ga et al., 2007). Eliciting LTR is important when inactivating TrPs and confirms that the needle was placed accurately into a TrP. Several studies have confirmed that an LTR can reduce or even eliminate the typical endplate noise and endplate spikes associated with TrPs, which suggests that DN inactivates TrPs (Hong, 1994; Hong & Torigoe, 1994; Chen et al., 2001; Hsieh et al., 2011; Liu et al., 2017). There is a positive correlation between the prevalence of endplate noise in a TrP region and the pain intensity of that TrP (Kuan et al., 2007b). Endplate noise and endplate spikes reflect a summation of miniature endplate potentials and are characteristic of TrPs (Simons et al., 1995, 2002; Hong & Simons, 1998; Simons, 2001, 2004). Moreover, eliciting LTRs appears to reduce the concentrations of many chemicals found in the immediate environment of active TrPs, such as calcitonin gene related peptide, substance P, serotonin, interleukins, and epinephrine, among others (Shah et al., 2003, 2005, 2008; Shah & Gilliams, 2008; Hsieh et al., 2014). Shah and colleagues (2008) had speculated that the drop in concentrations may be caused by a local increase in blood flow, by interference with nociceptor membrane channels, or by transport mechanisms associated with a briefly augmented inflammatory response. The decrease of concentrations of substance P and calcitonin gene-related peptide corresponds with the clinical observation of a reduction in pain after deep DN (Shah et al., 2008). Hsieh and colleagues (2012) confirmed that TrP-DN modulated the chemical mediators associated with pain and inflammation, such as substance P, β-endorphin, and tumour necrosis factor-α, among others. They also reported that modulating these chemical concentrations with TrP-DN is dose dependent, which implies that an excessive amount of DN may actually increase the concentrations. Liu and colleagues observed that TrP-DN with LTRs also reduced acetylcholine and acetylcholine receptor levels significantly in a well-executed rabbit study (Liu et al., 2017). The increased concentration of multiple chemicals is associated with a lowered pH as a result of ischaemia and hypoxia (Brückle et al., 1990; Sikdar et al., 2010; Ballyns et al., 2011). DN of the trapezius muscle increased the blood flow and oxygen saturation, which suggests another potential mechanism in support of DN (Cagnie et al., 2012).

LTRs are often visible with the naked eye and can be visualised with sonography (Gerwin & Duranleau, 1997; Lewis & Tehan, 1999; Rha et al., 2011). It is not known how many LTRs are required for a positive outcome or if there even is a correlation between the number and size of LTRs and therapeutic outcomes. A recent study reported no clinical differences on pain depending on the number of LTRs obtained in patients with neck pain (Fernández-Carnero et al., 2017). Nevertheless, individuals exhibited significant clinical improvement when eliciting the highest number (n = 6) of LTRs until exhaustion compared with not eliciting any (Fernández-Carnero et al., 2017). Koppenhaver and colleagues (2017) found no differences after 1 week between patients with low back pain experiencing LTR and those not experiencing LTR, although subjects who experienced a LTR reported a greater short-term improvement in the function of the lumbar multifidus muscle compared with those who did not. Discrepancies expressed in published studies have led some authors to question the need of LTRs during TrP-DN (Perreault et al., 2017). It appears that several DN studies do not resemble clinical practice, which may influence the findings and their utility. In the clinic, it would be highly unusual to stick a patient only once with a needle or treat only one muscle. Yet several studies exploring the efficacy of DN use a model with either one needle stick or a very limited number of muscles.

The efficacy of dry needling can be monitored with ultrasound imaging. Turo and colleagues (2015) visualised tissue changes after DN. Participants with at least one active TrP received a 3-week course of DN at their most active TrP. Grey-scale 2D B-mode and colour Doppler ultrasound images were taken at the TrP. A significant reduction in the heterogeneity of muscle stiffness was observed at those TrPs that responded to treatment even 8 weeks after the DN procedures. In addition, the TrP status changed from active to latent and eventually a complete resolution of pain symptoms in a significant number of cases (Turo et al., 2015). Gerber and colleagues (2015) confirmed that a few sessions of DN can effectively reduce pain for at least 6 weeks. Several clinical investigators are exploring whether DN can be used to decrease spasticity with promising results (see Chapter 4) (Salom-Moreno et al., 2014; Ansari et al., 2015; Calvo et al., 2016; Mendigutia-Gomez et al., 2016). Calvo and colleagues (2017) showed that DN had a positive effect on quantitative electroencephalographic activity, especially in both the frontal and prefrontal regions of two stroke patients.

The effects of superficial DN are often attributed to stimulation of Aδ sensory afferent fibres, which may outlast the stimulus for up to 72 hours (Baldry, 2005). It is true that stimulation of Aδ nerve fibres may activate enkephalinergic, serotonergic, and noradrenergic inhibitory systems (Bowsher, 1998); however, type I high-threshold Aδ nerve fibres are only activated by nociceptive mechanical stimulation, and type II Aδ fibres require cold stimuli (Millan, 1999). Because superficial DN is neither a painful mechanical nor a cold stimulus, it is unlikely that Aδ fibres would get activated (Dommerholt et al., 2006). When superficial DN is combined with rotation of the needle, the stimulus may activate the pain inhib-itory system associated with stimulation of Aδ fibres through segmental spinal and propriospinal hetero-segmental inhibition (Sandkühler, 1996). Deep DN can be also combined with rotation of the needle, after which the needle is left in place until relaxation of the muscle fibres has occurred (Dommerholt et al., 2006). The mechanical pressure exerted with the needle may electrically polarise muscle and connective tissue and transform mechanical stress into electrical activity, which is required for tissue remodelling (Liboff, 1997). It is also possible that superficial DN may activate mechanoreceptors coupled to slow conducting unmyelinated C fibre afferents. This could trigger a reduction of pain and a sense of progress and well-being through activation of the insular region and anterior cingulate cortex (Olausson et al., 2002; Mohr et al., 2005; Lund & Lundeberg, 2006).

Many clinicians combine superficial and deep DN with electrical stimulation through the needles (Mayoral & Torres, 2003; Mayoral-del-Moral, 2005; Dommerholt et al., 2006). Electrical stimulation can activate the endogenous opioid system, which likely has a facilitating effect of pain reduction (Han et al., 1984). In addition, it may activate the peri-aqueductal grey in some patients (Niddam et al., 2007). Modulating high- and low-frequency TENS produced better analgesia than either frequency by itself (DeSantana et al., 2008); however each application has specific effects. Only low-frequency TENS increased spinal concentrations of serotonin during and immediate after treatment (Sluka et al., 2006), which can reduce pain. Several rodent studies have shown that electrical acupuncture can modulate the expression of N-methyl-D-aspartate in primary sensory neurons (Choi et al., 2005; Wang et al., 2006). Only high-frequency TENS reduced spinal concentrations of glutamate and aspartate in rats with joint inflammation and activated delta-opioid receptors, possibly through spinal dorsal horn glial cells, as blocking the delta-opioid receptors with naltrindole caused a reduction in spinal concentrations (Gopalkrishnan & Sluka, 2000; Sluka et al., 2005). High-frequency TENS also reduced primary hyperalgesia to mechanical stimulation and heat (Gopalkrishnan & Sluka, 2000). It appears that combining high- and low-frequency TENS may give the best results, even though there is conflicting research (Lin et al., 2002; Barlas et al., 2006; Leon-Hernandez et al., 2016).

Unfortunately, there are no evidence-based guidelines of the optimal treatment parameters such as optimal amplitude, frequency, and duration. Stimulation frequencies between 2 and 4 Hz are thought to trigger the release of endorphins and enkephalin, whereas frequencies between 80 and 100 Hz may release gamma-aminobutyric acid, galanin, and dynorphin (Lundeberg & Stener-Victorin, 2002). The ideal needle placement for e-stim with DN has not been determined either. White and collagues (2000) recommended placing the needle-electrodes within the same dermatomes as the location of the lesion, whereas other clinicians recommended inserting two converging electrodes directly into a TrP at both sides of a TrP inside the taut band (Elorriaga 2000; Mayoral et al., 2004).

SUMMARY

A pain science approach to TrP-DN is without question the way of the future. Combining bottom–up and top–down interventions yields the best results. Where a decade ago, comparisons of DN to other modalities or treatment options frequently showed a lack of evidence for DN, more recently the evidence for DN and the quality of research are improving; however, more high-quality studies are still needed not only on its effectiveness, but more importantly, on the underlying mechanisms. TrPs are a constant source of nociceptive input especially in persistent pain conditions, but the details of their contributions remain an enigma. What is the role of conditioned pain modulation with TrP-DN? Which treatment parameters should clinicians use with DN electrotherapy? There are still more questions than answers.

REFERENCES

Affaitati, G., Costantini, R., Fabrizio, A., et al. (2011). Effects of treatment of peripheral pain generators in fibromyalgia patients. *European Journal of Pain, 15*, 61–69.

Arendt-Nielsen, L., Sluka, K. A., & Nie, H. L. (2008). Experimental muscle pain impairs descending inhibition. *Pain, 140*, 465–471.

Ansari, N. N., Naghdi, S., Fakhari, Z., Radinmehr, H., & Hasson, S. (2015). Dry needling for the treatment of poststroke muscle spasticity: a prospective case report. *NeuroRehabilitation, 36*(1), 61–65.

Baldry, P. E. (2005). *Acupuncture, trigger points and musculoskeletal pain.* Edinburgh: Churchill Livingstone.

Ballyns, J. J., Shah, J. P., Hammond, J., Gebreab, T., Gerber, L. H., & Sikdar, S. (2011). Objective sonographic measures for characterizing myofascial trigger points associated with cervical pain. *Journal of Ultrasound in Medicine, 30*, 1331–1340.

Bandura, A., O'Leary, A., Taylor, C. B., et al. (1987). Perceived self-efficacy and pain control: opioid and nonopioid mechanisms. *Journal of Personality and Social Psychology, 53*, 563–571.

Barlas, P., Ting, S. L., Chesterton, L. S., Jones, P. W., & Sim, J. (2006). Effects of intensity of electroacupuncture upon experimental pain in healthy human volunteers: a randomized, double-blind, placebo-controlled study. *Pain, 122*, 81–89.

Biella, G., Sotgiu, M. L., Pellegata, G., et al. (2001). Acupuncture produces central activations in pain regions. *NeuroImage, 14*, 60–66.

Bjorkedal, E., & Flaten, M. A. (2012). Expectations of increased and decreased pain explain the effect of conditioned pain modulation in females. *Journal of Pain Research, 5*, 289–300.

Bohlooli, N., Ahmadi, A., Maroufi, N., Sarrafzadeh, J., & Jaberzadeh, S. (2016). Differential activation of scapular muscles, during arm elevation, with and without trigger points. *Journal of Bodywork and Movement Therapies, 20*, 26–34.

Bowsher, D. (1998). Mechanisms of acupuncture. In J. Filshie & A. White (Eds.), *Western acupuncture, a Western scientific approach.* Edinburgh: Churchill Livingstone.

Brady, S., McEvoy, J., Dommerholt, J., & Doody, C. (2014). Adverse events following dry needling: a prospective survey of Chartered Physiotherapists. *The Journal of Manual & Manipulative Therapy, 22*, 134–140.

Brückle, W., Sückfull, M., Fleckenstein, W., Weiss, C., & Müller, W. (1990). Gewebe-Po2-Messung in der verspannten Rückenmuskulatur (m. erector spinae). *Zeitschrift für Rheumatologie, 49*, 208–216.

Butler, D. S. (1991). *Mobilisation of the nervous system.* Melbourne: Churchill Livingstone.

Cagnie, B., Barbe, T., De Ridder, E., Van Oosterwijck, J., Cools, A., & Danneels, L. (2012). The influence of dry needling of the trapezius muscle on muscle blood flow and oxygenation. *Journal of Manipulative and Physiological Therapeutics, 35*, 685–691.

Cagnie, B., Castelein, B., Pollie, F., Steelant, L., Verhoeyen, H., & Cools, A. (2015). Evidence for the use of ischemic compression and dry needling in the management of trigger points of the upper trapezius in patients with neck pain: a systematic review. *American Journal of Physical Medicine & Rehabilitation, 94*, 573–583.

Calandre, E. P., Hidalgo, J., Garcia-Leiva, J. M., & Rico-Villademoros, F. (2006). Trigger point evaluation in migraine patients: an indication of peripheral sensitization linked to migraine predisposition? *European Journal of Neurology, 13*, 244–249.

Carlson, C. R., Okeson, J. P., Falace, D. A., et al. (1993). Reduction of pain and EMG activity in the masseter region by trapezius trigger point injection. *Pain, 55*, 397–400.

Calvo, S., Navarro, J., Herrero, P., Del Moral, R., De Diego, C., & Marijuán, P. C. (2017). Electroencephalographic changes after application of dry needling [DNHS Technique] in two patients with chronic stroke. *MYOPAIN. online*, 1–6.

Calvo, S., Quintero, I., & Herrero, P. (2016). Effects of dry needling (DNHS technique) on the contractile properties of spastic muscles in a patient with stroke: a case report. *International Journal of Rehabilitation Research, 39*, 372–376.

Casale, R., Ceccherelli, F., Buttacchio, G., Calabrese, M., Labeeb, A., & Symeonidou, Z. (2017). Dry needling reverses vibration-induced changes in spinal motoneuronal pool: is there any basis for its action on muscle tone? *Journal of Pain Relief, 6*, 1000287.

Chaitow, L. (2004). Breathing pattern disorders, motor control, and low back pain. *Journal of Osteopathic Medicine, 7*, 33–40.

Chen, J. T., Chung, K. C., Hou, C. R., et al. (2001). Inhibitory effect of dry needling on the spontaneous electrical activity recorded from myofascial trigger spots of rabbit skeletal muscle. *American Journal of Physical Medicine & Rehabilitation, 80*, 729–735.

Choi, B. T., Lee, J. H., Wan, Y., & Han, J. S. (2005). Involvement of ionotropic glutamate receptors in low frequency electroacupuncture analgesia in rats. *Neuroscience Letters, 377*, 185–188.

Coppieters, M. W., Alshami, A. M., & Hodges, P. W. (2006). An experimental pain model to investigate the specificity of the neurodynamic test for the median nerve in the differential diagnosis of hand symptoms. *Archives of Physical Medicine and Rehabilitation, 87*, 1412–1417.

Cummings, M. (2003). Referred knee pain treated with electroacupuncture to iliopsoas. *Acupuncture in Medicine, 21*, 32–35.

DeSantana, J. M., Santana-Filho, V. J., & Sluka, K. A. (2008). Modulation between high- and low-frequency transcutaneous electric nerve stimulation delays the development of analgesic tolerance in arthritic rats. *Archives of Physical Medicine and Rehabilitation, 89*(4), 754–760.

Dexter, J. R., & Simons, D. G. (1981). Local twitch response in human muscle evoked by palpation and needle penetration of a trigger point. *Archives of Physical Medicine and Rehabilitation, 62*, 521.

Dilorenzo, L., Traballesi, M., Morelli, D., et al. (2004). Hemiparetic shoulder pain syndrome treated with deep dry needling during early rehabilitation: a prospective, open-label, randomized investigation. *Journal of Musculoskeletal Pain, 12*, 25–34.

Domingo, A., Mayoral, O., Monterde, S., & Santafe, M. M. (2013). Neuromuscular damage and repair after dry needling in mice. *Evidence-based Complementary and Alternative Medicine, 2013*, 260806.

Dommerholt, J., Mayoral, O., & Gröbli, C. (2006). Trigger point dry needling. *The Journal of Manual & Manipulative Therapy, 14*, E70–E87.

Dommerholt, J. (2011). Dry needling - peripheral and central considerations. *Journal of Manual & Manipulative Therapy., 19*(4), 223–227.

Dommerholt, J., & Stanborough, R. W. (2012). Muscle pain syndromes. In R. I. Cantu, A. J. Grodin, & R. W. Stanborough (Eds.), *Myofascial manipulation*. Austin: Pro-Ed.

Elorriaga, A. (2000). The 2-Needle Technique. *Medical Acupuncture, 12*, 17–79.

Escobar, P. L., & Ballesteros, J. (1988). Teres minor. Source of symptoms resembling ulnar neuropathy or C8 radiculopathy. *American Journal of Physical Medicine & Rehabilitation, 67*, 120–122.

Espejo-Antûnez, L., Fernández-Huertas Tejeda, J., Albornoz-Cabello, M., Rodrríguez-Mansilla, J., de la Cruz-Torres, B., Ribeiro, F., et al. (2017). Dry needling in the management of myofascial trigger points: a systematic review of randomized controlled trials. *Complementary Therapies in Medicine, 33*, 46–57.

Espi-Lopez, G. V., Serra-Ano, P., Vicent-Ferrando, J., Sanchez-Moreno-Giner, M., Arias-Buria, J. L., Cleland, J., et al. (2017). Effectiveness of inclusion of dry needling in a multimodal therapy program for patellofemoral pain: a randomized parallel-group trial. *The Journal of Orthopaedic and Sports Physical Therapy, 47*, 392–401.

Facco, E., & Ceccherelli, F. (2005). Myofascial pain mimicking radicular syndromes. *Acta Neurochir, 92*(Suppl), 147–150.

Fernandez-Carnero, J., La Touche, R., Ortega-Santiago, R., et al. (2010). Short-term effects of dry needling of active myofascial trigger points in the masseter muscle in patients with temporomandibular disorders. *Journal of Orofacial Pain, 24*, 106–112.

Fernandez-Carnero, J., Gilarranz-de-Frutos, L., Leon-Hernandez, J. V., Pecos-Martin, D., Alguacil-Diego, I., Gallego-Izquierdo, T., & Martin-Pintado-Zugasti, A. (2017). Effectiveness of different deep dry needling dosages in the treatment of patients with cervical myofascial pain: a pilot RCT. *American Journal of Physical Medicine & Rehabilitation, 96*(10), 726–733.

Fernández de las Peñas, C., & Dommerholt, J. (2014). Myofascial trigger points: peripheral or central phenomenon? *Current Rheumatology Reports, 16*(1), 395.

Fricton, J. R., Auvinen, M. D., Dykstra, D., & Schiffman, E. (1985). Myofascial pain syndrome electromyographic changes associated with local twitch response. *Archives of Physical Medicine and Rehabilitation, 66*, 314–317.

Furlan, A., Tulder, M., Cherkin, D., et al. (2005). Acupuncture and dry needling for low back pain: an updated systematic review with the framework of the Cochrane Collaboration. *Spine, 30*, 944–963.

Ga, H., Koh, H. J., Choi, J. H., & Kim, C. H. (2007). Intramuscular and nerve root stimulation vs lidocaine injection to trigger points in myofascial pain syndrome. *Journal of Rehabilitation Medicine, 39*, 374–378.

Gaspersic, R., Koritnik, B., Erzen, I., & Sketelj, J. (2001). Muscle activity-resistant acetylcholine receptor accumulation is induced in places of former motor endplates in ectopically innervated regenerating rat muscles. *International Journal of Developmental Neuroscience, 19*, 339–346.

Gattie, E., Cleland, J. A., & Snodgrass, S. (2017). The effectiveness of trigger point dry needling for musculoskeletal conditions by physical therapists: a systematic review and meta-analysis. *The Journal of Orthopaedic and Sports Physical Therapy, 47*, 133–149.

Ge, H. Y., Nie, H., Madeleine, P., et al. (2009). Contribution of the local and referred pain from active myofascial trigger points in fibromyalgia syndrome. *Pain, 147*, 233–240.

Ge, H. Y., Wang, Y., Danneskiold-Samsoe, B., et al. (2010). The predetermined sites of examination for tender points in fibromyalgia syndrome are frequently associated with myofascial trigger points. *The Journal of Pain, 11*, 644–651.

Ge, H. Y., Wang, Y., Fernández-de-las-Peñas, C., et al. (2011). Reproduction of overall spontaneous pain pattern by manual stimulation of active myofascial trigger points in fibromyalgia patients. *Arthritis Research & Therapy, 13*, R48.

Gerber, L. H., Shah, J., Rosenberger, W., Armstrong, K., Turo, D., Otto, P., et al. (2015). Dry needling alters trigger points in the upper trapezius muscle and reduces pain in subjects with chronic myofascial pain. *Physical Medicine and Rehabilitation, 7*, 711–718.

George, S. Z., Wittmer, V. T., Fillingim, R. B., & Robinson, M. E. (2010). Comparison of graded exercise and graded exposure clinical outcomes for patients with chronic low back pain. *The Journal of Orthopaedic and Sports Physical Therapy, 40*, 694–704.

Gerwin, R. D., & Duranleau, D. (1997). Ultrasound identification of the myofascial trigger point. *Muscle & Nerve, 20*, 767–768.

Giamberardino, M. A., Tafuri, E., Savini, A., et al. (2007). Contribution of myofascial trigger points to migraine symptoms. *The Journal of Pain, 8*, 869–878.

Gifford, L. S., & Butler, D. S. (1997). The integration of pain sciences into clinical practice. *Journal of Hand Therapy, 10*, 86–95.

Gonzalez-Perez, L. M., Infante-Cossio, P., Granados-Nunez, M., & Urresti-Lopez, F. J. (2012). Treatment of temporomandibular myofascial pain with deep dry needling. *Medicina Oral, Patología Oral y Cirugía Bucal, 17*, e781–785.

Gopalkrishnan, P., & Sluka, K. A. (2000). Effect of varying frequency, intensity, and pulse duration of transcutaneous electrical nerve stimulation on primary hyperalgesia in inflamed rats. *Archives of Physical Medicine and Rehabilitation, 81*, 984–990.

Han, J. S., Xie, G. X., Ding, X. Z., & Fan, S. G. (1984). High and low frequency electro-acupuncture analgesia are mediated by different opioids. *Pain, 2*, 543.

Hodges, P. W., & Tucker, K. (2011). Moving differently in pain: a new theory to explain the adaptation to pain. *Pain, 152*, S90–S98.

Hoeger Bement, M. K., & Sluka, K. A. (2015). The current state of physical therapy pain curricula in the United States: a faculty survey. *The Journal of Pain, 16*, 144–152.

Hong, C. Z. (1994). Lidocaine injection versus dry needling to myofascial trigger point. The importance of the local twitch response. *American Journal of Physical Medicine & Rehabilitation, 73*, 256–263.

Hong, C. Z., & Hsueh, T. C. (1996). Difference in pain relief after trigger point injections in myofascial pain patients with and without fibromyalgia. *Archives of Physical Medicine and Rehabilitation, 77*, 1161–1166.

Hong, C. Z., & Simons, D. G. (1998). Pathophysiologic and electrophysiologic mechanisms of myofascial trigger points. *Archives of Physical Medicine and Rehabilitation, 79*, 863–872.

Hong, C. Z., & Torigoe, Y. (1994). Electrophysiological characteristics of localized twitch responses in responsive taut bands of rabbit skeletal muscle. *J. Musculoskeletal Pain, 2*, 17–43.

Hong, C. Z., Kuan, T. S., Chen, J. T., & Chen, S. M. (1997). Referred pain elicited by palpation and by needling of myofascial trigger points: a comparison. *Archives of Physical Medicine and Rehabilitation, 78*, 957–960.

Hsieh, J. C., Belfrage, M., Stone-Elander, S., Hansson, P., & Ingvar, M. (1995). Central representation of chronic ongoing neuropathic pain studied by positron emission tomography. *Pain, 63*, 225–236.

Hsieh, J. C., Tu, C. H., Chen, F. P., et al. (2001). Activation of the hypothalamus characterizes the acupuncture stimulation at the analgesic point in human: a positron emission tomography study. *Neuroscience Letters, 307*, 105–108.

Hsieh, Y. L., Kao, M. J., Kuan, T. S., et al. (2007). Dry needling to a key myofascial trigger point may reduce the irritability of satellite MTrPs. *American Journal of Physical Medicine & Rehabilitation, 86*, 397–403.

Hsieh, Y. L., Chou, L. W., Joe, Y. S. et al. (2011). Spinal cord mechanism involving the remote effects of dry needling on the irritability of myofascial trigger spots in rabbit skeletal muscle. *Archives of Physical Medicine and Rehabilitation, 92*, 1098–1105.

Hsieh, Y. L., Yang, S. A., Yang, C. C., & Chou, L. W. (2012). Dry needling at myofascial trigger spots of rabbit skeletal muscles modulates the biochemicals associated with pain, inflammation, and hypoxia. *Evidence-based Complementary and Alternative Medicine, 2012*, 342165.

Hsieh, Y. L., Yang, S. A., Liu, S. Y., Chou, L. W., & Honc, C. Z. (2014). Remote dose-dependent effects of dry needling at distant myofascial trigger spots of rabbit skeletal muscles on reduction of substance P levels of proximal muscle and spinal cords. *BioMed Research International, 2014*, 982121.

Hui, K. K., Liu, J., Makris, N., et al. (2000). Acupuncture modulates the limbic system and subcortical gray structures of the human brain: evidence from fMRI studies in normal subjects. *Human Brain Mapping, 9*, 13–25.

Ilbuldu, E., Cakmak, A., Disci, R., & Aydin, R. (2004). Comparison of laser, dry needling, and placebo laser treatments in myofascial pain syndrome. *Photomedicine and Laser Surgery, 22*, 306–311.

Itoh, K., Katsumi, Y., & Kitakoji, H. (2004) Trigger point acupuncture treatment of chronic low back pain in elderly patients: a blinded RCT. *Acupuncture in Medicine, 22*, 170–177.

Itoh, K., Katsumi, Y., Hirota, S., & Kitakoji, H. (2007). Randomised trial of trigger point acupuncture compared with other acupuncture for treatment of chronic neck pain. *Complementary Therapies in Medicine, 15*, 172–179.

Joseph, L., Mohd Ali, K., Ramlia, A., Rajaduraia, S., Mohanc, V., Justine, M., et al. (2013). Fear of needles does not influence pain tolerance and sympathetic responses among patients during a therapeutic needling. *Polish, 20*, 1–7.

Jull, G., & Sterling, M. (2009). Bring back the biopsychosocial model for neck pain disorders. *Manual Therapy, 14*, 117–118.

Jull, G. A. (2012). Management of Cervical Spine Disorders: Where to Now? *Journal of Orthopaedic and Sport Physical Therapy., 42*(10), A1–A83.

Kamanli, A., Kaya, A., Ardicoglu, O., et al. (2005). Comparison of lidocaine injection, botulinum toxin injection, and dry needling to trigger points in myofascial pain syndrome. *Rheumatology International, 25*, 604–611.

Koppenhaver, S. L., Walker, M. J., Rettig, C., et al. (2017). The association between dry needling-induced twitch response and change in pain and muscle function in patients with low back pain: a quasi-experimental study. *Physiotherapy, 103*, 131–137.

Kuan, T. S., Hong, C. Z., Chen, J. T., Chen, S. M., & Chien, C. H. (2007a). The spinal cord connections of the myofascial trigger spots. *European Journal of Pain, 11*, 624–634.

Kuan, T. S., Hsieh, Y. L., Chen, S. M., et al. (2007b). The myofascial trigger point region: correlation between the degree of irritability and the prevalence of endplate noise. *American Journal of Physical Medicine & Rehabilitation, 86*, 183–189.

Legrain, V., Crombez, G., & Mouraux, A. (2011a). Controlling attention to nociceptive stimuli with working memory. *PLoS One, 6*, e20926.

Legrain, V., Crombez, G., Verhoeven, K., & Mouraux, A. (2011b). The role of working memory in the attentional control of pain. *Pain, 152*, 453–459.

Legrain, V., Iannetti, G. D., Plaghki, L., & Mouraux, A. (2011c). The pain matrix reloaded: a salience detection system for the body. *Progress in Neurobiology, 93*, 111–124.

Leon-Hernandez, J. V., Martin-Pintado-Zugasti, A., Frutos, L. G., Alguacil-Diego, I. M., de la Llave-Rincon, A. I., & Fernandez-Carnero, J. (2016). Immediate and short-term effects of the combination of dry needling and percutaneous TENS on post-needling soreness in patients with chronic myofascial neck pain. *Brazilian Journal of Physical Therapy, 20*, 422–431.

Lewis, J., & Tehan, P. (1999). A blinded pilot study investigating the use of diagnostic ultrasound for detecting active myofascial trigger points. *Pain, 79*, 39–44.

Lewit, K. (1979). The needle effect in the relief of myofascial pain. *Pain, 6*, 83–90.

Liboff, A. R. (1997). Bioelectromagnetic fields and acupuncture. *Journal of Alternative and Complementary Medicine, 3*, S77–S87.

Liu, L., Huang, Q. M., Liu, Q. G., Ye, G., Bo, C. Z., Chen, M. J., et al. (2015). Effectiveness of dry needling for myofascial trigger points associated with neck and shoulder pain: a systematic review and meta-analysis. *Archives of Physical Medicine and Rehabilitation, 96*, 944–955.

Liu, Q. G., Liu, L., Huang, Q. M., Nguyen, T. T., Ma, Y. T., & Zhao, J. M. (2017). Decreased spontaneous electrical activity and acetylcholine at myofascial trigger spots after dry needling treatment: a pilot study. *Evidence-based Complementary and Alternative Medicine, 2017*, 3938191.

Longo, M. R., Iannetti, G. D., Mancini, F., et al. (2012). Linking pain and the body: neural correlates of visually induced analgesia. *The Journal of Neuroscience, 32*, 2601–2607.

Louw, A. (2016). Treating the brain in chronic pain. In C. Fernández de las Peñas, J. Cleland, & J. Dommerholt (Eds.), *Manual therapy for musculoskeletal pain syndromes – an evidenced and clinical-informed approach* (pp. 66–75). Edinburgh: Churchill Livingstone (Elsevier).

Louw, A., Nijs, J., & Puentedura, E. J. (2017). A clinical perspective on a pain neuroscience education approach to manual therapy. *The Journal of Manual & Manipulative Therapy, 25*, 160–168.

Lucas, K. R., Polus, B. I., & Rich, P. S. (2004). Latent myofascial trigger points: their effects on muscle activation and movement efficiency. *Journal of Bodywork and Movement Therapies, 8*, 160–166.

Lucas, K. R., Rich, P. A., & Polus, B. I. (2010). Muscle activation patterns in the scapular positioning muscles during loaded scapular plane elevation: the effects of latent myofascial trigger points. *Clinical Biomechanics, 25*, 765–770.

Lund, I., & Lundeberg, T. (2006). Are minimal, superficial or sham acupuncture procedures acceptable as inert placebo controls? *Acupuncture in Medicine, 24*, 13–15.

Lundeberg, T., & Stener-Victorin, E. (2002). Is there a physiological basis for the use of acupuncture in pain? *International Congress Series, 1238*, 3–10.

Mahmoudzadeh, A., Rezaeian, Z. S., Karimi, A., & Dommerholt, J. (2016). The effect of dry needling on the radiating pain in subjects with discogenic low-back pain: a randomized control trial. *Journal of Research in Medical Sciences, 21*, 86.

Martín-Pintado Zugasti, A., Rodríguez-Fernández, Á.L., García-Muro, F., López-López, A., Mayoral, O., Mesa-Jiménez, J., & Fernández-Carnero, J. (2014). Effects of spray and stretch on postneedling soreness and sensitivity after dry needling of a latent myofascial trigger point. *Archives of Physical Medicine & Rehabiitation, 95*(10), 1925–1932.

Martín-Pintado-Zugasti, A., Pecos-Martin, D., Rodríguez-Fernández, Á.L., Alguacil-Diego, I. M., Portillo-Aceituno, A., Gallego-Izquierdo, T., & Fernandez-Carnero, J. (2015). Ischemic compression after dry needling of a latent myofascial trigger point reduces postneedling soreness intensity and duration. *PMR, 7*(10), 1026–1034.

Mason, J. S., Crowell, M., Dolbeer, J., Morris, J., Terry, A., Koppenhaver, S., et al. (2016). The effectiveness of dry needling and stretching vs. stretching alone on hamstring flexibility in patients with knee pain: a randomized controlled trial. *International Journal of Sports Physical Therapy, 11*, 672–683.

Mayoral-del-Moral, O. (2005). Fisioterapia invasiva del síndrome de dolor miofascial. *Fisioterapia, 27*, 69–75.

Mayoral, O., & Torres, R. (2003). Tratamiento conservador y fisioterápico invasivo de los puntos gatillo miofasciales. In *Patología de partes blandas en el hombro*. Madrid: Fundación MAPFRE Medicina.

Mayoral, O., De Felipe, J. A., & Martínez, J. M. (2004). Changes in tenderness and tissue compliance in myofascial trigger points with a new technique of electroacupuncture. Three preliminary cases report. *Journal of Musculokeletal Pain, 12*, S33.

McMillan, A. S., Nolan, A., & Kelly, P. J. (1997). The efficacy of dry needling and procaine in the treatment of myofascial pain in the jaw muscles. *Journal of Orofacial Pain, 11*, 307–314.

Melzack, R. (2001). Pain and the neuromatrix in the brain. *Journal of Dental Education, 65*, 1378–1382.

Mendigutia-Gomez, A., Martin-Hernandez, C., Salom-Moreno, J., & Fernandez-de-Las-Penas, C. (2016). Effect of dry needling on spasticity, shoulder range of motion, and Pressure Pain Sensitivity in patients with stroke: a crossover study. *Journal of Manipulative and Physiological Therapeutics, 39*(5), 348–358.

Mense, S. (2010). How do muscle lesions such as latent and active trigger points influence central nociceptive neurons? *Journal of Musculokeletal Pain, 18*, 348–353.

Mense, S., & Masi, A. T. (2011). Increased muscle tone as a cause of muscle pain. In S. Mense & R. D. Gerwin (Eds.), *Muscle pain, understanding the mechanisms*. Heidelberg: Springer.

Millan, M. J. (1999). The induction of pain: an integrative review. *Progress in Neurobiology, 57*, 1–164.

Milligan, E. D., & Watkins, L. R. (2009). Pathological and protective roles of glia in chronic pain. *Nature Reviews Neuroscience, 10,* 23–36.

Mohr, C., Binkofski, F., Erdmann, C., et al. (2005). The anterior cingulate cortex contains distinct areas dissociating external from self-administered painful stimulation: a parametric fMRI study. *Pain, 114,* 347–357.

Moreside, J. M., Vera-Garcia, F. J., & Mcgill, S. M. (2007). Trunk muscle activation patterns, lumbar compressive forces, and spine stability when using the bodyblade. *Physical Therapy, 87,* 153–163.

Moseley, G. L. (2003a). A pain neuromatrix approach to patients with chronic pain. *Manual Therapy, 8,* 130–140.

Moseley, L. (2003b). Unraveling the barriers to reconceptualization of the problem in chronic pain: the actual and perceived ability of patients and health professionals to understand the neurophysiology. *The Journal of Pain, 4,* 184–189.

Moseley, G. L., & Arntz, A. (2007). The context of a noxious stimulus affects the pain it evokes. *Pain, 133,* 64–71.

Moseley, G. L. (2012a). Teaching people about pain: why do we keep beating around the bush? *Pain Manage, 2,* 1–3.

Moseley, G. L. (2012b). Pain: why and how does it hurt? In P. Brukner & K. Khan (Eds.), *Brukner & Khan's clinical sports medicine. 4* (pp. 41–53). North Ryde: McGraw-Hill Australia.

Mueller, M., Bjorkedal, E., & Kamping, S. (2012). Manipulation of expectancy and anxiety in placebo research and their effects on opioid-induced analgesia. *The Journal of Neuroscience, 32,* 14051–14052.

Niddam, D. M., Chan, R. C., Lee, S. H., et al. (2007). Central modulation of pain evoked from myofascial trigger point. *The Clinical Journal of Pain, 23,* 440–448.

Niddam, D. M., Chan, R. C., Lee, S. H., et al. (2008). Central representation of hyperalgesia from myofascial trigger point. *NeuroImage, 39,* 1299–1306.

Nijs, J., Van Houdenhove, B., & Oostendorp, R. A. (2010). Recognition of central sensitization in patients with musculoskeletal pain: application of pain neurophysiology in manual therapy practice. *Manual Therapy, 15,* 135–141.

Olausson, H., Lamarre, Y., Backlund, H., et al. (2002). Unmyelinated tactile afferents signal touch and project to insular cortex. *Nature Neuroscience, 5,* 900–904.

Osborne, N. J., & Gatt, I. T. (2010). Management of shoulder injuries using dry needling in elite volleyball players. *Acupuncture in Medicine, 28,* 42–45.

Pecos-Martin, D., Montanez-Aguilera, F. J., Gallego-Izquierdo, T., Urraca-Gesto, A., Gomez-Conesa, A., Romero-Franco, N., et al. (2015). Effectiveness of dry needling on the lower trapezius in patients with mechanical neck pain: a randomized controlled trial. *Archives of Physical Medicine and Rehabilitation, 96,* 775–781.

Perez-Palomares, S., Olivan-Blazquez, B., Perez-Palomares, A., Gaspar-Calvo, E., Perez-Benito, M., Lopez-Lapena, E., et al. (2017). Contribution of dry needling to individualized physical therapy treatment of shoulder pain: a randomized clinical trial. *The Journal of Orthopaedic and Sports Physical Therapy, 47,* 11–20.

Perreault, T., Dunning, J., & Butts, R. (2017). The local twitch response during trigger point dry needling: is it necessary for successful outcomes? *Journal of Bodywork and Movement Therapies,* https://doi.org/10.1016/j.jbmt.2017.03.008.

Peyron, R., Garcia-Larrea, L., Gregoire, M. C., et al. (2000). Parietal and cingulate processes in central pain. A combined positron emission tomography (PET) and functional magnetic resonance imaging (fMRI) study of an unusual case. *Pain, 84,* 77–87.

Peyron, R., Laurent, B., & Garcia-Larrea, L. (2000). Functional imaging of brain responses to pain. A review and meta-analysis. *Neurophysiologie Clinique, 30,* 263–288.

Puentedura, E. L., & Louw, A. (2012). A neuroscience approach to managing athletes with low back pain. *Physical Therapy Sports, 13,* 123–133.

Rha, D. W., Shin, J. C., Kim, Y. K., et al. (2011). Detecting local twitch responses of myofascial trigger points in the lower-back muscles using ultrasonography. *Archives of Physical Medicine and Rehabilitation, 92,* 1576–1580.

Salom-Moreno, J., Sanchez-Mila, Z., Ortega-Santiago, R., Palacios-Cena, M., Truyol-Dominguez, S., & Fernandez-de-las-Penas, C. (2014). Changes in spasticity, widespread pressure pain sensitivity, and baropodometry after the application of dry needling in patients who have had a stroke: a randomized controlled trial. *Journal of Manipulative and Physiological Therapeutics, 37*(8), 569–579.

Salom-Moreno, J., Jiménez-Gómez, L., Gómez-Ahufinger, V., Palacios-Ceña, M., Arias-Buría, J. L., Koppenhaver, S. L., & Fernández-de-Las-Peñas, C. (2017). 2017. Effects of low-load exercise on postneedling-induced pain after dry needling of active trigger point in individuals with subacromial pain syndrome. *PMR, 9*(12), 1208–1216.

Sandkühler, J. (1996). The organization and function of endogenous antinociceptive systems. *Progress in Neurobiology, 50,* 49–81.

Sawamoto, N., Honda, M., Okada, T., et al. (2000). Expectation of pain enhances responses to nonpainful somatosensory stimulation in the anterior cingulate cortex and parietal operculum/posterior insula: an event-related functional magnetic resonance imaging study. *The Journal of Neuroscience, 20,* 7438–7445.

Shah, J., Phillips, T., Danoff, J. V., & Gerber, L. H. (2003). A novel microanalytical technique for assaying soft tissue demonstrates significant quantitative biomechanical differences in 3 clinically distinct groups: normal, latent and active. *Archives of Physical Medicine and Rehabilitation, 84,* A4.

Shah, J. P., Phillips, T. M., Danoff, J. V., & Gerber, L. H. (2005). An in-vivo microanalytical technique for measuring the local biochemical milieu of human skeletal muscle. *Journal of Applied Physiology, 99,* 1977–1984.

Shah, J. P., Danoff, J. V., Desai, M. J., et al. (2008). Biochemicals associated with pain and inflammation are elevated in sites near to and remote from active myofascial trigger points. *Archives of Physical Medicine and Rehabilitation, 89,* 16–23.

Shah, J. P., & Gilliams, E. A. (2008). Uncovering the biochemical milieu of myofascial trigger points using in vivo microdialysis: an application of muscle pain concepts to myofascial pain syndrome. *Journal of Bodywork and Movement Therapies*, *12*, 371–384.

Sikdar, S., Ortiz, R., Gebreab, T., Gerber, L. H., & Shah, J. P. (2010). In *Understanding the vascular environment of myofascial trigger points using ultrasonic imaging and computational modeling. Conference proceedings: Annual International Conference of the IEEE Engineering in Medicine and Biology Society IEEE Engineering in Medicine and Biology Society Conference. 1.*(pp. 5302–5305).

Simons, D. G. (2001). Do endplate noise and spikes arise from normal motor endplates? *American Journal of Physical Medicine & Rehabilitation*, *80*, 134–140.

Simons, D. G. (2004). Review of enigmatic MTrPs as a common cause of enigmatic musculoskeletal pain and dysfunction. *Journal of Electromyography and Kinesiology*, *14*, 95–107.

Simons, D. G., & Dexter, J. R. (1995). Comparison of local twitch responses elicited by palpation and needling of myofascial trigger points. *Journal of Musculoskeletal Pain*, *3*, 49–61.

Simons, D. G., Hong, C. Z., & Simons, L. (1995). Prevalence of spontaneous electrical activity at trigger spots and control sites in rabbit muscle. *Journal of Musculoskeletal Pain*, *3*, 35–48.

Simons, D. G., Hong, C. Z., & Simons, L. (2002). Endplate potentials are common to midfiber myofascial trigger points. *American Journal of Physical Medicine & Rehabilitation*, *81*, 212–222.

Sluka, K. A., Vance, C. G., & Lisi, T. L. (2005). High-frequency, but not low-frequency, transcutaneous electrical nerve stimulation reduces aspartate and glutamate release in the spinal cord dorsal horn. *Journal of Neurochemistry*, *95*, 1794–1801.

Sluka, K. A., Lisi, T. L., & Westlund, K. N. (2006). Increased release of serotonin in the spinal cord during low, but not high, frequency transcutaneous electric nerve stimulation in rats with joint inflammation. *Archives of Physical Medicine and Rehabilitation*, *87*(8), 1137–1140.

Srbely, J. Z., Dickey, J. P., Lee, D., & Lowerison, M. (2010). Dry needle stimulation of myofascial trigger points evokes segmental anti-nociceptive effects. *Journal of Rehabilitation Medicine*, *42*, 463–468.

Stoop, R., Clijsen, R., Leoni, D., Soldini, E., Castellini, G., Redaelli, V., et al. (2017). Evolution of the methodological quality of controlled clinical trials for myofascial trigger point treatments for the period 1978-2015: A systematic review. *Musculoskelet Science Practice*, *30*, 1–9.

Svensson, P., Minoshima, S., Beydoun, A., et al. (1997). Cerebral processing of acute skin and muscle pain in humans. *Journal of Neurophysiology*, *78*, 450–460.

Takeshige, C., Kobori, M., Hishida, F., Luo, C. P., & Usami, S. (1992a). Analgesia inhibitory system involvement in non-acupuncture point-stimulation-produced analgesia. *Brain Research Bulletin*, *28*(3), 379–391.

Takeshige, C., Nakamura, A., Asamoto, S., & Arai, T. (1992b). Positive feedback action of pituitary beta-endorphin on acupuncture analgesia afferent pathway. *Brain Research Bulletin.*, *29*(1), 37–44.

Téllez-García, M., de - la -Llave-Rincón, A. I., Salom-Moreno, J., Palacios-Ceña, M., Ortega-Santiago, R., & Fernández-de-las-Peñas, C. (2015). Neuroscience education in addition to trigger point dry needling for the management of patients with mechanical chronic low back pain: A preliminary clinical trial. *Journal of Bodywork and Movement Therapies*, *19*, 464–472.

Tsai, C. T., Hsieh, L. F., Kuan, T. S., et al. (2010). Remote effects of dry needling on the irritability of the myofascial trigger point in the upper trapezius muscle. *American Journal of Physical Medicine & Rehabilitation*, *89*, 133–140.

Turo, D., Otto, P., Hossain, M., Gebreab, T., Armstrong, K., Rosenberger, W. F., et al. (2015). Novel use of ultrasound elastography to quantify muscle tissue changes after dry needling of myofascial trigger points in patients with chronic myofascial pain. *Journal of Ultrasound in Medicine*, *34*, 2149–2161.

Vlaeyen, J. W., & Linton, S. J. (2000). Fear-avoidance and its consequences in chronic musculoskeletal pain: a state of the art. *Pain*, *85*, 317–332.

Wager, T. D., Rilling, J. K., Smith, E. E., et al. (2004). Placebo-induced changes in FMRI in the anticipation and experience of pain. *Science*, *303*, 1162–1167.

Wall, P. D., & Woolf, C. J. (1984). Muscle but not cutaneous C-afferent input produces prolonged increases in the excitability of the flexion reflex in the rat. *The Journal of Physiology*, *356*, 443–458.

Wang, F., & Audette, J. (2000). Electrophysiological characteristics of the local twitch response with active myofascial pain of neck compared with a control group with latent trigger points. *American Journal of Physical Medicine & Rehabilitation*, *79*, 203.

Wang, L., Zhang, Y., Dai, J., Yang, J., & Gang, S. (2006). Electroacupuncture (EA) modulates the expression of NMDA receptors in primary sensory neurons in relation to hyperalgesia in rats. *Brain Research*, *1120*, 46–53.

Watkins, L. R., Milligan, E. D., & Maier, S. F. (2001). Glial activation: a driving force for pathological pain. *Trends in Neurosciences*, *24*, 450–455.

Weiner, D. K., & Schmader, K. E. (2006). Postherpetic pain: more than sensory neuralgia? *Pain Medicine*, *7*, 243–249.

White, P. F., Craig, W. F., Vakharia, A. S., et al. (2000). Percutaneous neuromodulation therapy: does the location of electrical stimulation effect the acute analgesic response? *Anesthesia and Analgesia*, *91*, 949–954.

Wu, M. T., Hsieh, J. C., Xiong, J., et al. (1999). Central nervous pathway for acupuncture stimulation: localization of processing with functional MR imaging of the brain - preliminary experience. *Radiology*, *212*, 133–141.

Wu, M. T., Sheen, J. M., Chuang, K. H., et al. (2002). Neuronal specificity of acupuncture response: a fMRI study with electroacupuncture. *NeuroImage*, *16*, 1028–1037.

Zhang, Y., Ge, H. Y., Yue, S. W., et al. (2009). Attenuated skin blood flow response to nociceptive stimulation of latent myofascial trigger points. *Archives of Physical Medicine and Rehabilitation*, *90*, 325–332.

CHAPTER 3

Dry Needling for Fascia, Scar, and Tendon

CÉSAR FERNÁNDEZ-DE-LAS-PEÑAS • JOSÉ L. ARIAS-BURÍA • JAN DOMMERHOLT

INTRODUCTION

Although this textbook's primary focus is on trigger point (TrP) dry needling (DN), in clinical practice healthcare providers are using DN for several other indications, including fascial adhesions, scar tissue, tendinopathies, or enthesopathies. Already in 1979, Lewit described needling of many structures in the body (Lewit, 1979), and it is remarkable that it has taken a few decades before clinicians started using DN routinely for other conditions. There are only a few published case reports on fascial dry needling (Finnoff & Rajasekaran, 2016; Anandkumar & Manivasagam, 2017), but the theoretical basis for using needles in the treatment of fascial adhesions and scar tissue has developed sufficiently to consider its use in the clinic (Chiquet et al., 2003; Grinnell, 2003; Finando & Finando, 2011; Langevin et al., 2011). During the past decade, there has been a worldwide focus on fascial function and dysfunction with many new insights and clinical guidelines (Chaudhry et al., 2007; Huijing, 2009; Findley, 2012; Findley et al., 2012; Willard et al., 2012; Adstrum et al., 2017).

The literature of DN for tendinopathy is slightly more advanced compared with that for fascial needling; however, it is still in its infancy (Nagraba et al., 2013; Krey et al., 2015). There is poor consensus on possible mechanisms of tendon DN and on optimal treatment parameters, indications, and contraindications. Tendinopathies are very common, but there is little evidence for any of the commonly used therapeutic interventions, including eccentric loading (Camargo et al., 2014), manipulations and mobilisations (Pfefer et al., 2009), friction massage (Joseph et al., 2012), fascial manipulation (Pedrelli et al., 2009), ultrasound (Desmeules et al., 2015), laser therapy (Pfefer et al., 2009), orthotics (Simpson & Howard, 2009), or antiinflammatory and glucocorticoid injections (Andres & Murrell, 2008). Eccentric strengthening and low-level laser therapy look promising, but higher-quality studies are needed (Andres & Murrell, 2008; Haslerud et al., 2015). There is only anecdotal evidence for DN for enthesopathies. This chapter provides an overview of pertinent fascia, tendinopathy, and enthesopathy literature in the context of DN and describes needling procedures using solid filament needles.

FASCIA AND SCAR DRY NEEDLING
Introduction to Fascia

It is perhaps a bit surprising that there are no entries for the word 'fascia' in the index of Travell and Simons *Trigger Point Manuals*, even though Travell and Rinzler already realised the importance of fascia for myofascial pain conditions in the 1950s (Travell & Rinzler, 1952; Travell & Simons, 1992; Simons et al., 1999). To be fair to Travell, knowledge about fascia was practically non-existant when she developed the myofascial pain construct. Much has changed during the past decades, and today the role of fascia as a potential peripheral source of nociception is widely recognised (Tesarz et al., 2011).

During the 2015 4th Fascia Research Congress in Washington, DC, fascia was defined anatomically as 'a sheath, a sheet, or any number of other dissectible aggregations of connective tissue that forms beneath the skin to attach, enclose, separate muscles and internal organs' (Stecco & Schleip, 2016). This definition was not necessarily acceptable to all clinicians and researchers (Scarr, 2017); thus a new committee was formed to define 'the fascial system', which was described in 2017 as:

The fascial system consists of the three-dimensional continuum of soft, collagen-containing, loose and dense fibrous connective tissues that permeate the body. It incorporates elements such as adipose tissue, adventitia

and neurovascular sheaths, aponeuroses, deep and superficial fasciae, epineurium, joint capsules, ligaments, membranes, meninges, myofascial expansions, periostea, retinacula, septa, tendons, visceral fasciae, and all the intramuscular and intermuscular connective tissues including endo-/peri-/epi-mysium. The fascial system interpenetrates and surrounds all organs, muscles, bones and nerve fibres, endowing the body with a functional structure, and providing an environment that enables all body systems to operate in an integrated manner (Adstrum et al., 2017).

Dry needling (DN) and manual TrP therapy may alter the viscoelastic properties or behaviour of fascia tissue, which implies that manual fascial techniques should be incorporated into TrP therapy. As the definition of the fascial system indicates, fascia and muscles are intimately intertwined and connected. The epimysium surrounds all muscles, whereas individual muscle fibre bundles are situated within the perimysium, and individual muscle fibres are contained within the endomysium (Stecco et al., 2016a). The epimysium, perimysium, and endomysium are part of the deep fascia (Schleip et al., 2006; Roman et al., 2013), which must be distinguished from the superficial and visceral fascia (Stecco et al., 2016b).

Sensory Aspects of Fascia

It is noteworthy that the definition of the fascial system does not include any reference to the sensory aspects of fascia. Yet to be a source of pain, fascia must contain sensory fibres and nociceptors (Tesarz et al., 2011). In reviewing the myofascial pain literature, it may appear that muscles are the main source of nociception, but several studies point to fascia instead. Weinkauf and colleagues (2015) found that mechanical hyperalgesia was more pronounced in the tibial fascia than in the muscle after injecting nerve growth factor (NGF). NGF injections in the fascia of the erector spinae muscles also caused significant hyperalgesia, as well as a decreased pressure threshold and exercise-induced pain for 1 week and persistent sensitisation to chemical and mechanical stimuli for 2 weeks (Deising et al., 2012). The thoracolumbar fascia was more sensitive than the tibial fascia (Weinkauf et al., 2015). In another study comparing the tibial fascia with muscle, injections of hypertonic saline caused a greater delayed onset of muscle pain with anterior fascia injections compared with muscle injections (Gibson et al., 2009). Schilder and colleagues (2014) confirmed that hypertonic saline injections into the fascia resulted in significantly more pain than injections in the subcutis and muscle.

Danielson and colleagues (2009) found peptidergic sensory nerve endings with antibodies for calcitonin gene-related peptide (CGRP) and substance P in the loose connective tissue of the patellar tendon. Also of interest is that, under pathological conditions, fascia is able to establish new nociceptive fibres that are immunoreactive to substance P (Sanchis-Alfonso & Rosello-Sastre, 2000). Ruffini, Pacini and free nerve endings have been identified in the deep fascia, retinacula, and bicipital aponeurosis (Stilwell, 1957; Yahia et al., 1993; Sanchis-Alfonso & Rosello-Sastre, 2000; Stecco et al., 2008). There is some evidence that Pacinian receptors may be involved in high-velocity manipulation (Schleip, 2003), but there are no studies investigating whether manual TrP therapy or DN specifically target Pacinian receptors. The free nerve endings are likely mechanoreceptors.

Biomechanical Aspects of Fascia

Each muscle has specific connections with fascia (Stecco et al., 2007; Stecco et al., 2010, 2013b; Wilke et al., 2016); through these connections, force transmissions take place from muscles to bones and to deeper fascial layers. Close to 40% of muscle force is transmitted to adjacent structures and not through the muscle's tendon (Smeulders et al., 2005). Often, muscle fibres do not run from one end of the muscle to the other end and therefore frequently do not connect directly to the muscle's tendon. Instead, these fibres attach to other muscle fibres or to the intramuscular connective tissue (Hijikata & Ishikawa, 1997), which leads to epimuscular myofascial force transmission to connective tissues outside the muscle parameters (Huijing & Jaspers, 2005).

The contractile force distribution onto other fascial structures contributes to increased joint stability and facilitates movement involving adjacent muscles (Findley, 2011). Changes in fascial pliability can lead to altered movement patterns, local overuse, and a loss of strength and coordination. Considering the aponeurotic fascia such as the thoracolumbar fascia, decreased mobility between its fascial layers will lead to stiffness and limited mobility. The aponeurotic fascia consists of two or three layers of parallel collagen fibre bundles oriented in different directions (Stecco et al., 2013a) and is directly connected to muscles and tendons (Willard et al., 2012; Vleeming et al., 2014). The deep fascia contains multiple mechanoreceptors (Langevin, 2006), and the ability of fascia to process mechanoreceptive input is entirely dependent on structural relationship with bone tissue and muscles (van der Wal, 2009). It transmits forces over greater distances than the epimysial fascia (Huijing & Baan, 2008). Interestingly, Maas and Sandercock (2009) demonstrated that although the soleus muscle in a cat does have strong mechanical connections with synergistic muscles, the force transmission from the soleus muscle does not appear to be affected by length changes of its synergists, which means that apparently not all muscles use the same mechanisms for force transmission.

It is not possible to separate the epimysal fascia from the underlying muscle due to the many connections between the muscle and various fibrous septa of the epimysium, perimysium, and endomysium (Turrina et al., 2013). A decrease in flexibility of the epimysium may result in decreased mobility, especially in the elderly. The epimysium of older rats was much stiffer than the same structures in younger rats (Gao et al., 2008). Dense epimysium can restrict muscles in their function (Stecco et al., 2013a). Although the epimysium does not have any Pacini and Ruffini corpuscles, it plays an important role in proprioception because of its direct connections with muscle spindles (Maier, 1999). The perimysium can also increase muscle stiffness and appears to be more sensitive to changes in mechanical tension than the other intramuscular connective tissues, in spite of having direct connections with the epimysium and muscle fibres (Passerieux et al., 2007). Perimysium has a high density of fibroblasts (Schleip et al., 2006), which suggests that fascia may play a significant role in muscle contractibility and possibly in the formation of TrPs (Schleip et al., 2005, 2006).

Fibroblasts are located within the extracellular matrix and play a key role in the synthesis of collagen, ground substance, elastin, and reticulin. They register force-induced deformations in their extracellular matrix, and mechanical stretching of fibroblasts regulates key extracellular matrix genes by stimulating the release of multiple substances such as paracrine growth factor (Schleip et al., 2006). Langevin and colleagues showed that the effects of needling can at least partially be explained by mechanical stimulation of fibroblasts (Langevin et al., 2001a, 2010). Under high tension, fibroblasts feature stress fibres and focal adhesions and appear lamellar in shape, whereas under low stress, they are more or less rounded structures (Grinnell, 2003; Miron-Mendoza et al., 2008; Langevin et al., 2010). Lamellar fibroblasts can differentiate into myofibroblasts complete with a contractile apparatus of actin microfilaments and nonmuscle myosin (Tomasek et al., 2002). In other words, fascia is not just a passive structure but can perform very slow contractions (Schleip et al., 2008). In fact, fibroblasts are also involved in wound closure, muscle contractions (Yahia et al., 1992, 1993), and adhesions of scars.

Dry Needling of Fascia

There is a paucity of studies describing how DN may influence fascia. The work by Langevin and colleagues is exceptional in this regard as they evaluated the results of mechanical stimulation of fascia with an acupuncture needle (Langevin et al., 2001b, 2004, 2006). Rotating a needle causes tissue bundles, especially collagen, to adhere to the needle and create a mechanical bond between the needle and the tissue (Kimura et al., 1992; Langevin et al., 2002). Further rotating, or pistoning, the needle as is commonly used in DN will pull the tissues along the needling direction and create a mechanical stretch of the intermuscular connective tissue layers. Retaining the needle will provide a more continuous stretch of the fascia and muscle fibres and remodelling of the cytoskeleton. Langevin and colleagues (2001b) observed pulling of the subdermal tissue without structural changes in the dermis and muscle.

Collagen fibres in a particular layer are oriented in the same plane and direction; however, they are at a 78 degree angle with the fibre direction in adjacent layers (Purslow, 2010; Benetazzo et al., 2011). This may have implications for manual TrP therapy. Chaudhry and colleagues found that a greater fibre angle makes collagen fibres more resistant to longitudinal stretching (Chaudhry et al., 2007, 2008, 2012). Because the muscle fibre direction does not necessarily match the fascia fibre direction, further research should examine whether stretching exercises after manual TrP release or DN have evidence-based value and, if so, what the optimal stretching methods entails.

Rotating a needle that has been placed in a taut band or a TrP is often advocated in DN courses as the most direct method of stretching the taut band or muscle contracture (Gunn & Milbrandt, 1977). As every muscle fibre bundle is surrounded by fascial layers, the question emerges whether rotation of the needle actually stretches the taut band and muscle fibres or the deeper connective tissue fibres, or perhaps both muscle and fascia. In this context it is noteworthy that massage therapy can activate the mechano-transduction signaling pathways focal adhesion kinase (FAK) and extracellular signal–regulated kinase 1/2 (ERK1/2), potentiated mitochondrial biogenesis signaling (nuclear peroxisome proliferator–activated receptor g coactivator 1a [PGC-1a]) and increase mitochondrial biogenesis (Crane et al., 2012). Increasing the number of mitochondria would improve the energy metabolism in the muscle, which in turn may reduce focal adhesions (Jafri, 2014). It is not known whether DN triggers a similar response. Massage can also reduce the production of the inflammatory cytokines such as tumour necrosis factor-α and interleukin-6, which has also been described for DN (Shah & Gilliams, 2008). Stretching skeletal myocytes activates NADPH oxidase, which promotes the production of reactive oxygen species and accessibility of ryanodine receptors (Prosser et al., 2013; Jafri, 2014).

Dry Needling of Scar Tissue Adhesions

Empirically, adhesions of scar tissue can be treated effectively with DN by placing a needle directly into each adhesion or densification and rotating the needle unidirectional as much as possible to the pain tolerance level of the patient (Fig. 3.1). When the needle releases, periodic tightening is indicated until the adhesion has been resolved. Again, rotating the needle causes mechanical stress, which may restore the scar's mobility and pliability and immediately reduce the subject's hyperalgesia and allodynia. The torque increases exponentially with rotating the needle, which can be objectively measured up to several centimetres from the needle location (Langevin et al., 2004). Persistent adhesions are likely due to dysregulation of extracellular matrix proteins. Rotating the needle also inhibits Rho-dependent kinase and suppresses the induction of the tenascin-C gene. One of the best approaches to accomplish the transcription of the tenascin-C gene and to positively affect fibronectin and collagen XII is to cyclically stretch fibroblasts in the extracellular matrix. Fibroblasts feature integrins, which are critical for mechanical force patterning (Chiquet et al., 2003).

DRY NEEDLING AND TENDON
Clinical Reasoning for Tendon Needling

Tendinopathy is a common orthopaedic term that includes different conditions such as tendinitis, paratenonitis, and tendinosis. The most accepted term used to be tendinosis, which can be defined as an unsuccessful healing response within the tendon tissue (Khan et al., 2002); however, the term 'tendinopathy' is preferred as it does not imply a certain aetiology or pathology (Morrey et al., 2013).

The clinical presentation of a tendinopathy includes localised tendon pain (particularly with loading), local tenderness to palpation, and impaired function. Several changes can occur with repetitive overuse of the tendons and a subsequent development of tendin-

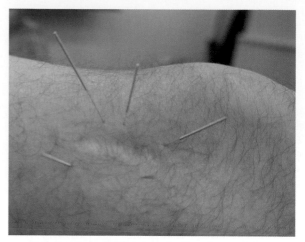

FIG. 3.1 Dry needling for adhesions in scar tissue.

opathy, including collagen disorientation, fibre disorganisation, fibre separation, increased concentration of proteoglycans, increased prominence of cells, focal area with neovascularisation, and even cell apoptosis (Cook et al., 2004). Nevertheless, structural changes of the tendon are not associated with pain. Therefore current theories suggest a role of altered nociceptive processing in pain associated with tendinopathies (Rio et al., 2014), which is supported by the presence of several algogenic substances and proinflammatory mediators in the pathological tendon (Danielson, 2009; Christensen et al., 2015).

Because tendon abnormalities observed in subjects with tendinopathy generally include degeneration and a disordered arrangement of collagen fibres, cell infiltration, tenocytes disruption, or vascularity changes, several therapeutic biological approaches have been proposed for the management of tendinopathy, including platelet-rich plasma (PRP) injections (Lee, 2016) and percutaneous electrolysis (EPE) (Arias-Buría et al., 2015) combined with biomechanical stimuli such as eccentric exercises. PRP injections use a volume of autologous plasma with a platelet concentration higher than the baseline. EPE is a newly developed treatment approach with a galvanic current stimulation delivered into the tendon via a needle.

Several questions arise regarding common biological interventions; for example, there is no agreement on the volume of PRP injections, platelet activation, the number of centrifugation steps during the preparation, the buffering of the PRP, and postinjection rehabilitation protocols (Peck et al., 2016). Similarly, no consensus exists on the dosage of galvanic electrical current with EPE, the optimal duration of treatments, or the frequency of the sessions. Furthermore, preliminary evidence suggests that injection of PRP or glucocorticoids is not superior to placebo injections for reducing pain in individuals with lateral epicondylalgia (Krogh et al., 2013a,b). Dunning and colleagues (2014) advocated using just a needle without the addition of biological agents for the treatment of tendons and connective tissues.

Needling Therapies for Tendons

Needling therapies for tendons include DN, sometimes referred to as tendon fenestration, and percutaneous needle tenotomy. Percutaneous needle tenotomy describes a technique using the bevel of a needle, usually referred to as a miniscalpel, to section or cut the affected tendon. Several researchers explored the effect of needle tenotomy using beveled needles of 20 to 22 gauge. A case series including individuals with chronic tendinopathy, who had failed physical therapy treatments, showed that ultrasound-guided percutaneous needle tenotomy, using a 22-gauge needle with a local anaesthetic, was effective for improving symptoms (Housner et al., 2009). In this study the patellar (n = 5) and Achilles (n = 4) tendons were the most affected (Housner et al., 2009), which was in agreement with the findings by Testa and colleagues (1999, 2002). Another study reported that ultrasound-guided percutaneous needle tenotomy combined with corticosteroid injections was also effective for patients with lateral elbow tendinosis for whom all other nonsurgical treatments had failed (McShane et al., 2006). Ultrasound-guided percutaneous needle tenotomy is recommended to ensure that the abnormal area of the tendon is accurately targeted with the needle. In fact, ultrasound identification of well-defined tendon abnormalities was a positive predictor for a successful ultrasound-guided needle tenotomy using a 22-gauge beveled needle (Kanaan et al., 2013). The presence or absence of hyperemia on Doppler imaging did not have the same predictive value.

On the contrary, tendon fenestration consists of repeated insertions with a solid needle into an abnormal tendon with the goal of converting a degenerative process into an acute inflammatory condition. With the appropriate treatment, the inflammatory condition may progress to proper tendon healing. Although some authors have proposed to use ultrasound guidance for tendon fenestrations with a solid needle, it is mostly indicated for tenotomies with beveled needles (Jacobson et al., 2016). It is interesting to note that as early as 1979, Lewit described the application of DN, not only for TrPs, but also for many other tissues, including ligaments, scars, periosteum, tendons, entheses, and even joints. This historic paper described the onset of immediate analgaesia in 87% of the painful structures after the insertion of a solid needle into the targeted tissue (Lewit, 1979). Several other case reports have suggested that tendon DN with an acupuncture needle, alone or combined with other injection modalities, was effective for calcifications in the elbow (Zhu et al., 2008a) and the supraspinatus (Zhu et al., 2008b). A more recent case study reported that ultrasound guided tendon DN combined with exercise was effective for an individual with a supraspinatus tendinopathy (Settergren, 2013). Lubojacky (2009) reported that needling therapy was as effective as arthroscopic surgery for rotator cuff tendinopathy.

Several high-quality studies of tendon needling therapies have been published in the past few years. Stenhouse and colleagues (2013) found that tendon needling with an acupuncture needle was equally effective to autologous conditioned plasma injections for decreasing pain and disability in subjects with refractory lateral elbow pain. Jacobson and colleagues (2015) recently found that ultrasound-guided tendon fenestration of gluteus medius, gluteus minimus, proximal hamstring, and tensor fascia latae tendon was effective for hip and pelvic pain.

A recent meta-analysis of the treatment of chronic tendinopathies highlighted significant advantages of PRP vs DN in the short term; however, no significant differences with placebo or DN were observed after 6 months (Tsikopoulos et al., 2016). The analysis included patients with rotator cuff, patellar, and lateral epicondyle tendinopathies. Interestingly, a subgroup analysis found marginal benefits of PRP in those with rotator cuff tendinopathy but not within patellar or lateral epicondyle tendons (Tsikopoulos et al., 2016). A review by Krey and colleagues (2015) concluded that tendon needling was effective for improving self-reported outcomes in subjects with lateral epicondyle, Achilles and rotator cuff tendinopathies. A 2017 systematic review of percutaneous tendon tenotomies in patients with lateral epicondylalgia did not identify any controlled trials comparing percutaneous tenotomy to placebo or conservative treatment, which means that the authors could not reach any conclusions about its effectiveness (Mattie et al., 2017).

Clinical Guidelines for Tendon Dry Needling

There is no consensus on the different technical aspects of tendon needling, including the number of insertions, the optimum dosage and frequency of treatment sessions, or the duration and the intensity of needling

(Krogh et al., 2013a,b). How many needles should be used? Should the needles be left in the tendon? Should needles be rotated as is commonly done with fascial DN?

Jacobson and colleagues (2015) recommended 20 to 40 needle passes, whereas Stenhouse and colleagues (2013) described 40 to 50 needle insertions through the long axis of the tendon. Mishra and colleagues (2014) found, however, that needling a tendon only five times was sufficient and effective for the majority of individuals with lateral epicondylalgia. Empirically, the number of insertions depends on the clinical presentation of the patient and the response of the tissue during the needling procedure, realising that there are no objective parameters to determine the optimum response pattern.

Similar to fascial needling, needles can be rotated with tendon needling to lengthen fibroblasts (Langevin et al., 2005) and reduce nociceptive input (Chiquet et al., 2003). Loyeung and Cobbin (2013) proposed needle retention for 21 minutes with manipulation of the needle every 3 minutes. Empirically, it is recommended to rotate the needle until the patient's symptoms are provoked.

Tendon needling can be performed with or without ultrasound guidance. As most clinicians do not have access to sonography, tendon needling will have to be based on the clinical presentation of the patient. Tenderness and pain with palpation are common with tendinopathy (Ramos et al., 2009). Placing the needle directly into the most painful region or spot of the tendon is recommended with or without needle rotation (Fig. 3.2). An alternative procedure is to insert the needle throughout the tendon, that is, parallel to the painful area (Fig. 3.3). With this approach, the needle can be either rotated or inserted over the tendon fibres.

Alternatively, the procedure can be performed with ultrasound guidance, which gives the clinician the opportunity to base the clinical decision on the evaluation of tendon fibres, the size of hypoechoic areas, the presence of lacerations, neovascularisation observed with colour Doppler, or tendon thickness (Nagraba et al., 2013). Once the affected area is visualised, the needle is inserted along the long axis of the tendon, parallel to the ultrasound transducer (Fig. 3.4). In fact, moving the needle across the transducer is the most accurate method as the needle can be visualised (Fig. 3.5). Once the needle has reached the tendon abnormality (visualised with ultrasound), it can be angled during the procedure to provide real-time visualisation of the insertions (Chiavaras & Jacobson, 2013).

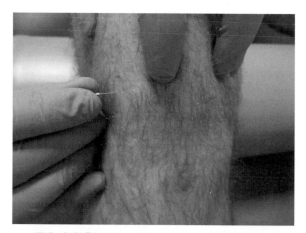

FIG. 3.3 Parallel needling of the patellar tendon.

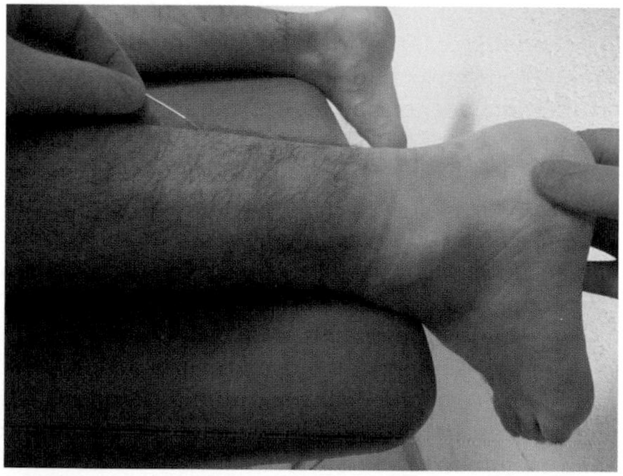

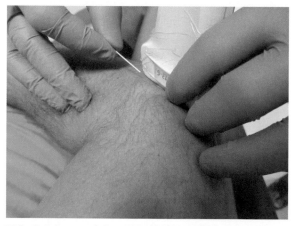

FIG. 3.4 Long-axis insertion of the needle in the lateral epicondyle tendon.

FIG. 3.2 Perpendicular needling of the Achilles tendon.

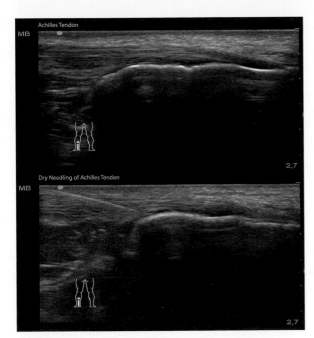

FIG. 3.5 Ultrasound visualisation of the needle in the lateral epicondyle tendon.

Mechanisms of Dry Needling for the Tendon

The mechanisms underlying tendon needling are poorly understood, but some hypotheses have been proposed. It seems that when a pathological tendon area is targeted with a needle, the procedure causes tendon trauma, bleeding and vasodilatation (James et al., 2007; Kubo et al., 2010), tenocyte disruption, collagen proliferation (Langevin et al., 2007), and a local inflammatory response with its subsequent increase in local growth factors and other substances. All these events will promote tendon healing (James et al., 2007). Histological changes have been confirmed in tendinopathy models of the Achilles tendon in animals (Kim et al., 2015).

Increased blood flow is particularly beneficial for tendons, which have poor vascularisation and heal slowly and inefficiently (Fenwick et al., 2002). The needle will cause small fenestrations on the surface of a degenerated tendon leading to a desirable increase in bleeding in the region of the newly produced microchannels. Although blood carries oxygen and nutrients, it also carries proinflammatory mediators. The latter can initiate local inflammatory reactions and growth factors directly influencing both regenerative and healing processes. Of importance is that granulocytes and macrophages reach the affected area within a few hours after a puncture and activate fibroblasts. As mentioned

previously, fibroblasts are essential in the synthesis of collagen, ground substance, elastin, and reticulin. The combined factors result in improved strengthening and regeneration of tendon structures (Nagraba et al., 2013). Therefore tendon needling appears to initiate a healing process causing remodeling within the tendon, which is the first step toward restoring its mechanical properties. Although tendon needling stimulates the tendon's biology and causes an initial inflammatory response during the repair phase, early controlled mechanical loading, particularly eccentric exercise and stretching, facilitates the process of collagen tissue proliferation thus improving the biomechanical properties of the tendon (Almeida Mdos et al., 2014).

REFERENCES

Adstrum, S., Hedley, G., Schleip, R., Stecco, C., & Yucesoy, C. A. (2017). Defining the fascial system. *Journal of Bodywork and Movement Therapies, 21*, 173–177.

Almeida Mdos, S., Guerra Fda, R., de Oliveira, L. P., et al. (2014). A hypothesis for the anti-inflammatory and mechanotransduction molecular mechanisms underlying acupuncture tendon healing. *Acupuncture in Medicine, 32*, 178–182.

Anandkumar, S. M., & Manivasagam, M. (2017). Effect of fascia dry needling on non-specific thoracic pain – A proposed dry needling grading system. *Physiotherapy Theory and Practice, 33*, 420–428.

Andres, B. M., & Murrell, G. A. (2008). Treatment of tendinopathy: what works, what does not, and what is on the horizon. *Clinical Orthopaedics and Related Research, 466*, 1539–1554.

Arias-Buría, J. L., Truyols-Domínguez, S., Valero-Alcaide, R., Salom-Moreno, J., Atín-Arratibel, M. A., & Fernández-de-las-Peñas, C. (2015). Ultrasound-guide percutaneous electrolysis and eccentric exercises for subacromial pain syndrome: a randomized clinical trial. *Evidence-based Complementary and Alternative Medicine, 2015*, 315219.

Benetazzo, L., Bizzego, A., De Caro, R., Frigo, G., Guidolin, D., & Stecco, C. (2011). 3D reconstruction of the crural and thoracolumbar fasciae. *Surgical and Radiologic Anatomy, 33*, 855–862.

Camargo, P. R., Alburquerque-Sendin, F., & Salvini, T. F. (2014). Eccentric training as a new approach for rotator cuff tendinopathy: review and perspectives. *World Journal of Orthopedics, 5*, 634–644.

Chaudhry, H., Huang, C.-Y., Schleip, R., Ji, Z., Bukiet, B., & Findley, T. (2007). Viscoelastic behavior of human fasciae under extension in manual therapy. *Journal of Bodywork and Movement Therapies, 11*, 159–167.

Chaudhry, H., Max, R., Antonio, S., & Findley, T. (2012). Mathematical model of fiber orientation in anisotropic fascia layers at large displacements. *Journal of Bodywork and Movement Therapies, 16*, 158–164.

Chaudhry, H., Schleip, R., Ji, Z., Bukiet, B., Maney, M., & Findley, T. (2008). Three-dimensional mathematical model for deformation of human fasciae in manual therapy. *The Journal of the American Osteopathic Association, 108,* 379–390.

Chiavaras, M. M., & Jacobson, J. A. (2013). Ultrasound-guided tendon fenestration. *Seminars in Musculoskeletal Radiology, 17,* 85–90.

Chiquet, M., Renedo, A. S., Huber, F., & Fluck, M. (2003). How do fibroblasts translate mechanical signals into changes in extracellular matrix production? *Matrix Biology, 22,* 73–80.

Christensen, J., Alfredson, H., & Andersson, G. (2015). Protease-activated receptors in the Achilles tendon: a potential explanation for the excessive pain signalling in tendinopathy. *Molecular Pain, 11,* 13.

Cook, J. L., Feller, J. A., Bonar, S. F., & Khan, K. M. (2004). Abnormal tenocyte morphology is more prevalent than collagen disruption in asymptomatic athletes' patellar tendons. *Journal of Orthopaedic Research, 22,* 334–338.

Crane, J. D., Ogborn, D. I., Cupido, C., Melov, S., Hubbard, A., Bourgeois, J. M., et al. (2012). Massage therapy attenuates inflammatory signaling after exercise-induced muscle damage. *Science Translational Medicine, 4,* 119ra13.

Danielson, P. (2009). Reviving the "biochemical" hypothesis for tendinopathy: new findings suggest the involvement of locally produced signal substances. *British Journal of Sports Medicine, 43,* 265–268.

Deising, S., Weinkauf, B., Blunk, J., Obreja, O., Schmelz, M., & Rukwied, R. (2012). NGF-evoked sensitization of muscle fascia nociceptors in humans. *Pain, 153,* 1673–1679.

Desmeules, F., Boudreault, J., Roy, J. S., Dionne, C., Fremont, P., & MacDermid, J. C. (2015). The efficacy of therapeutic ultrasound for rotator cuff tendinopathy: a systematic review and meta-analysis. *Physical Therapy in Sport, 16,* 276–284.

Dunning, J., Butts, R., Mourad, F., Young, I., Flannagan, S., & Perreault, T. (2014). DN: a literature review with implications for clinical practice guidelines. *The Physical Therapy Review, 19,* 252–265.

Findley, T. W. (2012). Fascia science and clinical applications: a clinician/researcher's perspectives. *Journal of Bodywork and Movement Therapies, 16,* 64–66.

Fenwick, S. A., Hazleman, B. L., & Riley, G. P. (2002). The vasculature and its role in the damaged and healing tendon. *Arthritis Research, 4,* 252–260.

Finando, S., & Finando, D. (2011). Fascia and the mechanism of acupuncture. *Journal of Bodywork and Movement Therapies, 15,* 168–176.

Findley, T. W. (2011). Fascia research from a clinician/scientist's perspective. *International Journal of Therapeutic Massage & Bodywork, 4,* 1–6.

Findley, T., Chaudhry, H., Stecco, A., & Roman, M. (2012). Fascia research—a narrative review. *Journal of Bodywork and Movement Therapies, 16,* 67–75.

Finnoff, J. T., & Rajasekaran, S. (2016). Ultrasound-guided, percutaneous needle fascial fenestration for the treatment of chronic exertional compartment syndrome: a case report. *PMR, 8,* 286–290.

Gao, Y., Kostrominova, T. Y., Faulkner, J. A., & Wineman, A. S. (2008). Age-related changes in the mechanical properties of the epimysium in skeletal muscles of rats. *Journal of Biomechanics, 41,* 465–469.

Gibson, W., Arendt-Nielsen, L., Taguchi, T., Mizumura, K., & Graven-Nielsen, T. (2009). Increased pain from muscle fascia following eccentric exercise: animal and human findings. *Experimental Brain Research, 194,* 299–308.

Grinnell, F. (2003). Fibroblast biology in three-dimensional collagen matrices. *Trends in Cell Biology, 13,* 264–269.

Gunn, C. C., & Milbrandt, W. E. (1977). The neurological mechanism of needle-grasp in acupuncture. *American Journal of Acupuncture, 5,* 115–120.

Haslerud, S., Magnussen, L. H., Joensen, J., Lopes-Martins, R. A., & Bjordal, J. M. (2015). The efficacy of low-level laser therapy for shoulder tendinopathy: a systematic review and meta-analysis of randomized controlled trials. *Physiotherapy Research International, 20*(2), 108–125.

Hijikata, T., & Ishikawa, H. (1997). Functional morphology of serially linked skeletal muscle fibers. *Acta Anatomica, 159,* 99–107.

Housner, J. A., Jacobson, J. A., & Misko, R. (2009). Sonographically guided percutaneous needle tenotomy for the treatment of chronic tendinosis. *Journal of Ultrasound in Medicine, 28,* 1187–1192.

Huijing, P. A. (2009). Epimuscular myofascial force transmission: a historical review and implications for new research. International Society of Biomechanics Muybridge Award Lecture, Taipei, 2007. *Journal of Biomechanics, 42,* 9–21.

Huijing, P. A., & Baan, G. C. (2008). Myofascial force transmission via extramuscular pathways occurs between antagonistic muscles. *Cells, Tissues, Organs, 188,* 400–414.

Huijing, P. A., & Jaspers, R. T. (2005). Adaptation of muscle size and myofascial force transmission: a review and some new experimental results. *Scandinavian Journal of Medicine & Science in Sports, 15,* 349–380.

Jacobson, J. A., Kim, S. M., & Brigido, M. (2016). Ultrasound-guided percutaneous tenotomy. *Seminars in Musculoskeletal Radiology, 20,* 414–421.

Jacobson, J. A., Rubin, J., Yablon, C. M., Kim, S. M., Kalume-Brigido, M., & Parameswaran, A. (2015). Ultrasound-guided fenestration of tendons about the hip and pelvis: clinical outcomes. *Journal of Ultrasound in Medicine, 34,* 2029–2035.

Jafri, M. S. (2014). *Mechanisms of Myofascial Pain.* International scholarly research notices.

James, S. L., Ali, K., Pocock, C., et al. (2007). Ultrasound guided DN and autologous blood injection for patellar tendinosis. *British Journal of Sports Medicine, 41,* 518–521.

Joseph, M. F., Taft, K., Moskwa, M., & Denegar, C. R. (2012). Deep friction massage to treat tendinopathy: a systematic review of a classic treatment in the face of a new paradigm of understanding. *Journal of Sport Rehabilitation, 21,* 343–353.

Kanaan, Y., Jacobson, J. A., Jamadar, D., Housner, J., & Caoili, E. M. (2013). Sonographically guided patellar tendon fenestration: prognostic value of preprocedure sonographic findings. *Journal of Ultrasound in Medicine, 32,* 771–777.

Khan, K. M., Cook, J., Kannus, P., Maffulli, N., & Bonar, S. (2002). Time to abandon the "tendinitis" myth. *BMJ (Clinical research ed.)*, 324, 626–627.

Kim, B. S., Joo, Y. C., Choi, B. H., Kim, K. H., Kang, J. S., & Park, S. R. (2015). The effect of DN and treadmill running on inducing pathological changes in rat Achilles tendon. *Connective Tissue Research*, 56, 452–460.

Kimura, M., Tohya, K., Kuroiwa, K., Oda, H., Gorawski, E. C., Hua, Z. X., et al. (1992). Electron microscopical and immunohistochemical studies on the induction of "Qi" employing needling manipulation. *The American Journal of Chinese Medicine*, 20, 25–35.

Krey, D., Borchers, J., & McCamey, K. (2015). Tendon needling for treatment of tendinopathy: a systematic review. *Physical Sports Medicine*, 43, 80–86.

Krogh, T. P., Bartels, E. M., Ellingsen, T., et al. (2013a). Comparative effectiveness of injections therapies in lateral epicondylitis: a systematic review and network meta-analysis of randomized controlled trials. *The American Journal of Sports Medicine*, 41, 1435–1446.

Krogh, T. P., Fredberg, U., Stengaard-Pedersen, K., Christensen, R., Jensen, P., & Ellingsen, T. (2013b). Treatment of lateral epicondylitis with platelet-rich plasma, glucocorticoid, or saline: a randomized, double-blind, placebo-controlled trial. *The American Journal of Sports Medicine*, 41, 625–635.

Kubo, K., Yajima, H., Takayama, M., Ikebukuro, T., Mizoguchi, H., & Takakura, N. (2010). Effects of acupuncture and heating on blood volume and oxygen saturation of human Achilles tendon in vivo. *European Journal of Applied Physiology*, 109, 545–550.

Langevin, H. M. (2006). Connective tissue: a body-wide signaling network? *Medical Hypotheses*, 66, 1074–1077.

Langevin, H. M., Bouffard, N. A., Badger, G. J., Churchill, D. L., & Howe, A. K. (2006). Subcutaneous tissue fibroblast cytoskeletal remodeling induced by acupuncture: evidence for a mechanotransduction-based mechanism. *Journal of Cellular Physiology*, 207, 767–774.

Langevin, H. M., Bouffard, N. A., Badger, G. J., Iatridis, J. C., & Howe, A. K. (2005). Dynamic fibroblast cytoskeletal response to subcutaneous tissue stretch ex vivo and in vivo. *American Journal of Physiology Cell Physiology*, 288, C747–756.

Langevin, H. M., Bouffard, N. A., Churchill, D. L., & Badger, G. J. (2007). Connective tissue fibroblast response to acupuncture: dose dependent effect of bidirectional needle rotation. *Journal of Alternative and Complementary Medicine*, 13, 355–360.

Langevin, H. M., Bouffard, N. A., Fox, J. R., Palmer, B. M., Wu, J., Iatridis, J. C., et al. (2011). Fibroblast cytoskeletal remodeling contributes to connective tissue tension. *Journal of Cellular Physiology*, 226, 1166–1175.

Langevin, H. M., Churchill, D. L., & Cipolla, M. J. (2001a). Mechanical signaling through connective tissue: a mechanism for the therapeutic effect of acupuncture. *The FASEB Journal*, 15, 2275–2282.

Langevin, H. M., Churchill, D. L., Fox, J. R., Badger, G. J., Garra, B. S., & Krag, M. H. (2001b). Biomechanical response to acupuncture needling in humans. *Journal of Applied Physiology*, 91, 2471–2478.

Langevin, H. M., Churchill, D. L., Wu, J., Badger, G. J., Yandow, J. A., Fox, J. R., et al. (2002). Evidence of connective tissue involvement in acupuncture. *The FASEB Journal*, 16, 872–874.

Langevin, H. M., Konofagou, E. E., Badger, G. J., Churchill, D. L., Fox, J. R., Ophir, J., et al. (2004). Tissue displacements during acupuncture using ultrasound elastography techniques. *Ultrasound in Medicine & Biology*, 30, 1173–1183.

Langevin, H. M., Storch, K. N., Snapp, R. R., Bouffard, N. A., Badger, G. J., Howe, A. K., et al. (2010). Tissue stretch induces nuclear remodeling in connective tissue fibroblasts. *Histochemistry and Cell Biology*, 133, 405–415.

Lee, K. S. (2016). Ultrasound-guided platelet-rich plasma treatment: application and technique. *Seminars in Musculoskeletal Radiology*, 20, 422–431.

Lewit, K. (1979). The needle effect in the relief of myofascial pain. *Pain*, 6, 83–90.

Loyeung, B. Y., & Cobbin, D. (2013). Investigating the effects of three needling parameters (manipulation, retention time, and insertion site) on needling sensation and pain profiles: a study of eight deep needling interventions. *Evidence-based Complementary and Alternative Medicine*, 2013, 136763.

Lubojacky, J. (2009). Kalkareozni tendinitida ramene—needling. *Acta Chirurgiae Orthopaedicae et Traumatologiae Cechoslovaca*, 76, 225–231.

Maas, H., & Sandercock, T. G. (2009). Are skeletal muscles independent actuators? Force transmission from soleus muscle in the cat. In P. A. Huijing, P. Hollander, T. Findley, & R. Schleip (Eds.), *Fascia research II; Basic science and implications for conventional and complementary health care* (pp. 69–81). Munich: Urban & Fischer.

Maier, A. (1999). Proportions of slow myosin heavy chain-positive fibers in muscle spindles and adjoining extrafusal fascicles, and the positioning of spindles relative to these fascicles. *Journal of Morphology*, 242, 157–165.

Mattie, R., Wong, J., McCormick, Z., Yu, S., Saltychev, M., & Laimi, K. (2017). Percutaneous needle tenotomy for the treatment of lateral epicondylitis: a systematic review of the literature. *PM & R: The Journal of Injury, Function, and Rehabilitation*, 9, 603–611.

McShane, J. M., Nazarian, L., & Harwood, M. (2006). Sonographically guided percutaneous needle tenotomy for treatment of common extensor tendinosis in the elbow. *Journal of Ultrasound in Medicine*, 25, 1281–1289.

Miron-Mendoza, M., Seemann, J., & Grinnell, F. (2008). Collagen fibril flow and tissue translocation coupled to fibroblast migration in 3D collagen matrices. *Molecular Biology of the Cell*, 19, 2051–2058.

Mishra, A. K., Skrepnik, N. V., Edwards, S. G., et al. (2014). Efficacy of platelet-rich plasma for chronic tennis elbow: a double-blind, prospective, multicenter, randomized controlled trial of 230 patients. *The American Journal of Sports Medicine*, 42, 463–471.

Morrey, M. E., Dean, B. J. F., Carr, A. J., & Morrey, B. F. (2013). Tendinopathy: same disease different results—why? *Operative Techniques in Orthopaedics*, 23, 39–49.

Nagraba, L., Tuchalska, J., Mitek, T., Stolarczyk, A., & Deszczynski, J. (2013). Dry needling as a method of tendinopathy treatment. *Ortopedia, Traumatologia, Rehabilitacja, 15,* 109–116.

Passerieux, E., Rossignol, R., Letellier, T., & Delage, J. P. (2007). Physical continuity of the perimysium from myofibers to tendons: involvement in lateral force transmission in skeletal muscle. *Journal of Structural Biology, 159,* 19–28.

Peck, E., Jelsing, E., & Onishi, K. (2016). Advanced ultrasound-guided interventions for tendinopathy. *Physical Medicine and Rehabilitation Clinics of North America, 27,* 733–748.

Pedrelli, A., Stecco, C., & Day, J. A. (2009). Treating patellar tendinopathy with Fascial Manipulation. *Journal of Bodywork and Movement Therapies, 13,* 73–80.

Pfefer, M. T., Cooper, S. R., & Uhl, N. L. (2009). Chiropractic management of tendinopathy: a literature synthesis. *Journal of Manipulative and Physiological Therapeutics, 32,* 41–52.

Prosser, B. L., Khairallah, R. J., Ziman, A. P., Ward, C. W., & Lederer, W. J. (2013). X-ROS signaling in the heart and skeletal muscle: stretch-dependent local ROS regulates [Ca^{2+}]i. *Journal of Molecular and Cellular Cardiology, 58,* 172–181.

Purslow, P. P. (2010). Muscle fascia and force transmission. *Journal of Bodywork and Movement Therapies, 14,* 411–417.

Ramos, L. A., Carvalho, R. T., Garms, R., Navarro, M. S., Abdalla, R. J., & Cohen, M. (2009). Prevalence of pain on palpation of the inferior pole of the patella among patients with complaints of knee pain. *Clinics, 64,* 199–202.

Rio, E., Moseley, L., Purdam, C., Samiric, T., Kidgell, D., Pearce, A. J., et al. (2014). The pain of tendinopathy: physiological or pathophysiological? *Sports Medicine, 44,* 9–23.

Roman, M., Chaudhry, H., Bukiet, B., Stecco, A., & Findley, T. W. (2013). Mathematical analysis of the flow of hyaluronic acid around fascia during manual therapy motions. *The Journal of the American Osteopathic Association, 113,* 600–610.

Sanchis-Alfonso, V., & Rosello-Sastre, E. (2000). Immunohistochemical analysis for neural markers of the lateral retinaculum in patients with isolated symptomatic patellofemoral malalignment. A neuroanatomic basis for anterior knee pain in the active young patient. *The American Journal of Sports Medicine, 28,* 725–731.

Scarr, G. (2017). Comment on 'Defining the fascial system'. *Journal of Bodywork and Movement Therapies, 21,* 178.

Schilder, A., Hoheisel, U., Magerl, W., Benrath, J., Klein, T., & Treede, R. D. (2014). Sensory findings after stimulation of the thoracolumbar fascia with hypertonic saline suggest its contribution to low back pain. *Pain, 155,* 222–231.

Schleip, R. (2003). Fascial plasticity: a new neurobiological explanation: Part 1. *Journal of Bodywork and Movement Therapies, 7,* 11–19.

Schleip, R., Klingler, W., & Lehmann-Horn, F. (2005). Active fascial contractility: fascia may be able to contract in a smooth muscle-like manner and thereby influence musculoskeletal dynamics. *Medical Hypotheses, 65,* 273–277.

Schleip, R., Klingler, W., & Lehmann-Horn, F. (2006). Fascia is able to contract in a smooth muscle-like manner and thereby influence musculoskeletal mechanics. *Journal of Biomechanics, 39,* S488.

Schleip, R., Klingler, W., & Lehmann-Horn, F. (2008). Faszien besitzen eine der glatten Muskulatur vergleichbare Kontraktionsfähigkeit und können so die muskoskelettale Mechanik beeinflussen. *Osteopathische Medizin, Zeitschrift für ganzheitliche Heilverfahren, 9,* 19–21.

Shah, J. P., & Gilliams, E. A. (2008). Uncovering the biochemical milieu of myofascial trigger points using in vivo microdialysis: an application of muscle pain concepts to myofascial pain syndrome. *Journal of Bodywork and Movement Therapies, 12,* 371–384.

Simons, D. G., Travell, J. G., & Simons, L. S. (1999). *Travell and Simons' myofascial pain and dysfunction; the trigger point manual* (2 ed.). Baltimore: Williams & Wilkins.

Simpson, M. R., & Howard, T. M. (2009). Tendinopathies of the foot and ankle. *American Family Physician, 80,* 1107–1114.

Smeulders, M. J., Kreulen, M., Hage, J. J., Huijing, P. A., & van der Horst, C. M. (2005). Spastic muscle properties are affected by length changes of adjacent structures. *Muscle & Nerve, 32,* 208–215.

Stecco, C., Gagey, O., Macchi, V., Porzionato, A., De Caro, R., Aldegheri, R., et al. (2007). Tendinous muscular insertions onto the deep fascia of the upper limb. First part: anatomical study. *Morphologie, 91,* 29–37.

Stecco, C., Macchi, V., Porzionato, A., Morra, A., Parenti, A., Stecco, A., Delmas, V., De Caro, R. (2010). The ankle retinacula: morphological evidence of the proprioceptive role of the fascial system. *Cells Tissues Organs, 192*(3):200–210.

Stecco, A., Gesi, M., Stecco, C., & Stern, R. (2013a). Fascial components of the myofascial pain syndrome. *Current Pain and Headache Reports, 17,* 352.

Stecco, A., Gilliar, W., Hill, R., Fullerton, B., & Stecco, C. (2013b). The anatomical and functional relation between gluteus maximus and fascia lata. *Journal of Bodywork and Movement Therapies, 17,* 512–517.

Stecco, C., Porzionato, A., Lancerotto, L., Stecco, A., Macchi, V., Day, J. A., et al. (2008). Histological study of the deep fasciae of the limbs. *Journal of Bodywork and Movement Therapies, 12,* 225–230.

Stecco, C., & Schleip, R. (2016a). A fascia and the fascial system. *Journal of Bodywork and Movement Therapies, 20,* 139–140.

Stecco, A., Stern, R., Fantoni, I., De Caro, R., & Stecco, C. (2016b). Fascial disorders: implications for treatment. *PM & R: The Journal of Injury, Function, and Rehabilitation, 8,* 161–168.

Stenhouse, G., Sookur, P., & Watson, M. (2013). Do blood growth factors offer additional benefit in refractory lateral epicondylitis? A prospective, randomized pilot trial of DN as a stand-alone procedure versus DN and autologous conditioned plasma. *Skeletal Radiology, 42,* 1515–1520.

Stilwell DL, Jr. (1957). Regional variations in the innervation of deep fasciae and aponeuroses. *The Anatomical Record, 127,* 635–653

Tesarz, J., Hoheisel, U., Wiedenhofer, B., & Mense, S. (2011). Sensory innervation of the thoracolumbar fascia in rats and humans. *Neuroscience, 194,* 302–308.

Testa, V., Capasso, G., Benazzo, F., & Maffulli, N. (2002). Management of Achilles tendinopathy by ultrasound-guided percutaneous tenotomy. *Medicine and Science in Sports and Exercise, 34*, 573–580.

Testa, V., Capasso, G., Maffulli, N., & Bifulco, G. (1999). Ultrasound-guided percutaneous longitudinal tenotomy for the management of patellar tendinopathy. *Medicine and Science in Sports and Exercise, 31*, 1509–1515.

Tomasek, J. J., Gabbiani, G., Hinz, B., Chaponnier, C., & Brown, R. A. (2002). Myofibroblasts and mechano-regulation of connective tissue remodelling. *Nature Reviews Molecular Cell Biology, 3*, 349–363.

Travell, J., & Rinzler, S. H. (1952). The myofascial genesis of pain. *Postgraduate Medicine, 11*, 425–434.

Travell, J. G., & Simons, D. G. (1992). *Myofascial pain and dysfunction: the trigger point manual.* Baltimore: Williams & Wilkins.

Settergren, R. (2013). Treatment of supraspinatus tendinopathy with ultrasound guided DN. *Journal of Chiropractic Medicine, 12*, 26–29.

Tsikopoulos, K., Tsikopoulos, I., Simeonidis, E., Papathanasiou, E., Haidich, A. B., Anastasopoulos, N., et al. (2016). The clinical impact of platelet-rich plasma on tendinopathy compared to placebo or DN injections: a meta-analysis. *Physical Therapy in Sport, 17*, 87–94.

Turrina, A., Martinez-Gonzalez, M. A., & Stecco, C. (2013). The muscular force transmission system: role of the intramuscular connective tissue. *Journal of Bodywork and Movement Therapies, 17*, 95–102.

Vleeming, A., Schuenke, M. D., Danneels, L., & Willard, F. H. (2014). The functional coupling of the deep abdominal and paraspinal muscles: the effects of simulated paraspinal muscle contraction on force transfer to the middle and posterior layer of the thoracolumbar fascia. *Journal of Anatomy, 225*, 447–462.

van der Wal, J. (2009). The architecture of the connective tissue in the musculoskeletal system-an often over-looked functional parameter as to proprioception in the locomotor apparatus. *International Journal of Therapeutic Massage & Bodywork, 2*, 9–23.

Weinkauf, B., Deising, S., Obreja, O., Hoheisel, U., Mense, S., Schmelz, M., et al. (2015). Comparison of nerve growth factor-induced sensitization pattern in lumbar and tibial muscle and fascia. *Muscle & Nerve, 52*, 265–272.

Wilke, J., Engeroff, T., Nurnberger, F., Vogt, L., & Banzer, W. (2016). Anatomical study of the morphological continuity between iliotibial tract and the fibularis longus fascia. *Surgical and Radiologic Anatomy, 38*, 349–352.

Willard, F. H., Vleeming, A., Schuenke, M. D., Danneels, L., & Schleip, R. (2012). The thoracolumbar fascia: anatomy, function and clinical considerations. *Journal of Anatomy, 221*, 507–536.

Yahia, L. H., Pigeon, P., & DesRosiers, E. A. (1993). Viscoelastic properties of the human lumbodorsal fascia. *Journal of Biomedical Engineering, 15*, 425–429.

Yahia, L., Rhalmi, S., Newman, N., & Isler, M. (1992). Sensory innervation of human thoracolumbar fascia. An immunohistochemical study. *Acta Orthopaedica Scandinavica, 63*, 195–197.

Zhu, J., Hu, B., Xing, C., & Li, J. (2008a). Ultrasound-guided, minimally invasive, percutaneous needle puncture treatment for tennis elbow. *Advances in Therapy, 25*, 1031–1036.

Zhu, J., Jiang, Y., Hu, Y., Xing, C., & Hu, B. (2008b). Evaluating the long-term effect of ultrasound-guided needle puncture without aspiration on calcifying supraspinatus tendinitis. *Advances in Therapy, 25*, 1229–1234.

CHAPTER 4

Dry Needling for Neurological Conditions

JAIME SALOM MORENO • CÉSAR FERNÁNDEZ-DE-LAS-PEÑAS

INTRODUCTION

Neurological conditions are chronic, progressive, and lifelong diseases accounting for about 6% of the global burden of diseases and resulting in a substantial effect on healthcare use (World Health Organization, 2006). In fact, the burden of neurological diseases is expected to increase as the population ages (Gaskin et al., 2017; Gooch et al., 2017). Raggi and Leonardi (2015) found that the years lived with a disability and costs of neurological conditions were lower in southern European countries, whereas prevalence was lower in northern European countries, However, no statistical differences were observed. Danila and colleagues (2014) reported that neurological conditions with the highest estimated prevalence in various Canadian settings, including home care, nursing homes, complex continuing care, and psychiatric hospitals, were: Alzheimer disease and related dementias (9%–25%); Parkinson disease (2%–8%); epilepsy (3%–8%); and traumatic brain injury (3%–6%). Additionally, cerebral vascular accidents (Feigin et al., 2017) and multiple sclerosis (Adelman et al., 2013) are important neurological causes of related disability and burden with a prevalence of nearly 5% (Favate & Younger, 2016; Howard et al., 2016). Although stroke has dropped from being the third main leading cause of death to the fourth cause in the United States and Europe (Burke et al., 2012), patients with this disease exhibit higher rates of related disability. This chapter will discuss the presence of spasticity and pain as potential causes of disability in subjects with neurological conditions and their management with needling therapies.

SPASTICITY AND MUSCLE TONE

One of the main causes leading to physical disability in neurological conditions is the presence of spasticity. The prevalence of spasticity is around 65% in patients with multiple sclerosis (Oreja-Guevara et al., 2013), 65% in patients with spinal cord injury (Holtz et al., 2017), and 40% in patients who had suffered a stroke (Wissel et al., 2013). Not surprisingly, there is a significant correlation between increasing severity of spasticity and worsening of symptoms. Patients with spasticity exhibit lower motor activity performance than patients who do not have spasticity (Sommerfeld et al., 2004; Milinis & Young, 2015); the presence of spasticity, in this case in the lower extremity, is associated with a fourfold increase in direct care costs during the first year poststroke (Lundstrom et al., 2010).

Spasticity was originally defined by Lance as 'a motor disorder characterised by a velocity-dependent increase in tonic stretch reflexes (muscle tone) with exaggerated tendon jerks, resulting from hyperexcitability of the stretch reflex, as a component of upper motor neuron syndrome' (Lance, 1990). The upper motor neuron syndrome is associated with positive and negative symptoms. Negative signs include weakness and loss of dexterity such as during the acute phase after a stroke. Positive signs are characterised mainly by muscle overactivity such as excessive muscle contractions or other inappropriate muscle activity. Lance's descriptive definition has been questioned because the term spasticity can also include several other clinical syndromes, including spasms, clonus, and hypertonia. In clinical practice, it is not very common to see spasticity as a primary hypertonic, velocity-dependent increase in tonic stretch reflexes. Burridge and colleagues (2005) proposed that spasticity features 'disordered sensory-motor control, resulting from an upper motor neuron lesion, and presenting as intermittent or sustained involuntary activation of muscles', which is a broader and clinically more applicable definition.

Current hypotheses of the potential mechanisms of spasticity suggest two main mechanisms: a neural hypothesis involving the cortex, brainstem and spinal cord; and a muscular hypothesis. Potential neural mechanisms include hyperexcitability of the stretch reflex due to an imbalance between excitatory and inhibitory cortical mechanisms on spinal cord circuits (Sheean, 2002) and the release of primitive reflexes or the development of pathological new reflexes; however, these hypotheses are controversial (Sheean, 2002). Not all patients with spasticity exhibit signs of hyperreflexia (Sinkjaer & Magnussen, 1994), which suggests that the neural hypothesis is incomplete by itself.

Although the primary lesion is probably neural in origin, there is emerging evidence of secondary changes in the soft tissues such as changes in muscles at the protein, single-fibre, and whole-muscle levels (Foran et al., 2005). Spastic musculature features: decreased mitochondrial volume fraction; an appearance of intracellular amorphous material; a reduction in muscle fibre length; and a decrease in the number of serial sarcomeres (Lieber et al., 2004; Olsson et al., 2006). This suggests that the increased muscle tone in subjects with spasticity could be caused by structural changes in the musculature (Gracies, 2005). The degree to which each proposed mechanism may be responsible for the development of spasticity is not currently known, partially due to the great variability between individuals.

PAIN IN NEUROLOGICAL CONDITIONS

In addition to spasticity, pain is one of the most disabling symptoms experienced by subjects with neurological conditions. The prevalence of pain has been estimated to be: 20% to 70% in stroke (Harrison & Field, 2015); 60% to 70% in spinal cord injury (Siddall et al., 2003); 50% to 60% in multiple sclerosis (Foley et al., 2013a); and 30% to 50% in Parkinson disease (Fil et al., 2013).

Patients with spasticity after a stroke, with multiple sclerosis, or with a spinal cord injury may suffer from nociceptive and neuropathic pain. In fact, different types of pain can be present at the same time. For example, patients who have suffered a stroke may suffer central poststroke pain, complex regional pain syndrome, and musculoskeletal or spasticity-related pain, among other types of pain (Paolucci et al., 2016a). Management of pain in individuals with spasticity involves both pharmacological and nonpharmacological interventions. In this chapter, the focus is on nociceptive pain in subjects who have suffered a stroke because this condition is the most studied in the context of indications for dry needling.

The most common form of nociceptive pain is hemiplegic shoulder pain, which is present in up to 54% of patients who have suffered a stroke (Coskun Benlidayi & Basaran, 2014). Additionally, musculoskeletal pain

is observed in approximately 25% of stroke survivors, and a recent study showed an overall prevalence of 29.5% being 14.1% in the acute phase, 42.7% in the subacute, and 31.9% in the chronic phase (Paolucci et al., 2016b).

Hemiplegic shoulder pain has been referred to by different diagnostic terms such as tendinitis, rotator-cuff tear, shoulder subluxation, adhesive capsulitis, or spasticity; however, the contribution of these factors is disputed (Lee et al., 2009). It is interesting to note that, although typically pain is located mainly in the shoulder area, it can also involve additional areas of the upper extremity (Dromerick et al., 2008), suggesting the presence of sensitisation mechanisms. Zeilig and colleagues (2013) confirmed that poststroke shoulder pain is likely related to central sensitisation. Poststroke shoulder pain is currently considered a specific subtype of central poststroke syndrome with both nociceptive and neuropathic influences. It is conceivable that needling therapies can address the nociceptive aspects of hemiplegic (poststroke) shoulder pain.

BOTULINUM TOXIN A FOR SPASTICITY AND RELATED PAIN

Several therapeutic approaches have been proposed for the management of spasticity in patients with neurological conditions, with intramuscular botulinum toxin A (BTX-A) injections among the most popular (Ghasemi et al., 2013) and recognised in clinical practice guidelines for stroke (European Stroke Organization Executive Committee, 2008). BTX-A works primarily by preventing the release of acetylcholine and blocking cholinergic transmission at the neuromuscular junction for a limited period of time of approximately 3 to 4 months (Brown et al., 2014).

Different meta-analyses have found that the application of BTX-A in patients who have experienced a stroke is associated with both moderate improvements in upper extremity performance (Foley et al., 2013b) and function and muscle tone in the lower extremity (Wu et al., 2016). In addition, BTX-A is used for treating spasticity-related pain. Although the underlying mechanisms are still unclear, some hypothesis are proposed, including: blocking nociceptor transduction, reduction of neurogenic inflammation by inhibiting neural substances and neurotransmitters such as substance P, calcitonin gene-related peptide, and glutamate; and prevention of peripheral and central sensitisation (Durham et al., 2004; Bach-Rojecky et al., 2010; Paterson et al., 2014). The review by Baker and Pereira (2013) found that the use of BTX-A was effective for upper and lower extremity spasticity, but its effects on spasticity-related pain were rather limited. A more recent meta-analysis found that BTX-A resulted in small to moderate pain relief and in an increase in range of motion in patients with chronic hemiplegic shoulder pain (Wu et al., 2015). The most common targeted muscles for treatment of hemiplegic shoulder pain included the pectoralis major, teres major, subscapularis, biceps brachii, and infraspinatus muscles (Yelnik et al., 2007; Marciniak et al., 2012).

Currently, the dosages of BTX-A vary considerably in clinical practice and are frequently based on the personal experience of the practitioner, expert opinions, the formulation and brand of the type of BTX-A, and the individual patient's response (Yablon et al., 2011). Yablon and colleagues reported the estimated doses of BTX-A to produce a mean one-point decrease in the Ashworth scale for the flexor carpi radialis (22.5U), the flexor carpi ulnaris (18.4U), the flexor digitorum superficialis (66.3U), and the flexor digitorum profundus (42.5U) muscles. Significant drawbacks of BTX-A therapy are its high cost, the transient nature of the toxin, and the possibility, although very rare, of the development of neurotoxicity (Intiso et al., 2015).

Finally, it is important to consider that BTX-A should not be clinically applied as an isolated intervention. Kinnear and associates (2014) found that therapy combined with BTX-A was slightly more effective than BTX-A alone. In fact, several rehabilitation interventions are applied in combination with BTX-A: ergometer cycling, electrical stimulation, stretching exercises, constraint-induced movement therapy, task-specific motor training, and exercise programs (Kinnear et al., 2014).

DRY NEEDLING FOR NEUROLOGICAL CONDITIONS

Considering the disadvantages of BTX-A injections, needling therapy with solid filament needles may be a reasonable and worthy alternative. Several studies have investigated the effects of acupuncture on poststroke spasticity; however, the results are conflicting. Some observed that acupuncture was effective for reducing spasticity (Mukherjee et al., 2007; Zhao et al., 2009), but others did not find any significant effect (Fink et al., 2004; Wayne et al., 2005). A recent meta-analysis showed that acupuncture or electroacupuncture was associated with a decrease in wrist, knee, and elbow spasticity in patients after stroke, although a subgroup analysis did not reveal significance (Lim et al., 2015). A review of 24 systematic reviews suggested that acupuncture can be effective for stroke rehabilitation and

stroke related disorders (Zhang et al., 2014); another review concluded that acupuncture combined with exercise was effective for shoulder pain after stroke (Lee et al., 2012).

Discrepancies between published studies appear to exist because of different methodologies and point selection. Although in most acupuncture studies, classical acupuncture points were the target, in other studies the needle was directed to the region of spastic muscles or entirely outside the affected area. In the latter scenario, the needle placement was therefore remote from the spastic musculature. Dry needling with the needle placed directly into the spastic muscles may offer an alternative intervention for the spastic musculature.

Evidence for the effects of dry needling in neurological conditions is slowly emerging (Uttam, 2015). Two recent case reports discussed dry needling for poststroke spasticity of the upper extremity (Ansari et al., 2015) and for quadriparesis of a 4-year-old child (Gallego & del Moral, 2007), respectively. In the first case report, Ansari and associates applied dry needling to the pronator teres, the flexor carpi radialis, and the flexor carpi ulnaris muscles. In the second report, Gallego and del Moral applied dry needling to the opponens pollicis, the flexor carpi radialis, the flexor digitorum superficialis, and the biceps brachii muscles. A recent case series that included 29 patients with poststroke spasticity observed an improvement of spasticity, alpha motor neuron excitability, range of motion, and hand dexterity 1 hour after the application of a single session of dry needling into the wrist flexor muscles (Fakari et al., 2017). Mendigutia-Gómez and colleagues (2016) conducted the only clinical trial to date investigating changes in spasticity in the upper extremity with dry needling, which included a control group. In this study, patients with poststroke spasticity received three sessions of dry needling in the shoulder girdle muscles combined with a multimodal rehabilitation program. The results showed significant improvements in shoulder range of motion, pressure pain thresholds, and spasticity in the external rotator muscles such as the infraspinatus muscle (Mendigutia-Gómez et al., 2016).

There is only one study investigating the effects of dry needling in hemiplegic shoulder pain. The study by DiLorenzo and associates (2004) found that inclusion of dry needling into a rehabilitation program was effective for improving hemiparetic shoulder pain. In this study, patients experienced pain in the anterior and lateral parts of the shoulder area, the deltoid and rotator cuff muscles, and the lateral aspect of the upper extremity. This pain pattern resembles the referred pain from TrPs in the shoulder girdle muscles (Simons et al., 1999). The supraspinatus, infraspinatus, anterior deltoid, middle deltoid, and levator scapulae were the most painful muscles with the dry needling intervention. Dry needling was effective for reducing severe pain during sleep and providing more comfort overall in the wheelchairs, in bed, and during their physiotherapy treatment (DiLorenzo et al., 2004). Subjects receiving dry needling reduced their pain medicine intake (DiLorenzo et al., 2004).

Evidence for the application of dry needling in the lower extremity is similar to the upper limb. A single case study reported that dry needling was able to decrease local muscle stiffness assessed by tensiomyography in a patient with chronic poststroke spasticity (Calvo et al., 2016). In this report, the treated muscles included the biceps and triceps brachii, rectus femoris, semitendinous, biceps femoris, and medial and lateral gastrocnemius (Calvo et al., 2016). The only randomised clinical trial investigating the immediate effects of dry needling on spasticity in the lower extremity found a decrease in spasticity in the ankle plantar-flexor muscles and improvements in pressure pain sensitivity in individuals with poststroke spasticity (Salom-Moreno et al., 2014). In this clinical trial, agonist (i.e., gastrocnemius) and antagonist (i.e., tibialis anterior) muscles received a single session of dry needling (Salom-Moreno et al., 2014). There were significant improvements in support surface of the affected and unaffected feet, which suggest that dry needling may improve gait parameters in poststroke subjects (Salom-Moreno et al., 2014).

A recent case study report including two poststroke patients reported specific electroencephalographic changes after dry needling of TrPs. The first subject was a 51-year-old male with an ischaemic stroke affecting the left side. The researchers used dry needling for TrPs within the pronator teres, medial and lateral gastrocnemius, soleus, and peroneus longus muscles. The second subject was a 56-year-old male with a haemorrhagic stroke affecting the right side, who received dry needling targeting TrPs in the pectoralis major, biceps brachii, brachialis, latissimus dorsi, teres major, pronator teres, flexor digitorum superficialis and profundus, adductor pollicis, medial and lateral gastrocnemius, soleus, semitendinosus, semimembranosus, and the long head of biceps femoris muscles. The researchers observed an improvement in the regional brain activity, especially in alpha waves, and changes in the cordance of the frontal/prefrontal regions, using quantitative electroencephalographic activity and electroencephalographic cordance. This is the first demonstration that the results of peripherally applied dry needling can be objectively assessed with electroencephalographic outcome measures.

In conclusion, dry needling is an emerging therapeutic intervention for the management of spasticity in patients with neurological conditions; however, current evidence has only investigated the short-term effects and has focused mainly on patients who suffered a stroke. Several questions about the use of repetitive treatments, appropriate dosage, the combination with other pharmacological and nonpharmacological agents the combination with other physical therapy approaches, and the longer-term duration of the effects of dry needling remain to be elucidated.

CLINICAL REASONING FOR DRY NEEDLING IN NEUROLOGICAL CONDITIONS

The application of dry needling in spastic muscles is based on the similarities between structural changes observed in spastic muscles, changes observed in muscles with myofascial trigger points (TrPs), and the similarities between the neurophysiological mechanisms of dry needling and BTX-A injections.

There is clear evidence that muscle contractures secondary to spasticity are due to a reduction in muscle fibre length, an increase in the number of cross bridges, an increase in collagen tissue, and an increase in active muscle stiffness. In fact, the muscle fibres from patients with spasticity are more than twice as stiff as the fibres from patients without spasticity (Fridén & Lieber, 2003). It is interesting to note that current pathophysiological theories explaining the formation of TrPs also involve a reduction of muscle fibres (Bron & Dommerholt, 2012) and an increase in stiffness in the taut band, which involves the TrP (Chen et al., 2016) (see Chapter 1). In addition, TrPs can also contribute to movement alterations observed in patients with neurological conditions because they promote accelerated fatigue, altered patterns of intramuscular activity, an increase antagonist coactivation, and altered muscle activation patterns (Lucas et al., 2004; Ibarra et al., 2011; Ge et al., 2012, 2014; Bohlooli et al., 2016).

Both dry needling and BTX-A interventions target dysfunctional motor end-plate zones. In an animal model, Domingo and associates (2013) observed that the application of dry needling induces a destruction of the neuromuscular junction, including damage of the axonal area. On the other hand, BTX-A blocks the release of acetylcholine at the neuromuscular endplate, and BTX-A injections are also used in the management of myofascial pain syndrome (Zhou & Wang, 2014).

A recent Cochrane review concluded that BTX-A injections were only effective for patients with epicondylalgia (Soares et al., 2014). The efficacy of BTX-A injections for myofascial pain is not entirely clear, which may be due to a wide variety of factors such as an incomplete treatment of a regional myofascial pain syndrome, inappropriate or confounding control populations or treatments, inappropriate time periods for assessment of outcomes, and a misinterpretation of the timeframe of action of BTX-A (Gerwin, 2012).

The presence of pain is another clinical application of dry needling for patients with neurological conditions. De Oliveira and colleagues (2012) reported that burning was the most common descriptor used by 70% of patients for describing postcentral stroke pain. In this sample of patients, active TrPs reproducing their symptoms were found in up to 65% of the sample, especially in the upper trapezius (50%), splenius (30%), supraspinatus (30%), semispinalis (25%), and infraspinatus (20%) muscles (De Oliveira et al., 2012). In this scenario, active TrPs can serve as peripheral generators of nociceptive input that may alter pain perception in a subgroup of patients with stroke. At the same time, spasticity and altered central descending pain modulation observed in poststroke patients (Roosink et al., 2011) may induce overload to the affected muscles and contribute to the development of TrPs. It is conceivable that a vicious cycle may exist between the development of TrPs, spasticity, and sensitisation.

CLINICAL GUIDELINES FOR DRY NEEDLING IN SPASTICITY
Diagnostic Clinical Decision
It is important to consider whether a clinician aims to reduce spasticity or pain as the main objective of dry needling with patients with neurological conditions. If the objective is to reduce spasticity or muscle tone, patients with spasticity but without pain may not experience the phenomenon of referred pain that is observed commonly in patients suffering from musculoskeletal pain due to sensory disturbances. For these cases, the clinical reasoning process for the application of dry needling should not be based on the same diagnostic criteria as used in patients with musculoskeletal pain.

Of interest is whether the term 'TrP dry needling' should be used in individuals with spasticity, as many patients do not exhibit any sensory symptom usually associated with myofascial pain. Because spasticity is related to an increase in muscle tone, perhaps the mere presence of a taut band and hypersensitive spots in the spastic muscle would be more relevant clinical criteria.

In patients showing sensory disturbances without being able to clearly discriminate the most sensitive spot, the clinician may need to rely on palpation and locate the tightest spot within a spastic contracture, which would be similar to locating active TrPs in individuals without spasticity (Turo et al., 2013). The identification of taut bands in a spastic muscle is usually more difficult than in a nonspastic muscle and requires excellent palpatory skills.

Another reason to consider dry needling clinically is to improve the commonly observed resistance to passive movement. To address this clinical issue, clinicians must understand the specific spastic pattern of each individual patient. Once the individual pattern has been determined, therapists must decide which muscles will be included in the actual dry needling treatment.

Based on clinical experience, we recommend this cluster of clinical diagnostic criteria:
- palpable (if possible) taut band in a spastic muscle;
- hypersensitive (thicker) spot in the taut band; and
- an increase in resistance to passive movement.

For patients with primary complaints of spasticity-related local and referred pain, who recognise elicited sensory (pain) symptoms, the more standard criteria for myofascial pain would apply.

Dry Needling Procedure
When needling patients with neurological conditions, the clinical criteria and the actual needling procedures differ from needling patients with just musculoskeletal pain.

1. In patients with musculoskeletal pain syndromes, dry needling is usually applied with the affected muscle in a relaxed position. In patients with neurological conditions, due to the presence of spasticity, the technique will be applied in a prestretched (submaximal stretched) position. In this prestretched position, the taut band is located within the spastic muscle and the needle placed on it (Fig. 4.1).
2. The needle will be inserted into the spastic taut band looking for local twitch responses, as it is commonly done in clinical practice with the 'fast-in and fast-out' technique (Hong, 1994). Local twitch responses can be elicited in both nonspastic and spastic muscles, but in individuals with neurological conditions, sometimes the twitch can involve the entire muscle. This has been called the 'global twitch response'. This global response of the spastic muscle is expected, because these muscles are related to a hyperexcitability of the neural pathways. Additionally, in some patients the twitch responses can appear in the antagonist

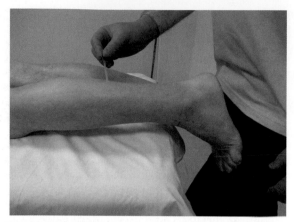

FIG. 4.1 Dry needling over the soleus with the muscle placed in a prestretched (submaximal stretched) position.

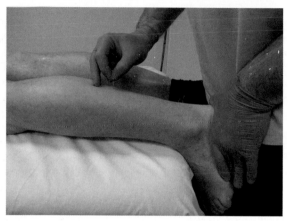

FIG. 4.2 Control of the spastic area receiving dry needling for avoiding involuntary or unexpected movements.

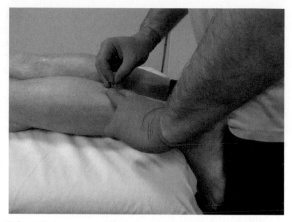

FIG. 4.3 Increase in stretching of the spastic muscle during the dry needling procedure.

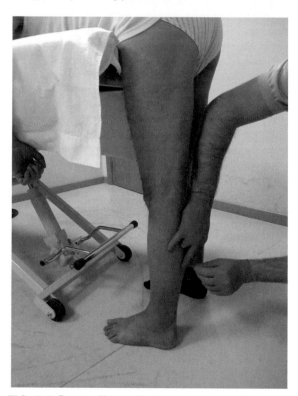

FIG. 4.4 Dry needling applied over the soleus with the patient in standing.

muscles due to the neural component of spasticity. During this procedure, it is important that the therapist controls the position of the region of the patient receiving the procedure for better control of the intervention (Fig. 4.2).

3. Once the clinician experienced a release of the taut band or a decrease in tone of the spastic muscle (usually related to fact of obtaining twitch responses with the needle), the muscle will be stretched until a new barrier is engaged (Fig. 4.3).

4. The procedure is repeated two or three times, depending on the patient's tolerance.

In some patients, when the gastrocnemius and soleus are the targeted muscles, dry needling can be applied when standing to use the weight of the patient's body (Fig. 4.4). This can be used in patients with high muscle tone when passive stretching of the muscle by the therapist is difficult.

MECHANISMS OF DRY NEEDLING ON NEUROLOGICAL CONDITIONS

Irrespective of whether patients have a neurological condition, the underlying mechanisms of dry needling in this population can be considered from a mechanical and neurophysiological perspective (Chou et al., 2012; Cagnie et al., 2013). The mechanical effects of dry needling include disruption of muscle contraction knots, localised stretch of the contractured cytoskeletal structures, and a reduction of the overlap between actin and myosin filaments (Chapter 2). Therefore the improvements after dry needling of spastic muscles may be explained biomechanically through changes occurring at the local muscle and connective tissue levels. Mechanical manipulation with the needle likely disrupts the integrity of the soft tissue contractures locally, leading to an immediate reduction of resistance felt when stretching the spastic muscle. Dry needling can reduce muscle stiffness assessed by ultrasound shear wave elastography (Maher et al., 2013), and local tissue changes may continue for at least 8 weeks after a dry needing intervention (Turo et al., 2015). Because an increased resistance in spastic muscles appears to be related to the inability of the fascicles to elongate (Barber et al., 2011), the restoration of sarcomere length and the decrease in stiffness of spastic taut bands may, at least in part, explain the decrease of poststroke spasticity observed in patient receiving dry needling. This mechanical effect would explain why dry needling should be applied preferably in a prestretched (submaximal) position to decrease the stiffness and elongate the spastic muscle.

Dry needling could also exert a potential neural effect. It is conceivable that dry needling may modulate motor neuron activity and modify synaptic transmission from muscle afferents to spinal motor neuron by different reflex mechanisms because increased motor neuron excitability induced by an increased excitatory synaptic input, and reduced interneuron inhibition or alteration in intrinsic neuron properties are neural components of spasticity (Nielsen et al., 2007). In this mechanism, the local or global twitch response would be a key element. We know that the local twitch response is an involuntary spinal reflex resulting from mechanical stimulation of a taut band with a needle, which occurs in response to altered sensory spinal processing related to the modulation of the myotatic reflex (Hsieh et al., 2011). Because dry needling has a positive inhibitory effect on spontaneous electrical activity of muscle motor neurons when local twitch responses are elicited during the technique (Chen et al., 2001), it is possible that their elicitation in individuals with neurological conditions can modulate motor neuron excitability at the spinal cord. This mechanism may be more evident when global twitch responses are elicited; however, this needs to be confirmed in future studies.

The effects of dry needling might not be restricted to just the needled area, but may influence the central nervous system of individuals with neurological conditions. Mechanical sensory stimulation after needling might trigger events, both locally and centrally, leading to the neuromodulation of the spasticity. Because dry needling can activate nociceptors that may lead to pain, the relaxing effects found on spastic muscles could be related to activation of the noxious inhibitory control systems and inhibition of excitatory control systems. This central mechanism may help to restore the imbalance between inhibitory and excitatory fibres due to upper motor neuron lesion related to spasticity and poststroke central pain (Roosink et al., 2012). Therefore dry needling may be able to contribute to this process by modulating the central nervous system through an antinociceptive effect (Srbely et al., 2010) involving peripheral and central mechanisms (Dommerholt, 2011). More research is needed to further elucidate the underlying mechanisms.

CLINICAL CONSIDERATIONS

Because the application of dry needling in neurological conditions represents a recent use of the technique, there are several clinical questions and considerations that need to be explored in more detail.

It is not really known what the optimal dosage is of dry needling in neurological conditions. It appears that several treatment sessions are required to achieve clinically significant improvements in spasticity and function and in the ability to execute task-specific movements. The number of dry needling sessions applied in trials or case reports ranges from one to three, but it is likely that in clinical practice more sessions are required. Successive applications of dry needling will more effectively modulate sensitisation mechanisms in neurological conditions and may prevent the development of spasticity-related pain. Regarding the frequency of the dry needling sessions, we have concluded empirically that at least 7 days between sessions are needed to avoid excessive damage to the muscle. Again, more studies are clearly needed.

Clinical evidence suggests that, although changes in spasticity can be observed immediately after dry needling, changes in function need more time to be apparent. It is currently not known how long the effects of dry needling on spasticity and pain will last. To date, studies have investigated only the short-term effects of dry needing, and there is no available data about the mid- and long-term effects of dry needling.

As with dry needling for other conditions, dry needling to reduce spasticity should not be applied in isolation of other interventions. To further improve the effects of dry needling, active exercises or other therapeutic interventions after dry needling may enhance the gains achieved with the technique.

In conclusion, dry needling is an emerging technique for the management of muscle tone, spasticity, and spasticity related-pain in patients with neurological conditions. However, further research is clearly needed to determine its effectiveness, mainly concerning BTX-A. Dry needling should always be applied as part of a more comprehensive treatment program and should not become the sole intervention for patients with spasticity or spasticity-related pain.

REFERENCES

Adelman, G., Rane, S. G., & Villa, K. F. (2013). The cost burden of multiple sclerosis in the United States: a systematic review of the literature. *Journal of Medical Economics, 16,* 639–647.

Ansari, N. N., Naghdi, S., Fakhari, Z., Radinmehr, H., & Hasson, S. (2015). Dry needling for the treatment of post-stroke muscle spasticity: A prospective case report. *NeuroRehabilitation, 36,* 61–65.

Bach-Rojecky, L., Salkovic-Petrisic, M., & Lackovic, Z. (2010). Botulinum toxin type A reduces pain supersensitivity in experimental diabetic neuropathy: bilateral effect after unilateral injection. *European Journal of Pharmacology, 633,* 10–14.

Baker, J. A., & Pereira, G. (2013). The efficacy of Botulinum Toxin A for spasticity and pain in adults: a systematic review and meta-analysis using the Grades of Recommendation, Assessment, Development and Evaluation approach. *Clinical Rehabilitation, 27,* 1084–1096.

Barber, L., Barrett, R., & Lichtwark, G. (2011). Passive muscle mechanical properties of the medial gastrocnemius in young adults with spastic cerebral palsy. *Journal of Biomechanics, 44,* 2496–2500.

Bohlooli, N., Ahmadi, A., Maroufi, N., Sarrafzadeh, J., & Jaberzadeh, S. (2016). Differential activation of scapular muscles, during arm elevation, with and without trigger points. *Journal of Bodywork and Movement Therapies, 20,* 26–34.

Bron, C., & Dommerholt, J. D. (2012). etiology of myofascial trigger points. *Current Pain and Headache Reports, 16,* 439–444.

Brown, E. A., Schütz, S. G., & Simpson, D. M. (2014). Botulinum toxin for neuropathic pain and spasticity: An overview. *Pain Management, 4,* 129–151.

Burke, J. F., Lisabeth, L. D., Brown, D. L., Reeves, M. J., & Morgenstern, L. B. (2012). Determining stroke's rank as a cause of death using multicause mortality data. *Stroke, 43,* 2207–2211.

Burridge, J. H., Wood, D. E., Hermens, H. J., et al. (2005). The practical and methodological considerations in the measurement of spasticity. *Disability and Rehabilitation, 27,* 69–80.

Cagnie, B., Dewitte, V., Barbe, T., Timmermans, F., Delrue, N., & Meeus, M. (2013). Physiologic effects of dry needling. *Current Pain and Headache Reports, 17,* 348.

Calvo, S., Quintero, I., & Herrero, P. (2016). Effects of dry needling (DNHS technique) on the contractile properties of spastic muscles in a patient with stroke: a case report. *International Journal of Rehabilitation Research, 39,* 372–376.

Chen, J. T., Chung, K. C., Hou, C. R., Kuan, T. S., Chen, S. M., & Hong, C. Z. (2001). Inhibitory effect of dry needling on the spontaneous electrical activity recorded from myofascial trigger spots of rabbit skeletal muscle. *American Journal of Physical Medicine & Rehabilitation, 80,* 729–735.

Chen, Q., Wang, H. J., Gay, R. E., Thompson, J. M., Manduca, A., An, K. N., et al. (2016). Quantification of myofascial taut bands. *Archives of Physical Medicine and Rehabilitation, 97,* 67–73.

Chou, L. W., KAo, M. J., & Lin, J. G. (2012). Probable mechanisms of needling therapies for myofascial pain control. *Evidence-based Complementary and Alternative Medicine, 705327.*

Coskun Benlidayi, I., & Basaran, S. (2014). Hemiplegic shoulder pain: a common clinical consequence of stroke. *Practical Neurology, 14,* 88–91.

Danila, O., Hirdes, J. P., Maxwell, C. J., Marrie, R. A., Patten, S., Pringsheim, T., et al. (2014). Prevalence of neurological conditions across the continuum of care based on interRAI assessments. *BMC Health Services Research, 14,* 29.

De Oliveira, R. A., de Andrade, D. C., Machado, A. G., & Teixeira, M. J. (2012). Central post-stroke pain: somatosensory abnormalities and the presence of associated myofascial pain syndrome. *BMC Neurology, 12,* 89.

DiLorenzo, L., Traballesi, M., Morelli, D., Pompa, A., Brunelli, S., Buzzi, M. G., et al. (2004). Hemiparetic shoulder pain syndrome treated with deep dry needling during early rehabilitation: A prospective, open-label, randomized investigation. *Journal of Musculoskeletal Pain, 12,* 25–34.

Domingo, A., Mayoral, O., Monterde, S., & Santafé, M. M. (2013). Neuromuscular damage and repair after dry needling in mice. *Evidence-based Complementary and Alternative Medicine, 260806.*

Dommerholt, J. (2011). Dry needling: peripheral and central considerations. *The Journal of Manual & Manipulative Therapy, 19,* 223–237.

Dromerick, A. W., Edwards, D. F., & Kumar, A. (2008). Hemiplegic shoulder pain syndrome: frequency and characteristics during inpatient stroke rehabilitation. *Archives of Physical Medicine and Rehabilitation, 89,* 1589–1593.

Durham, P. L., Cady, R., & Cady, R. (2004). Regulation of calcitonin gene-related peptide secretion from trigeminal nerve cells by botulinum toxin type A: implications for migraine therapy. *Headache, 44,* 35–42.

European Stroke Organisation (ESO) Executive Committee. (2008). ESO Writing Committee Guidelines for management of ischaemic stroke and transient ischaemic attack 2008. *Cerebrovascular Diseases, 25,* 457–507.

Fakhari, Z., Ansari, N. N., Naghidi, S., Mansouri, K., & Radinmehr, H. (2017). A single group, pretest-posttest clinical trial for the effects of dry needling on wrist flexors spasticity after stroke. *NeuroRehabilitation, 40,* 325–336.

Favate, A. S., & Younger, D. S. (2016). Epidemiology of ischemic stroke. *Neurologic Clinics, 34,* 967–980.

Feigin, V. L., Norrving, B., & Mensah, G. A. (2017). Global Burden of Stroke. *Circulation Research, 120,* 439–448.

Fil, A., Cano-de-la-Cuerd, R., Muñoz-Hellín, E., Vela, L., Ramiro-González, M., & Fernández-de-las-Peñas, C. (2013). Pain in Parkinson disease: a review of the literature. *Parkinsonism & Related Disorders, 19,* 285–294.

Fink, M., Rollnik, J. D., Bijak, M., Borstädt, C., Däuper, J., Guergueltcheva, V., et al. (2004). Needle acupuncture in chronic poststroke leg spasticity. *Archives of Physical Medicine and Rehabilitation, 85,* 667–672.

Foley, P. L., Vesterinen, H. M., Laird, B. J., Sena, E. S., Colvin, L. A., Chandran, S., et al. (2013a). Prevalence and natural history of pain in adults with multiple sclerosis: systematic review and meta-analysis. *Pain, 154,* 632–642.

Foley, N., Pereira, S., Salter, K., Fernandez, M. M., Speechley, M., Sequeira, K., et al. (2013b). Treatment with botulinum toxin improves upper-extremity function post stroke: a systematic review and meta-analysis. *Archives of Physical Medicine and Rehabilitation, 94,* 977–989.

Foran, J. R., Steinman, S., Barash, I., Chambers, H. G., & Lieber, R. L. (2005). Structural and mechanical alterations in spastic skeletal muscle. *Developmental Medicine and Child Neurology, 47,* 713–717.

Fridén, J., & Lieber, R. L. (2003). Spastic muscle cells are shorter and stiffer than normal cells. *Muscle & Nerve, 27,* 157–164.

Gallego, P. H., & del Moral, O. M. (2007). A case study looking at the effectiveness of deep dry needling for the management of hypertonia. *Journal of Musculoskeletal Pain, 15,* 55–60.

Gaskin, J., Gomes, J., Darshan, S., & Krewski, D. (2017). Burden of neurological conditions in Canada. *Neurotoxicology, 61,* 2–10.

Ge, H. Y., Arendt-Nielsen, L., & Madeleine, P. (2012). Accelerated muscle fatigability of latent myofascial trigger points in humans. *Pain Medicine, 13,* 957–964.

Ge, H. Y., Monterde, S., Graven-Nielsen, T., & Arendt-Nielsen, L. (2014). Latent myofascial trigger points are associated with an increased intramuscular electromyographic activity during synergistic muscle activation. *The Journal of Pain, 15,* 181–187.

Gerwin, R. (2012). Botulinum toxin treatment of myofascial pain: a critical review of the literature. *Current Pain and Headache Reports, 16,* 413–422.

Ghasemi, M., Salari, M., Khorvash, F., & Shaygannejad, V. (2013). A literature review on the efficacy and safety of botulinum toxin: an injection in post-stroke spasticity. *International Journal of Preventive Medicine, 4,* S147–158.

Gooch, C. L., Pracht, E., & Borenstein, A. R. (2017). The burden of neurological disease in the United States: A summary report and call to action. *Annals of Neurology, 81,* 479–484.

Gracies, J. M. (2005). Pathophysiology of spastic paresis. I: Paresis and soft tissue changes. *Muscle & Nerve, 31,* 535–551.

Harrison, R. A., & Field, T. S. (2015). Post stroke pain: identification, assessment, and therapy. *Cerebrovascular Diseases, 39,* 190–201.

Holtz, K. A., Lipson, R., Noonan, V. K., Kwon, B. K., & Mills, P. B. (2017). Prevalence and effect of problematic spasticity following traumatic spinal cord injury. *Archives of Physical Medicine and Rehabilitation, 98,* 1132–1138.

Hong, C. Z. (1994). Lidocaine injection versus dry needling to myofascial trigger point: The importance of the local twitch response. *American Journal of Physical Medicine & Rehabilitation, 73,* 256–263.

Howard, J., Trevick, S., & Younger, D. S. (2016). Epidemiology of multiple sclerosis. *Neurologic Clinics, 34,* 919–939.

Hsieh, Y. L., Chou, L. W., Joe, Y. S., & Hong, C. Z. (2011). Spinal cord mechanism involving the remote effects of dry needling on the irritability of myofascial trigger spots in rabbit skeletal muscle. *Archives of Physical Medicine and Rehabilitation, 92,* 1098–1105.

Ibarra, J., Ge, H. Y., Wang, C., Martínez-Vizcaíno, V., Graven-Nielsen, T., & Arendt-Nielsen, L. (2011). Latent myofascial trigger points are associated with an increased antagonistic muscle activity during agonist muscle contraction. *The Journal of Pain, 12,* 1282–1288.

Intiso, D., Basciani, M., Santamato, A., Intiso, M., & Di Rienzo, F. (2015). Botulinum Toxin Type A for the treatment of neuropathic pain in neuro-rehabilitation. *Toxins, 7,* 2454–2480.

Kinnear, B. Z., Lannin, N. A., Cusick, A., Harvey, L. A., & Rawicki, B. (2014). Rehabilitation therapies after botulinum toxin-A injection to manage limb spasticity: a systematic review. *Physical Therapy, 94,* 1569–1581.

Lance, J. W. (1990). What is spasticity? *Lancet, 335,* 606.

Lee, I. S., Shin, Y. B., Moon, T. Y., Jeong, Y. J., Song, J. W., & Kim, D. H. (2009). Sonography of patients with hemiplegic shoulder pain after stroke: correlation with motor recovery stage. *American Journal of Roentgenology, 192,* 40–44.

Lee, J. A., Park, S. W., Hwang, P. W., Lim, S. M., Kook, S., Choi, K. I., et al. (2012). Acupuncture for shoulder pain after stroke: a systematic review. *Journal of Alternative and Complementary Medicine, 18,* 818–823.

Lieber, R. L., Steinman, S., Barash, I. A., & Chambers, H. (2004). Structural and functional changes in spastic skeletal muscle. *Muscle & Nerve, 29,* 615–627.

Lim, S. M., Yoo, J., Lee, E., Kim, H. J., Shin, S., Han, G., et al. (2015). Acupuncture for spasticity after stroke: a systematic review and meta-analysis of randomized controlled trials. *Evidence-based Complementary and Alternative Medicine,* 870398.

Lucas, K. R., Polus, B. I., & Rich, P. S. (2004). Latent myofascial trigger points: their effects on muscle activation and movement efficiency. *Journal of Bodywork and Movement Therapies, 8,* 160–166.

Lundstrom, E., Smits, A., Borg, J., & Terent, A. (2010). Fourfold increase in direct costs of stroke survivors with spasticity compared with stroke survivors without spasticity: the first year after the event. *Stroke, 41,* 319–324.

Maher, R. M., Hayes, D. M., & Shinohara, M. (2013). Quantification of dry needling and posture effects on myofascial trigger points using ultrasound shear-wave elastography. *Archives of Physical Medicine and Rehabilitation, 94,* 2146–2150.

Marciniak, C. M., Harvey, R. L., Gagnon, C. M., et al. (2012). Does botulinum toxin type A decrease pain and lessen disability in hemiplegic survivors of stroke with shoulder pain and spasticity? A randomized, double-blind, placebo-controlled trial. *American Journal of Physical Medicine & Rehabilitation, 91*, 1007–1019.

Mendigutia-Gómez, A., Martín-Hernández, C., Salom-Moreno, J., & Fernández-de-las-Peñas, C. (2016). Effect of dry needling on spasticity, shoulder range of motion, and pressure pain sensitivity in patients with stroke: A crossover Study. *Journal of Manipulative and Physiological Therapeutics, 39*, 348–358.

Milinis, K., & Young, C. A. (2015). Trajectories of outcome in neurological conditions (TONiC) study: Systematic review of the influence of spasticity on quality of life in adults with chronic neurological conditions. *Disability and Rehabilitation, 29*, 1–11.

Mukherjee, M., McPeak, L. K., Redford, J. B., Sun, C. M., & Liu, W. (2007). The effect of electro-acupuncture on spasticity of the wrist joint in chronic stroke survivors. *Archives of Physical Medicine and Rehabilitation, 88*, 159–166.

Nielsen, J. B., Crone, C., & Hultborn, H. (2007). The spinal pathophysiology of spasticity: from a basic science point of view. *Acta Physiologica, 189*, 171–180.

Olsson, M. C., Krüger, M., Meyer, L. H., Ahnlund, L., Gransberg, L., Linke, W. A., et al. (2006). Fibre type-specific increase in passive muscle tension in spinal cord-injured subjects with spasticity. *The Journal of Physiology, 577*, 339–352.

Oreja-Guevara, C., González-Segura, D., & Vila, C. (2013). Spasticity in multiple sclerosis: results of a patient survey. *The International Journal of Neuroscience, 123*, 400–408.

Paolucci, S., Martinuzzi, A., Scivoletto, G., et al. (2016a). Assessing and treating pain associated with stroke, multiple sclerosis, cerebral palsy, spinal cord injury and spasticity. Evidence and recommendations from the Italian Consensus Conference on Pain in Neurorehabilitation. *European Journal of Physical and Rehabilitation Medicine, 52*, 827–840.

Paolucci, S., Iosa, M., Toni, D., Barbanti, P., Bovi, P., Cavallini, A., et al. (2016b). Prevalence and time course of post-stroke pain: A multicenter prospective hospital-based study. *Pain Medicine, 17*, 924–930.

Paterson, K., Lolignier, S., Wood, J. N., McMahon, S. B., & Bennett, D. L. (2014). Botulinum toxin-A treatment reduces human mechanical pain sensitivity and mechano-transduction. *Annals of Neurology, 75*, 591–596.

Raggi, A., & Leonardi, M. (2015). Burden and cost of neurological diseases: a European North-South comparison. *Acta Neurologica Scandinavica, 132*, 16–20.

Roosink, M., Renzenbrink, G. J., Buitenweg, J. R., van Dongen, R. T., Geurts, A. C., & Ijzerman, M. J. (2011). Somatosensory symptoms and signs and conditioned pain modulation in chronic post-stroke shoulder pain. *The Journal of Pain, 12*, 476–485.

Roosink, M., Renzenbrink, G. J., Geurts, A. C., & Ijzerman, M. J. (2012). Towards a mechanism-based view on post-stroke shoulder pain: theoretical considerations and clinical implications. *NeuroRehabilitation, 30*(2), 153–165.

Salom-Moreno, J., Sánchez-Mila, Z., Ortega-Santiago, R., Palacios-Ceña, M., Truyol-Domínguez, S., & Fernández-de-las-Peñas, C. (2014). Changes in spasticity, widespread pressure pain sensitivity, and baropodometry after the application of dry needling in patients who have had a stroke: a randomized controlled trial. *Journal of Manipulative and Physiological Therapeutics, 37*, 569–579.

Sheean, G. (2002). The pathophysiology of spasticity. *European Journal of Neurology, 9*, S3–S9.

Siddall, P. J., McClelland, J. M., Rutkowski, S. B., & Cousins, M. J. (2003). A longitudinal study of the prevalence and characteristics of pain in the first 5 years following spinal cord injury. *Pain, 103*, 249–257.

Simons, D. G., Travell, J. G., & Simons, L. S. (1999). *Myofascial pain and dysfunction: the trigger point manual. Vol. 1.* Philadelphia: Lippincott William & Wilkins.

Sinkjaer, T., & Magnussen, I. (1994). Passive, intrinsic and reflex-mediated stiffness in the ankle extensors of hemiparetic patients. *Brain, 117*, 355–363.

Soares, A., Andriolo, R. B., Atallah, A. N., & da Silva, E. M. (2014). Botulinum toxin for myofascial pain syndromes in adults. *Cochrane Database of Systematic Reviews, 7*, CD007533.

Sommerfeld, D. K., Eek, E. U., Svensson, A. K., et al. (2004). Spasticity after stroke: its occurrence and association with motor impairments and activity limitations. *Stroke, 35*, 134–139.

Srbely, J. Z., Dickey, J. P., Lee, D., & Lowerison, M. (2010). Dry needle stimulation of myofascial trigger points evokes segmental anti-nociceptive effects. *Journal of Rehabilitation Medicine, 42*, 463–468.

Turo, D., Otto, P., Shah, J. P., Heimur, J., Gebreab, T., Zaazhoa, M., et al. (2013). Ultrasonic characterization of the upper trapezius muscle in patients with chronic neck pain. *Ultrasonic Imaging, 35*, 173–187.

Turo, D., Otto, P., Hossain, M., Gebreab, T., Armstrong, K., Rosenberger, W. F., et al. (2015). Novel use of ultrasound elastography to quantify muscle tissue changes after dry needling of myofascial trigger points in patients with chronic myofascial pain. *Journal of Ultrasound in Medicine, 34*, 2149–2161.

Uttam, M. (2015). To explore the literature on the effects of dry needling on muscle spasticity: a scoping review. *Research and Reviews: J Neuroscience, 5*, 40–42.

Wayne, P. M., Krebs, D. E., Macklin, E. A., Schnyer, R., Kaptchuk, T. J., Parker, S. W., et al. (2005). Acupuncture for upper-extremity rehabilitation in chronic stroke: a randomized sham-controlled study. *Archives of Physical Medicine and Rehabilitation, 86*, 2248–2255.

Wissel, J., Manack, A., & Brainin, M. (2013). Toward an epidemiology of post-stroke spasticity. *Neurology, 80*, S13–19.

World Health Organization (2006). *Neurological Disorders: Public Health Challenges.* Geneva, Switzerland: World Health Organization.

Wu, T., Fu, Y., Song, H. X., Ye, Y., Dong, Y., & Li, J. H. (2015). Effectiveness of botulinum toxin for shoulder pain treatment: A systematic review and meta-analysis *Archives of Physical Medicine and Rehabilitation, 96*, 2214–2220.

Wu, T., Li, J. H., Song, H. X., & Dong, Y. (2016). Effectiveness of Botulinum Toxin for lower limbs spasticity after stroke: A systematic review and meta-analysis. *Topics in Stroke Rehabilitation, 23,* 217–223.

Yablon, S., Brin, M., VanDenburgh, A., et al. (2011). Dose response with onabotulinumtoxin A for post-stroke spasticity: a pooled data analysis. *Movement Disorders, 26,* 209–215.

Yelnik, A. P., Colle, F. M., Bonan, I. V., & Vicaut, E. (2007). Treatment of shoulder pain in spastic hemiplegia by reducing spasticity of the subscapular muscle: a randomised, double blind, placebo controlled study of botulinum toxin A. *Journal of Neurology, Neurosurgery, and Psychiatry, 78,* 845–848.

Zeilig, G., Rivel, M., Weingarden, H., Gaidoukov, E., & Defrin, R. (2013). Hemiplegic shoulder pain: evidence of a neuropathic origin. *Pain, 154,* 263–271.

Zhang, J. H., Wang, D., & Liu, M. (2014). Overview of systematic reviews and meta-analyses of acupuncture for stroke. *Neuroepidemiology, 42,* 50–58.

Zhao, J. G., Cao, C. H., Liu, C. Z., Han, B. J., Zhang, J., Li, Z. G., et al. (2009). Effect of acupuncture treatment on spastic states of stroke patients. *Journal of the Neurological Sciences, 276,* 143–147.

Zhou, J. Y., & Wang, D. (2014). An update on botulinum toxin A injections of trigger points for myofascial pain. *Current Pain and Headache Reports, 18,* 386.

CHAPTER 5

Trigger Point Dry Needling: Safety Guidelines

JOHNSON McEVOY

SAFETY CONSIDERATIONS

Introduction

Dry needling (DN) is an invasive procedure that poses certain risks, in part, not generally associated with other physical therapy or chiropractic treatments. The focal point of this chapter is on safety issues associated with DN. DN can be divided into superficial dry needling (SDN) and trigger point dry needling (TrP-DN). Ultimately, the health and welfare of the patient should be the first consideration (World Health Association, 2006), but the welfare of healthcare workers (HCWs) and third parties should not be overlooked. Guidelines and checklists have been employed to improve the quality and safety of complex systems and practices in, for example, aviation, engineering, medicine, and surgery (Gawande, 2009). A practice guideline is a formal statement about a defined task or function in clinical practice (Barlow-Pugh, 2000). DN practice guidelines have been developed in Australia (ASAP, 2007), Canada (CPTA, 2007), and Ireland (McEvoy et al., 2012), among others. The main focus of this chapter is on patient safety, but HCWs and third party risks are also recognised.

DN is the use of a solid filament needle for the treatment of pain and dysfunction of various body tissues. DN is an invasive technique within the scope of practice of multiple disciplines such as physical therapy, chiropractic, medicine, dentistry, and acupuncture. There are a variety of conceptual models as outlined in other chapters of this book, including TrP-DN and SDN, which are commonly employed to treat pain and dysfunction associated with myofascial TrPs as described by Travell and Simons (Travell & Simons, 1983, 1992; Simons et al., 1999). Clinicians may employ one or a combination of conceptual models in clinical practice.

TrP-DN is practiced by physical therapists in many countries, including Australia, Canada, Ireland, the Netherlands, South Africa, Spain, Switzerland, the UK, and the US (Dommerholt et al., 2006). An increasing number of states in the US, the American Physical Therapy Association, and the American Academy of Orthopaedic Manual Physical Therapists have ruled DN to be under the scope of physical therapy practice (APTA, 2012). Other disciplines also employ TrP-DN such as chiropractors in the UK and in several US states, myotherapists in Australia, and dentists in various countries, among others. With the increase in DN among clinicians internationally, it is important to focus on safety, which must be considered the number one priority. In this chapter, DN is approached from a physical therapy perspective, but the safety precautions are of course applicable to all HCWs. Acronyms used throughout this chapter are listed in Box 5.1.

TRIGGER POINT DRY NEEDLING: SAFETY

TrP-DN poses potential risks to patients, HCWs, and third parties. Many of these risks are not associated with traditional noninvasive physical therapy treatments and may include bruising, pneumothorax, infection, internal tissue damage, and bleeding. The term *adverse event* (AE) is used to describe any ill effect of a treatment, no matter how small, that is unintended and nontherapeutic (White et al., 1997). The severity of AEs can be graded as mild (minor), significant, and serious (White et al., 2001, 2008). A mild AE is considered of short duration, reversible, and does not particularly inconvenience the patient; a significant AE requires medical attention or interferes with the patient's activities; a serious AE requires hospital admission with potential persistent or significant disability or death (White et al., 2008). Quantification and qualification grading of AEs has been proposed to objectify risk, and this is invaluable for patient education and informed consent. AEs can be categorised into very common, common, uncommon, rare, and very rare with corresponding quantification (Table 5.1) (Witt et al., 2009). This grading is helpful when reviewing AE studies.

TABLE 5.1 Qualification and Quantification of Adverse Events				
Very Common	**Common**	**Uncommon**	**Rare**	**Very Rare**
≥ 10%	≥ 1–10%	≥ 0.1% –1%	≥ 0.01% – 0.1%	< 0.01%
> 1–10	1–10/100	1–10/1000	1–10/10 000	< 1/10 000

Adapted from: Witt et al. (2009). Safety of acupuncture: results of a prospective observational study with 229,230 patients and introduction of a medical information and consent form. *Forsch Komplementmed*, 16, 91–97.

BOX 5.1
Glossary of Acronyms

AE: Adverse event
DN: Dry needling
HAI: Healthcare associated infection
HCWs: Healthcare workers
NMES: Neuromuscular electrical stimulation
NSI: Needlestick injury
PENS: Percutaneous electrical nerve stimulation
PNS: Postneedling soreness
SDN: Superficial dry needling
TENS: Transcutaneous electrical nerve stimulation
TRP: Myofascial trigger points
TRPDN: Trigger point dry needling
USCDC: United States Centers for Disease Control and Prevention
WHO: World Health Organization

(Adapted from McEvoy et al., 2012)

Safety of DN is of significant importance. Individual cases of significant injury have been reported, including cervical spine haematoma (Lee et al., 2011), pneumothorax (Cummings et al., 2014), hemiplegia (Ji et al., 2015), and infection (Callan et al., 2016; Steentjes et al., 2016). Despite this, significant TrP-DN AEs are rare. Nevertheless, there is a need for more high quality TrP-DN AE studies to quantify risk in different settings, among clinicians with different levels of experience, for example.

A prospective TrP-DN AE study among physiotherapists was carried out in Ireland (Brady et al., 2014). The study was adapted from a previous study on AE in acupuncture by healthcare clinicians (White et al., 2001). Thirty-nine physiotherapists who had undertaken 63 hours of TrP-DN training completed the study over a 10-month period, totaling 7629 treatments. No significant AEs were reported. Common minor AEs included bruising (7.55%), bleeding (4.65%), pain during treatment (3.01%), and pain after treatment (2.19%). Uncommon minor AEs included aggravation of symptoms (0.88%), drowsiness (0.26%), headache (0.14%), and nausea (0.13%). Reported rare minor AEs were fatigue (0.04%), altered emotions (0.04%), shaking, itching, claustrophobia, and numbness, all 0.01%. Minor AEs were common (19.18%). Although no significant AEs were recorded, utilising Hanley's rule of three (Hanley & Lippman-Hand, 1983), the upper risk rate for significant AEs was estimated at less than or equal to 0.04%. The authors concluded that the sample size may limit the results for more rare occurrences such as pneumothorax or infection. For pneumothorax and infection, larger scale acupuncture studies may assist in quantifying risk (see later in this chapter).

Although TrP-DN and acupuncture differ in terms of historical, philosophical, indicative, and practical contexts, similarities do exist in terms of solid filament needle skin penetration to varying depths within the body. In this context, acupuncture AE studies assist in identifying TrP-DN risks. Notwithstanding the differences between traditional acupuncture and TrP-DN, clinicians practicing TrP-DN should familiarise themselves with acupuncture AE studies to optimise safe practice and also for patient informed consent. Acupuncture is considered one of the safer forms of medical treatment (Vincent, 2001; White et al., 2008). Despite this safety statement, AEs do occur. Peuker and Gronemeyer (2001) grouped acupuncture AEs into five categories including delayed or missed diagnosis, deterioration of disorder under treatment, autonomic reactions, infections, and trauma to tissues or organs (Table 5.2).

A significant number of acupuncture safety and AE studies have been published. Three studies are of particular interest to TrP-DN as they were carried out on physiotherapists and medical doctors and may best reflect clinicians with Western medical training. A summary of the main AEs is presented in Table 5.3.

White and colleagues (2001) reported AEs related to acupuncture in a prospective clinician survey of 32,000 treatments of 78 British physiotherapists and medical doctors. Common minor AEs included bleeding and needling pain; uncommon minor AEs included aggravation of symptoms, faintness, drowsiness, a stuck or

TABLE 5.2 Acupuncture Adverse Events	
Adverse Event Category	**Example**
Delayed or missed diagnosis	Cancer
Deterioration of disorder under treatment	Increased pain
Vegetative reactions	Autonomic type reaction, nausea etc.
Bacterial and viral infections	Hepatitis B
Trauma of tissue and organs	Pneumothorax, nerve lesion

Categories adapted from: Peuker E, Gronemeyer D (2001). Rare but serious complication of acupuncture: traumatic lesions. *Acupunct Med*, 19, 103–108.

bent needle, and headache. Significant AEs were rare or very rare (n = 43) and included administrative problems (forgotten needle, forgotten patient), issues at the application site (cellulitis, needle allergy, needle site pain), cardiovascular problem (fainting), gastrointestinal problem (nausea, vomiting), neurological and psychiatric problem (anxiety, panic, euphoria, hyperesthesia, headache, slurred speech), or exacerbation of symptoms (back pain, fibromyalgia, shoulder pain, vomiting, migraine). No serious AE was reported in the 32,000 treatments surveyed. It was concluded that acupuncture in skilled hands is one of the safer forms of medical intervention (White et al., 2001).

Witt and associates (2009) reported AEs related to acupuncture in a prospective 229,230 patient based survey consisting of 2.2 million treatments delivered by German physician acupuncturists. AEs were reported per patient (n = 229,230) and not per treatment (n = 2.2 million); this should be taken into account when comparing with White et al. (2001), who reported AE per treatment (n = 32,000). A noteworthy 8.6% of patients reported at least one AE, in which 2.2% of patients required medical treatment (significant or serious AE). Common side effects included bleeding and haematoma (n = 14,083; 6.1%) and pain (n = 4681; 2%). Uncommon side effects included strong pain during needling (n = 490; 0.2%), autonomic symptoms (n = 1663; 0.7%), and nerve irritation and injury (n = 601; 0.26%). Rare and very rare side effects included local infection (n = 31; 0.014%), systemic infection (n = 5; 0.002%), and pneumothorax (n = 2; 0.001%). As this is arguably the most comprehensive AE acupuncture study, clinicians should familiarise themselves with this study and the expansive quantification of side effects.

Melchart and associates (2004) reported AE after acupuncture in a prospective clinician-based survey of 97,733 patients (760,000 treatments) delivered by German physician acupuncturists. Again, similar to the results of Witt et al. (2009), the incidence of AE was reported per patient and not per treatment. Nonserious AEs were seen in 7.10% of patients and included needling pain (3.28%), haematoma (3.19%), and bleeding (1.3%). Serious AE were reported in 6 of 97,733 patients, including exacerbation of depression, acute hypertensive crisis, vasovagal reaction, asthma attack with hypertension, angina, and pneumothorax in two cases.

Despite the generally good safety of acupuncture, a review of acupuncture systematic reviews from 2000

TABLE 5.3 Selected Qualification and Quantification Risks Associated with Acupuncture				
Very Common	**Common**	**Uncommon**	**Rare**	**Very Rare**
≥ 10%	≥ 1–10%	≥ 0.1%–1%	≥ 0.01%–0.1%	< 0.01%
> 1–10	1–10/100	1–10/1000	1–10/10 000	< 1/10 000
	Bleeding Hematoma Needling site pain	Inflammation Swelling Strong pain during treatment Nerve irritation Nerve injury Headache Fatigue Vertigo Nausea	Local infection Redness Itching Sweating Blood pressure changes Unconsciousness Tachycardia Breathing difficulties Vomiting	Pneumothorax Broken needle Forgotten needle Systemic infection Affected speech Disorientation

See these references for further information: White et al. (2001), Melchart et al. (2004), and Witt et al. (2009).

onwards identified 95 cases of severe AEs including five fatalities (Ernst et al., 2011). Peuker and Gronemeyer (2001) reported on rare but serious complications of acupuncture due to traumatic lesions in a review of the literature from 1965 onwards. According to the authors, all traumatic lesions described could be avoided if clinicians had better anatomical knowledge or applied existing knowledge.

HYGIENE

DN is an invasive procedure that poses infection risks to patients, clinicians, and third parties, which are not normally associated with manual treatments. In 2002 US healthcare-associated infections (HAI) amounted to 1.7 million recorded incidents with 98,987 deaths (Klevens et al., 2007). As many as 1 in 10 patients acquire a HAI (HSE, 2009). Infectious agents include bacteria (e.g., S*taphylococcus, E. coli*), viruses (e.g., hepatitis B and C, human immunodeficiency virus [HIV]), fungi (e.g., tinea pedis, *Candida albicans*), protozoa (e.g., toxoplasmosis), and prions (e.g., Creutzfeldt–Jakob disease). The *chain of infection* is a six-element way of describing infectious disease transmission (HSE, 2009) and consists of an infectious agent, a reservoir (infectious agent area), a portal of exit (from infected person), a means of transmission, a portal of entry (to target person), and a susceptible host.

Standard Precautions are clinical guidelines to prevent transmission of infectious agents and are published by the United States Centers for Disease Control and Prevention (USCDC) (Siegel et al., 2007; HSE, 2009). The purpose of Standard Precautions is to break the chain of infection by focusing particularly, but not exclusively, on the mode of transmission, portal of entry, and susceptible hosts (HSE, 2009). Standard precautions require HCWs to assume that every person is potentially infected or colonised with an organism that could be transmitted in the healthcare setting and apply a set of work practices to minimise the risk of contamination (HSE, 2009). Work practices relevant to DN include attention to hand hygiene, glove usage, skin preparation, management of needles and medical waste, and needle-stick injuries (NSI) (Dommerholt, 2011).

Hand Hygiene

Hand hygiene is considered the single most important intervention to prevent transmission of infection (SARI, 2005). Hand hygiene activity recommendations have been evidenced-categorised.

- Category I: supported by experimental, clinical, or epidemiological studies based on strong theoretical basis

- Category II: supported by suggestive clinical or epidemiological studies or a theoretical-based rationale
- Category III: recommended by healthcare experts from experience

For hand hygiene preparation, nails should be kept short and cut smoothly (II) with the avoidance of false nails or extenders (I) and nail polish (III). All wrist and hand jewelry except plain wedding bands should be removed (II), and sleeves should be short or turned up (III).

Hand decontamination should be carried out with suitable soap and water or, if hands are visibly clean of contaminant, with appropriate alcohol-based hand rub or gel. Hand decontamination is recommended for these situations.

1. When the hands are visibly soiled with dirt, soil, or organic material (I), they should be washed thoroughly to remove the contaminant.
2. Before and after each patient contact (II).
3. At the beginning and end of each work shift (III).
4. After removing gloves (I).
5. After moving from a contaminated area (II).
6. After handling soiled equipment, materials, or environment (II).
7. After personal bodily functions (e.g., blowing nose, after using the toilet) (I).
8. Before handling food (I).

Hand hygiene and decontamination is a learned skill and should be a quality standard in all healthcare institutions (SARI, 2005). It may appear rudimentary, but attention to hand decontamination technique is important and often practiced poorly by HCWs. Handwashing with regular soap can remove dirt but is generally ineffective in preventing antimicrobial activity, whereas alcohol-based hand rub is generally effective (Ehrenkranz & Alfonso, 1991). Antimicrobial soap is somewhat more efficient than nonantimicrobial soap and produces a statistically significant reduction in microbial activity compared with nonantimicrobial soap (Montville & Schaffner, 2011). However, the use of alcohol in either soap or gel is more effective than antimicrobial or bland soap without alcohol (Paulson et al., 1999).

Handwashing with soap

1. Wet hands with water.
2. Apply an amount of suitable soap to the hands as recommended by the product manufacturer.
3. Rub hands vigorously for at least 15 seconds encompassing all surfaces of the hands and fingers.
4. Rinse hands with water.

5. Dry hands with a good quality, single use, disposable paper towel.
6. Use towel to turn off faucet and dispose of it in pedal bin.
7. Avoid using hot water as this may increase skin dryness and dermatitis (Boyce & Pittet, 2002; SARI, 2005; HSE, 2009).

Multiple-use cloth towel, either roll type or hanging style are not appropriate for the healthcare setting (Boyce & Pittet, 2002).

Hand decontamination with alcohol-based hand rub

Hands can be decontaminated with suitable alcohol-based hand rub or gel once the hands are visibly clean. Alcohol-based hand rub can be inactivated by organic material and therefore if hands are visibly soiled, they should be washed per the previous recommendations. Alcohol-based hand sanitiser is usually recommended at a 70% concentration by weight of isopropanol, ethanol, or n-propanol. Higher concentrations may increase the risk of skin dryness and dermatitis. The US Centers for Disease Control and Prevention recommend hand-washing with soap after every 5 to 10 applications of alcohol-based hand gel due to build-up of emollients on the hands (Boyce & Pittet, 2002). Manufacturer's instructions of such products should be noted.

1. Apply product to palm of one hand and rub hands together.
2. Cover all surfaces of hands and fingers.
3. Rub for at least 15 seconds and until hands are dry.

As HCWs wash and decontaminate their hands up to 30 times per shift (Boyce & Pittet, 2002), there is a significant risk of skin irritation and dermatitis. Irritant dermatitis is a nonimmunological inflammatory skin response to an external agent and may leave the skin more prone to harbor microorganisms (SARI, 2005). Prevention and management of all forms of dermatitis is important for the safety of patients and HCWs. The USCDC recommends the addition of 1% to 3% glycerol to alcohol-based hand gel as this can reduce or eliminate the drying effect of the alcohol (Boyce & Pittet, 2002). Advice for the prevention of occupational dermatitis in the healthcare setting includes (SARI, 2005):

1. Follow manufacturer's recommendations on use of hand hygiene product.
2. Use products with low irritation potential and when able with emollient.
3. Receive feedback from HCWs on products used.
4. Use alcohol-based hand rubs with emollients.
5. Promote the use of suitable hands lotions to assist in skin hydration and replace skin lipids.

Gloves

Gloves are the main protective equipment employed during DN. Gloves should be worn without exception at least on the palpating hand or, if so preferred or legally required, on both hands. Guidelines vary in different countries and jurisdictions. There are potential arguments against the use of gloves that may include the effect on kinesthetic feedback, awkwardness, time consuming, or lack of evidence for reducing NSI. These objections are muted, however, by the requirements of Standard Precautions that require gloves to be worn for all activities when it can be reasonably anticipated to have hand contact with blood, bodily fluids, or other potentially infectious materials, mucous membranes, and nonintact skin (HSE, 2009). According to regulations (Standards 29 CFR) published by the United States Occupational Safety and Health Administration (OSHA, 2011):

> 'Gloves shall be worn when it can be reasonably anticipated that the employee may have hand contact with blood, other potentially infectious materials, mucous membranes, and non-intact skin....'

Due to the fact that clinicians need to compress the needle site after removal of the needle and that bleeding is the most common side effect of DN, the use of gloves is consistent with OSHA regulations. Nevertheless, some physician and acupuncture organisations, including the American Academy of Medical Acupuncture, do not recommend using gloves with needling procedures.

Gloves should be single use, disposable, and conform to international community standards. Latex-free gloves should be available for clinicians and used with patients with known latex allergies. Latex-free surgical gloves are being used more frequently due to latex hypersensitivity in HCWs and patients; however, some may not offer the same protection as latex gloves (Boyce & Pittet, 2002; Aldlyami et al., 2010). The Food and Drug Administration has approved several powdered and powdered-free latex gloves with reduced protein contents and synthetic gloves for latex-sensitive HCWs (Boyce & Pittet, 2002). Nitrile gloves are usually preferable, especially for individuals with latex allergy concerns. Gloves should be donned immediately before and removed immediately after the DN procedure is completed and, if contaminated with blood or body fluids, should be disposed of in appropriate healthcare waste. Wearing gloves provides an ideal environment for bacterial growth, and hands should be washed after removal of gloves.

Patient Skin Preparation

Patient skin disinfection is not usually required before DN if the skin is visibly clean, which is in line with the World Health Organization's (WHO) best practice for intradermal, subcutaneous, and intramuscular needle injections (Hoffman, 2001; Hutin et al., 2003; Baldry, 2005; BAC, 2006; ASAP, 2007; White et al., 2008). Resident skin bacteria are unlikely to lead to infection if host immunity is not compromised (Hoffman, 2001). Many countries do not have formal regulations regarding skin disinfection for needling procedures, but it is required in some jurisdictions (Dommerholt, 2011). The National Acupuncture Foundation recommends disinfecting the skin with 70% isopropyl alcohol before needling (Given, 2009). The British Acupuncture Council Code of Safe Practice recommends using 70% isopropyl alcohol or products that contain 0.5% chlorhexidine before needling in 'areas of the body where moisture or exudates may collect, such as the groin and genital area, ears, feet, under arms and the area below the breasts, near the mouth, nose, scalp and other hair covered areas'. In contrast, Dutch guidelines (WIP, 2008; Dommerholt, 2011) in line with WHO do not recommend disinfecting the skin, except when using semipermanent needling or performing ear acupuncture. If the skin is visibly soiled it should be washed with warm water and soap and dried accordingly before DN. Clinicians should not needle into joints or bursae. During DN the clinicians should only touch the needle at the handle and should avoid touching the needle shaft. If this occurs the needle should be removed, disposed of, and replaced with a fresh sterile needle. Multipack needles are not recommended for DN as their use increases the likelihood of touching the needle shaft.

Immunocompromised patients may not be suitable for DN and special consideration is required. If DN is considered suitable, skin preparation with a sterilising solution such as 2% iodine in 70% alcohol should be used and left on the skin to dry for a minimum time of 2 minutes (ASAP, 2007).

Needle and Medical Waste Disposal

Needle and medical waste disposal should be done in accordance with local jurisdictional policies and procedures. Clinicians should be knowledgeable with local laws and regulations as standards differ internationally. In the US, regulated medical waste is material derived from animal or human sources or from biomedical research as described by UN-3291 (USDA, 2009). All sharps and blood or bodily fluid soiled waste from DN needs to be disposed of in suitable waste disposal per local jurisdictional policies. Used needles are disposed of in a regulated 'sharps container' meeting regulatory standards such as UN-3291. Medical waste such as soiled gloves or blood swabs (but no sharps objects) is placed in a suitable clinical waste bag. Both sharps containers and clinical waste bags should be disposed in accordance with local laws and procedures, which may entail the use of a licensed medical waste company.

Workstations should be designed to ensure sharps containers and medical waste bags are within easy reach. Follow the instructions in relation to sharps containers and do not fill above the permitted 'fill line' as this may pose a risk of NSI. Ensure such items are kept out of reach of children.

Needlestick Injury

NSI is a common occupational injury among HCWs. In the UK 37% of nurses reported a prevalence of NSI (Yang & Mullan, 2011). In Ireland medical interns reported a 26% incidence of NSI in the first 8 months of work with only 26% commonly using gloves in phlebotomy-like tasks (O'Sullivan et al., 2011). Medical students based in the US reported a 59% NSI rate during their training (Sharma et al., 2009). It has been estimated that over 20 bloodborne pathogens can be transmitted from contaminated needles, including hepatitis B (HBV), hepatitis C (HCV), and human immunodeficiency virus (HIV) (Yang & Mullan, 2011), and therefore NSI creates a serious risk for HCWs. Surprisingly, NSIs commonly go unreported. In one study, only 17.5% of incidences were reported (Hettiaratchy et al., 1998). The associated risk of infection transmission of HIV after a hollow needle NSI is about 0.3%, compared with 3% for HCV and 30% for HBV (Parsons, 2000). Exposure risk increases with a larger quantity of blood, for example, when the needle is visibly contaminated with the patient's blood (Rodts & Benson, 1992). Furthermore, hepatitis B virus can survive for 1 week in dried blood, which underpins the importance of good hygiene techniques and needle and waste disposal (Bond et al., 1981). Other factors that increase NSI infection transmission include piercing deeply or directly into an artery or vein with the contaminated needle (CDC, 1995). The risk of NSI infection with a solid filament needle would be expected to be less than a hollow needle; however, NSI risk should be taken seriously. If a NSI occurs, the USCDC recommends immediately washing the punctured area with soap and water, reporting the incident to the appropriate line manager, and seeking medical assessment as soon as possible (CDC, 2011). HCWs should have hepatitis A and B vaccinations as required.

To prevent NSI related to DN practice, clinicians should account for all needles and ensure adequate disposal into the sharps container. Keep the sharps container within easy reach of the treatment area and do not overfill the box. Avoid rushing and interruptions, and do not needle when tired. Gloves should be worn—although they may not fully protect against an NSI, they may offer some level of protection, especially from contact with blood and bodily fluids.

The risk of NSI may extend to patients, patient family members, visitors, and other staff from a lost or forgotten needle. Clinicians should ensure that all needles are accounted for and safely discarded and that workstation design and access minimises risk to third parties.

CONTRAINDICATIONS AND PRECAUTIONS

It is important to recognise contraindications, relative contraindications, and special precautions for safe DN practice (WHO, 1999; Batavia, 2006; ASAP, 2007; White et al., 2008). Patients should be routinely screened for current or historical presence of contraindications or precautions. Special attention should be paid to medical diagnoses and comorbidities (e.g., a patient with low immune function and history of diabetes). Further, when a contraindication is present, it is important that the clinician is not persuaded to needle by an enthusiastic patient (White et al., 2008).

Absolute Contraindications

DN therapy is contraindicated and should be avoided in patients under these circumstances (ASAP, 2007; White et al., 2008).
1. In a patient with needle phobia.
2. Patient unwilling—fear, patient belief.
3. Unable to give consent—communication, cognitive, age-related factors.
4. Medical emergency or acute medical condition.
5. Over an area or limb with lymphedema as this may increase the risk of infection/cellulitis and the difficulty of fighting the infection if one should occur (Filshie, 2001; Goodman et al., 2003).
6. With severe neutropenia or thrombocytopenia—for example, in patients undergoing chemotherapy, in which case consultation with the treating oncologist is indicated.
7. Inappropriate for any other reason.

Relative Contraindications

When absolute contraindications have been ruled out, clinicians should consider the relative contraindications and precautions for patient selection. This should be done in relation to the patient's characteristics and medical history, clinical reasoning, likely benefits of treatment, and whether the goals can be met with non-invasive treatments. It is the clinician's responsibility to discuss the relative risks and benefits of DN therapy with patients (White et al., 2008).

Abnormal bleeding tendency

Bleeding and bruising are among the most common side effects of needling therapies. Therefore caution should be noted with patients with thrombocytopenia for any reason (e.g., haemophilia, blood thinning medication, chemotherapy, etc.). These patients may not be suitable for DN other than by experienced clinicians, or light needling technique may be advisable initially as a trial. As mentioned previously, severe thrombocytopenia is an absolute contraindication. It is essential to apply pressure hemostasis after needling.

Compromised immune system

Patients with a compromised immune system for any reason may be more susceptible to infection and therefore be at a greater risk of local or systemic infection from DN (ASAP, 2007; White et al., 2008). Patients who may be vulnerable to infection include:
1. Disease related immunocompromised patients (e.g., bloodborne diseases, cancer, HIV, hepatitis, endocarditis, incompetent heart valve, or valve replacements, etc.).
2. Immunocompromised patients from immunosuppression therapy (e.g., drug cancer therapy). Consultation with the treating oncologist is critical as below certain laboratory values, neutropenia is an absolute contraindication.
3. Acute immune disorders (e.g., acute states of rheumatoid arthritis, current infection—local or systemic, etc.).
4. Debilitated patients and those with chronic illness, among others.

Vascular disease

Patients with vascular disease may be more susceptible to haematoma, bleeding, tissue trauma, infection, among other conditions.

Diabetes

Patients with diabetes may have compromised tissue healing capabilities, sensory deficits, and poor peripheral circulation. Patients with diabetes may be more susceptible to cellulitis (Goodman et al., 2003). The presence of diabetes may influence the decision to needle or which needling techniques to use (e.g., SDN versus TrP-DN) and may determine the intensity of the treatment.

Pregnancy

The use of DN therapy during pregnancy needs to be discussed thoroughly with the patient and should be used with caution especially in the first trimester (ASAP, 2007). Clinicians should be aware that 20% to 25% of pregnancies may naturally terminate in the first trimester (ASAP, 2007) and therefore erroneous connections between such occurrences and DN are possible. There is conflicting opinion of the ability of acupuncture to induce labour or spontaneous abortion (WHO, 1999; ASAP, 2007; White et al., 2008). In a controlled trial of women with pregnancy-related nausea (n = 593), acupuncture in early pregnancy did not alter the pregnancy outcomes or health of the child (Smith et al., 2002). Carr provided an excellent summary of 15 clinical studies and concluded that there is a well-supported lack of evidence of harm (Carr, 2015). The rates of miscarriage, preterm birth and labour, and other possible complications of pregnancy were comparable with untreated controls or consistent with their anticipated incidence (Carr, 2015). The European Guidelines for the Diagnosis and Treatment of Pelvic Girdle Pain consider the use of acupuncture for low back and pelvic pain during pregnancy (Vleeming et al., 2008).

1. Contraindications, precaution, risks, and benefits of treatment are considered in the usual manner.
2. Education and informed consent are of significant importance.
3. It is wise to avoid strong treatment that may threaten the patient.

Children

In addition to gaining informed consent from persons under 18 years old, parental or guardian consent must be sought when treating children under the age of 18. Follow local laws in regard to consent issues. Ensure that younger patients do not have a needle phobia and are cooperative to the procedure. It would be judicious to avoid deep DN with children under the age of 13 to 15, dependent on the maturity of the child, due to the ability to understand and follow the procedure.

Frail patients

Infirm or frail patients may not tolerate DN therapy well. This includes anorexic and bulimic patients (Steinberg, 2014).

Patients with epilepsy

In patients with epilepsy, caution should be taken due to tolerance of strong sensory stimulation. Patients with epilepsy should not be left unattended when needles are in situ.

Psychological status

Some patients with psychological disorders or distress may not be optimal candidates for DN. Anxiety and emotional distress may affect the ability to safely apply DN and for patients to rationally understand, tolerate treatment, or follow treatment instructions. High stress may reduce the likelihood of response to treatment (Huang et al., 2011) and may increase risk of adverse psychological or physical response to DN.

Patient allergies

Patients allergic to metals may react to metals used in monofilament needles, particularly to nickel and chromium (Romaguera & Grimalt, 1979; Fisher, 1986; Castelain et al., 1987). A typical monofilament needle contains approximately 8% to 10% nickel and 11% chromium. Relevant risks should be discussed with the patient before treatment. Allergic reactions to needles are very rare. DN treatments can still be administered by using silver- or gold-plated needles. DN should be discontinued if allergic reactions still occur. Allergies to latex, as found in latex gloves, are possible, and alternative gloves should be used for these patients. Latex allergies can be severe. Nitrile gloves are generally better tolerated, but some patients and HCWs may still have allergic reactions.

Patient medication

Clinicians should be aware of a patient's medical and medication history. Medications may alert the clinician to relative contraindications and may include immune suppressive drugs, psychotropic or mood altering medication, and blood thinning agents, among others.

Unsuitable patient for any reason

The clinician is privy to the overall patient characteristics and should identify other potential contraindications or safety precautions that may affect the suitability of DN. Patient characteristics may change and clinicians need to remain cognisant of this. If there is a specific reason to suggest a patient is unsuitable for DN therapy, then DN should be avoided and reconsidered as appropriate.

ANATOMICAL CONSIDERATIONS

Dry needling poses potential risks to anatomical structures including organs, such as the lungs, nerves, and blood vessels. Clinicians require excellent academic and practical knowledge of anatomy. All serious needling related traumatic complications, described by Peuker and Gronemeyer (2001), could have been avoided if clinicians had better anatomical knowledge or had applied existing anatomical knowledge better. It is imperative that practical anatomy skills are applied as part of routine DN practice. Clinicians should ensure they limit DN to anatomical regions they are familiar with and have been trained in. Furthermore, it may be wise to limit treatment to one side of the thorax only to prevent the unlikely but serious effect of bilateral pneumothorax. Anatomical considerations include:

Pleura and lung

Pneumothorax is a rare but serious complication of DN and has been reported in the acupuncture literature (Peuker & Gronemeyer, 2001; Melchart et al., 2004; Peuker, 2004; Witt et al., 2009) and DN (Cummings et al., 2014). The risk of pneumothorax is very small if proper consideration of practical anatomy and application of needling techniques are employed. Consideration of pleural and lung anatomy is essential and clinicians should remain aware of anatomical landmarks (Standring & Gray, 2008).

DN should be performed in such a manner to avoid needling towards the lung or intercostal space. When able, a pincher grip should be used such as with needling TrPs in the upper and lower trapezius, pectoral muscles, levator scapulae, and latissimus dorsi muscles. A second consideration is to needle towards bone such as the rib or scapula to avoid needling into the pleural space. With this technique it is vitally important to ensure the hand placement over the bone to avoid inadvertently entering the pleura. Clinicians should remain aware of anatomical anomalies. When a pincher grip and needling over bony structures is not feasible, a third option is to block the intercostal space with the fingers of the palpating hand, for example, when needling TrPs in the serratus anterior or rhomboid muscles.

The risk of pneumothorax is very rare when needling is practiced by well-trained clinicians skillfully applying practical anatomy.

Blood vessels

Anatomical knowledge of the vascular system is important as there is a potential to puncture blood vessels during needling. Application of practical anatomical knowledge is important. Clinicians should inspect for location of superficial veins and avoid needling these. Palpating for a pulse, where accessible, may be helpful to locate an artery. Haemostasis is important after withdrawing the needle. Special attention and caution should be paid to those with thrombocytopenia (see previous section).

Nerves

Anatomical knowledge of the nervous system is important as there is a potential for injury to nerves. Needling should be performed slowly and carefully and, when not sure, should be avoided in the vicinity of nerves. If a sharp electrical-type pain is felt distally from the needling site, the needle may have encountered a nerve. Special attention needs to be given in relation to the spinal cord (Yazawa et al., 1998; Lee et al., 2011) and the posterior suboccipital area due to potential brainstem access through the foramen magnum (Nelson & Hoffman, 1998). Several case studies described acute cervical and thoracic epidural haematomae as a complication of DN (Chen et al., 2006; Lee et al., 2011).

Organs

Anatomical knowledge of internal organs is important. There is potential for internal organ penetration such as the kidney with needling of TrPs in the psoas major and quadratus lumborum muscles or organs within the peritoneal cavity with needling of TrPs in the abdominal muscles or pelvic floor muscles such as the coccygeus and iliococcygeus muscles.

Joints

Anatomical knowledge of joint anatomy, including capsule and bursa, is important to avoid needling into joints through the joint capsule or bursae. Although needling the capsule or bursae would not necessarily be problematic, it is not the objective of dry needling.

Prosthetic implants

Some physicians feel that needling should be avoided into or close to joint or limb prosthetics, including internal and external fixation devices to avoid any kind of infection (Steentjes, 2016; Callan et al., 2016); however, there is no evidence that needling would increase the risk of infection. As a side note, both case reports by Steentjes (2015) and Callan and associates (2016) erroneously blamed a physical therapist for causing a postsurgical infection, even though the infection was with a high degree of medical probability a delayed surgical site complication (Lewkonia et al., 2016). By definition, surgical site infections are infections occurring within 30 days of surgery or 90 days if a prosthesis is involved (Mockford & O'Grady, 2017); delayed infections are a rare, but very serious complication (Lewkonia et al., 2016).

Implanted devices

Clinicians should avoid needling in the vicinity of implanted devices, including catheters, drug delivery systems, cosmetic breast, buttocks, calves, and other implants, electrical devices and wires associated with such devices as spinal cord stimulators, pacemakers, and defibrillators.

Other

Clinicians should avoid needling into pathological sites such as areas with acute inflammation or infected sites, varicose veins, cysts, tumours, and skin lesions, among others.

PROCEDURAL SAFETY ISSUES

As DN is an invasive procedure, it raises the potential for procedural adverse events. Recognising the potential for these adverse events is important. Patient education and communication are central to good needling practice. Patient education is carried out before, during, and after DN. Although obvious, it is worth stressing that patients should not carry out DN on themselves.

Painful treatment

Postneedling soreness (PNS) from DN is common for 1 to 2 days after treatment. On occasion this may prolong to 3 to 4 days. This is common with TrPDN and unlikely with SDN. PNS is usually felt in the vicinity of the needled site and may at times be felt in the referral zone of the muscle. It may feel similar to delayed onset of muscle soreness after exercise. Patients should be educated on PNS and be prepared to avoid unnecessary distress and worry. DN should be carried out to the patient's tolerance and ability by monitoring the response by verbal and nonverbal communication. Do not encourage patients to tolerate pain during DN. Also, consider limiting the number of muscles treated initially to test the patient's response. Timing of treatment should suit patient's lifestyle, work, and social commitments. As an example, consider the issues surrounding the application of DN to a 'needle-naïve' athlete before a sporting event or a musician before a recital.

On the initial insertion of the needle under the skin, if the patient experiences sharp continuing pain the needle should be withdrawn and inserted again slightly away from the original site. It is likely that the needle is in close vicinity of a free nerve ending and provides an Aδ sensory nerve stimulus. If the patient feels a sharp, burning electrical or lancing pain, penetration of a nerve or blood vessel may have occurred. The needle should be withdrawn immediately and haemostasis by manual pressure should be applied for at least 10 seconds. This may attenuate muscle bleeding and therefore PNS. Consider the use of thermal modalities,

active pain free range of motion, stretching, muscle reeducation, and posture training after treatment as DN is usually part of a multimodal plan of care.

Bruising and bleeding

Bruising is a common side effect of DN, which patients should be made aware of. Care should be taken to avoid penetrating blood vessels. Haemostasis by manual pressure is important after DN, and this may assist in reducing bruising and PNS. If bleeding occurs on the skin site, pressure with a cotton swab until stopped and discard the swab in medical waste disposal as appropriate. An ice application can be used over the site.

Fainting and autonomic responses

Fainting during or after DN treatment is possible and may occur for a variety of reasons such as pain, psychological stress, needle averse or phobic patients, or autonomic lability. Therefore it is important to treat the patient in a recumbent position. In patients with needle aversion, DN is contraindicated, unless the patient can be educated and coached into tolerating needling. If DN is experienced as a threatening stimulus, it is no longer therapeutic. SDN may be the initial choice of treatment. Avoid aggressive DN technique and maintain verbal and nonverbal communication with the patient to assess response. Watch for autonomic signs including clamminess, sweating, dizziness, increased tension, and light-headedness, among others. If these symptoms occur or the patient faints, remove the needle(s) and consider raising the patient's legs. Offer reassurance. Symptoms should abate after resting. If symptoms were to persist or if there is any concern about the patient, driving a car should be delayed, and the patient may require medical assessment. Such responses will influence the decision to carry out DN in the future.

Needle issues

Needles should be of good quality and used before the printed expiration date. Needles may bend, break, or be forgotten about. These adverse procedural issues can easily be avoided. Needles should be of suitable thickness and length to suit the patient and area being treated.

Bending of the needle may occur from contacting harder tissue such as bone, fascia, or a stiffened TrP zone or from a nonoptimal needling technique by curving the needle. Patients should be needled in a relaxed and optimal position. Avoid curving the needle during dynamic DN techniques. If a needle bends, it should be removed, discarded, and replaced with a new needle.

Needle breakage is rare, but may occur with poor quality needles or from repeated bending due to poor needling technique. In the past, when needles were sterilised repeatedly with autoclaving, needle breakage may have been more common due to metal fatigue. Therefore DN should be performed only with good quality single use sterile needles. It is recommended to avoid inserting the needle to the handle so that in the event of a breakage at the hub, the needle can be removed by tweezers. In the unlikely event of needle breakage, inform the patient to stay still and remove the needle with fingers or tweezers if accessible. If not visible, press the surrounding tissues gently to see if the needle exposes through the tissue, and if so, then remove with tweezers. If not, mark around the site of insertion with a marker or pen to locate the needle site and seek medical attention as the needle may require surgical removal.

Clinicians should account for all needles used. A forgotten needle could cause tissue damage, such as a pneumothorax. This is more likely with static needling techniques and especially if treating several body areas simultaneously. It is advisable not to rush to avoid time pressure mistakes. Consider using a 'count them in, count them out' policy aloud, which is useful to the clinician and reassuring to the patient. Tally needle packets with needles withdrawn.

There is differing opinion on whether a needle may be used more than once on the same patient in a treatment session (Dommerholt, 2011). The US National Acupuncture Foundation recommends never reusing a needle on the same patient in the same treatment session to avoid autogenous infection (Given, 2009). In contrast, the British Acupuncture Council Code of Safe Practice advises to 'use a fresh needle for every point needled during a treatment, or if reusing the same needle, only do so where all of the sites to be needled have been swabbed before needling and where the needle (and guide tube, if used) is not placed on any other surface in between separate insertions' (BAC, 2006). In this regard, clinicians should be guided by local jurisdictional rules and regulations.

Forgotten patient

If using a static needling technique and leaving the patient alone in a treatment room or cubicle, it is important not to forget the patient. Patients with needles in situ are unable to move and therefore are vulnerable. Be sure that the patient has the ability to alert the clinician verbally or with the use of a call bell. Clinicians should delineate procedures to avoid this stressful and embarrassing situation.

Infection

DN involves a marginal risk of infection. There are no valid studies or case reports of infections as a result of

DN. Every time a needle is entered through the skin, the body will respond with an inflammatory reaction; however, in patients with a functional immune response, this should not lead to any noticeable signs of inflammation. Nevertheless, clinicians should follow hygiene guidelines as outlined previously and appropriately select the patient. Before DN, the area and skin should be inspected for any signs of infection before initial and follow-up treatments. Infection signs may include pain, swelling, redness, heat, and tenderness and may be associated with fever and malaise. DN should be avoided with any suggestion of local or systemic infection and medical assessment sought immediately.

Pneumothorax

When needling in the vicinity of the thorax and lung fields, it is important to be aware of the rare but potential risk of pneumothorax. This has been discussed in the previous section under anatomical considerations. The symptoms of a pneumothorax may include shortness of breath, chest pain, coughing, and decreased breath sounds on auscultation or percussion. Pneumothorax symptoms may not occur for several hours after treatment. Should a pneumothorax be suspected, the patient should urgently be sent to the nearest emergency department.

Drowsiness and fatigue

A small percentage of patients may report feeling tired, fatigued, or sleepy after DN. Should this occur the patient should be advised not to drive or operate machinery until this feeling has subsided. In individual patients, if there is a history of DN-related drowsiness or fatigue, it may be best to avoid DN or, when appropriate, to time treatment around the patient's lifestyle. It would be important for the patient to be driven home.

GENERAL GUIDELINES FOR PRINCIPLES OF PRACTICE

This section presents general guidelines for principles of practice. There are many factors relating to safe needling practice. Individual jurisdictional rules and regulations may have specific requirements and these should be taken into account when drafting local DN guidelines. The following guidelines are therefore offered as a general outline. Ultimately the responsibility of patient care solely rests with the individual clinician. These general recommendations are advised (McEvoy et al., 2012).

1. Clinicians should ensure that DN falls under the scope of practice of their profession, for example, physical therapy, chiropractic, among others.

2. Clinicians should follow the rules of professional conduct of their professional organisation and be guided by practice guidelines and ethics.

3. Clinicians should confirm they are insured for the practice of DN and remain insured.

4. Clinicians should ensure that DN teaching programs meet the requirements for practicing within their jurisdiction.

5. Clinicians should confine themselves to DN practice in body areas they have been trained during appropriate postgraduate training.

6. Clinicians should stay up to date with research and trends in DN practice and meet the continuing professional development requirements for their jurisdiction.

7. Clinicians should ensure they have informed consent from patients before DN therapy. Again, clinicians should follow local professional policies and procedures related to informed consent.

8. Clinicians should implement local guidelines as applicable when practicing DN.

9. Clinicians should recognise they are responsible for patient welfare and maintain high safety standards at all times.

10. Clinicians should complete an appropriate clinical assessment before DN and ascertain whether DN is suitable for the individual patient and the condition to be treated. Contraindications and safety precautions should be noted and DN should be avoided as appropriate.

11. Clinicians should practice DN in a sensible and reasonable manner and apply professional judgement and adequate patient selection criteria (see appropriate section).

12. Clinicians should consider DN therapy as part of a comprehensive rehabilitation program and recognise the importance of correcting perpetuating factors. Multimodal and multidisciplinary care may be required to address the complexities of patient presentations. Furthermore, clinicians should remain aware of other treatment options that may be appropriate and discuss the treatment approach and options with the patient as part of the informed consent process.

13. Clinicians should consider DN in the light of evidence-informed practice, scientific research, clinical reasoning, and patient goals (Cicerone, 2005).

14. Clinicians should comply with best practice hygiene practices such as standard precautions (Siegel et al., 2007; HSE, 2009) and any other additional requirements of the local jurisdiction and employer or local workplace policy.

15. Clinicians should comply with waste disposal rules and requirements for needles and body fluid and blood contaminated waste for their local jurisdiction.

16. Clinicians should comply with occupational requirements set out in safety health and welfare at work acts and policies and procedures for their local jurisdiction.

17. Clinicians should comply with best practice requirements for the management of NSI and adverse reactions and comply with local policies and procedures for their jurisdiction.

PATIENT SELECTION

Choosing the correct patient for TrP-DN is a skill based upon balancing the benefits of treatment with the patient's characteristics and presentation. The selection criteria may vary from patient to patient and in various situations and contexts. One of the fundamental safety principles is the understanding of the patient's contraindications and precautions to particular treatments and understanding the potential risks (Batavia, 2006). Healthcare clinicians such as physical therapists routinely use patient selection and clinical reasoning skills in practice to enhance safe practice. As an example, consider the selection criteria for the use of neck traction, manipulation, and use of electrophysical agents such as ultrasound, among others. Many of these skills are developed throughout the physical therapist's training program and further enhanced from experience in clinical practice.

Patient selection criteria for TrP-DN have been recommended by the College of Physical Therapists of Alberta (CPTA), Canada (CPTA, 2007). Appropriate patient selection should involve consideration of the following.

1. The patient's physical therapy diagnosis and dysfunction.
2. Expectation of a reasonable benefit from DN therapy.
3. The patient's medical conditions and history and recognise conditions that require precaution or contraindication (e.g., pregnancy, low immune dysfunction, blood thinners, needle phobia).
4. The patient's ability to understand the rationale for treatment, give informed consent, provide feedback and communication to the therapist, and be able to follow instructions (e.g., lying still).
5. Capacity for the safe application and management of precautions and side effects.

Furthermore the CPTA recommends consideration of patient characteristics, including the patient's cultural background, functional and physical abilities, language and communication skills, psychological profile (e.g., fear of needles, stress response), and age (CPTA, 2007). As an example of the importance of patients' disease characteristics and demographic profile, a study for TrP-DN for myofascial pain syndrome, demonstrated that negative prognostic predictors included long duration of pain, high intensity of pain, poor quality of sleep, and repetitive stress (Huang et al., 2011).

PRINCIPLES OF DRY NEEDLING APPLICATION

DN is a learned skill and standards and safety are promoted by routine approach to practice. This section outlines principles to promote a rational and uniform approach to practice. These principles can be modified to develop guidelines, policies, and procedures. It is assumed that the clinician has selected the patient appropriately and determined that DN is appropriate. The principles of DN application include patient education and consent, procedural education, and practical application such as positioning, palpation, technique, and aftercare (McEvoy et al., 2012).

Patient Education and Consent

Before the application of DN, it is important to educate the patient on the rationale for the procedure and what to expect. The clinician should ascertain whether the patient has undergone DN therapy in the past, and if so, what was their personal experience. Informed consent should be sought from each patient. This is an excellent time for the clinician to make the patient feel at ease by demonstrating knowledge and confidence. Clinician confidence is important to reduce patient anxiety. The clinician can also gauge the patient's comfort level and answer patient's questions. Appropriate education should include elements of the following.

1. Explanation of the indication and aim of treatment.
2. A brief explanation of how the chosen DN technique potentially works (e.g., SDN or TrP-DN).
3. Explanation that DN is an invasive procedure with insertion of a monofilament needle into the skin, subcutaneous tissues, and muscle as appropriate.
4. The risks of DN therapy should be clearly explained to the patient as appropriate, thus allowing the patient to offer informed consent. This should be done in such a manner to impart knowledge to the patient, but avoid instilling fear of the procedure. The patient should be informed that single use disposable needles will be utilised during treatment. Local jurisdiction informed consent policies and procedures must be followed.

5. The patient should be informed of post-treatment soreness as this may be common at the local needling site for several days after treatment.
6. The patient should be given the opportunity to ask questions.
7. Persons under 18 should also have informed consent from a parent or guardian. Clinicians should follow local jurisdiction rules.
8. Patient education should outline that DN when administered by a clinician does not constitute the practice of acupuncture unless the clinician is an acupuncturist or is qualified to deliver acupuncture within the jurisdiction.

Procedural Education

DN requires an optimum interaction between the patient and clinician and communication should be encouraged during the procedure. Before any DN application these steps are recommended.

1. The patient is asked and encouraged to provide feedback and communicate with the clinician during treatment.
2. The patient is asked to remain still during the procedure.
3. The patient is aware that he can withdraw from treatment at any time.
4. In the case of TrP-DN, the patient should be made aware of the local twitch response (LTR) which may be perceived similar to an electric shock, cramp, or other sensation. The patient should be made aware that reproduction of the LTR is the aim of TrP-DN.
5. If static needling technique is employed, where the needle is statically in the muscle for a period of time, the patient should be informed not to move, as this may pose a risk of further penetration and tissue damage, such as a pneumothorax, among others.
6. If the patient is left resting during static needling technique, the patient should be able to call or alert the clinician easily.
7. Any further education or advice before, during or after treatment that may be important for an individual patient, should be given as part of the overall plan of care.

Practical Application
Positioning

1. The patient should be treated reclined to avoid difficulty if fainting should occur.
2. The patient should be positioned suitably to allow easy palpation and access to the muscle(s) being treated.

3. Positions may include supine, prone, sidelying or a combination of these positions. It is important that the patient is comfortable and relaxed. Pillows, rolls, or similar items can be used for positioning.

4. It is helpful to be able to see the patient's face, but this may not always the possible. Verbal communication should be ongoing to assess the patient's response to DN procedures.

5. Clinicians should position themselves ergonomically, comfortably and ensure good body mechanics to reduce the risk of work related disorders and to assure that they are in control of the DN process.

6. Parents and guardians of children or care takers and other individuals accompanying the patient should be comfortable during DN procedures. It is not uncommon to see fainting or other autonomic symptoms in on-lookers when observing DN.

Palpation

Skilled palpation is the key element for identifying TrPs and for the application of safe DN. Clinicians should have excellent knowledge of practical anatomy including: muscle attachments, bony landmarks, muscle fibre directions, muscles layers, neurovascular structures, organs (e.g., pleura and lungs), joints and capsules, among others.

1. The muscle(s) being treated along with anatomical landmarks should be located by skilled visual observation and palpation.

2. The clinician should be cognisant of other anatomical structures that need to be avoided including neurovascular structures, lungs, among others, and should at all times aim to avoid needling into these structures. The directive "when in doubt, stay out" applies.

3. TrPs are identified by skilled palpation using relevant criteria (Simons et al., 1999; McEvoy & Huijbregts, 2011) and the muscle is positioned to allow optimal tension for palpation and treatment. The muscles can be contracted to assist in locating fibre direction and differentiating from other muscles.

4. Flat palpation or pincer grip techniques are used as indicated. For safety, pincer grip is likely to improve safety and is preferable when appropriate. Should the clinician's hands be removed from the patient to prepare the needle, the muscle and bony landmarks should be identified again.

5. Ensure that the patient and muscle is relaxed before starting the DN procedure.

6. Should the clinician not be sure of the needle tip location or is unsure of the topographical anatomy,

DN should be avoided. This could occur for example in obese patients. Again, when in doubt, stay out.

Technique

There are various DN conceptual models and techniques and clinicians may use a combination of techniques during clinical practice. Equipment required includes needles, gloves, hand sanitiser, alcohol wipes (as required), needle disposal box, cotton swabs for bleeds, and a waste disposal bag or can. General guidelines for technique are as follows.

1. Single use, sterile, suitable monofilament needles are employed. Needles should be high quality and may be tubed or untubed. We recommend DN with tubed needles only as they reduce the risk of touching the needle shaft and increase the likelihood of painful needle insertion. Needles should be stored and used per the manufacturer's guidelines and be within date. Needle length and thickness is chosen on the basis of patient size, muscle to be needled and expected depth of penetration. When choosing needle length, clinicians should bear in mind that needles should not be inserted all the way to the handle.

2. A hygiene protocol is carried out as previously recommended and gloves are worn on at least the palpating hand or, if so preferred or required, on both hands.

3. The muscle being needled is identified and a flat or pincer grip technique is employed by the palpating hand. The needling hand holds the needle by the handle only.

4. The needle is inserted across the skin using the guide tube. The guide tube is then removed. The needle shaft should not be touched to prevent contamination.

5. The clinician should be cognisant of anatomical structures within the treatment area that are vulnerable to DN, for example, neurovascular structures and the lung, and ensure that the needling technique avoids penetration vulnerable anatomical structures. Also, voluntary and involuntary patient movement may compromise safe DN, which is why the needling hand should always rest on the patient's body.

6. For SDN the needle is inserted to the depth for superficial needling as has been recommended by Baldry (2002, 2005) (see Chapter 12) or to a depth to engage the TrP in TrP-DN.

7. TrP-DN involves a relatively slow but deliberate steady lancing motion in and out of the muscle, which is considered a dynamic needling technique (Simons et al., 1999; Dommerholt et al., 2006). The needle

is brought out to the edge of the myofascia into the subdermal tissue and moved back into the muscle. The main aim of this treatment is to elicit LTRs.

8. Sharp pain of a stinging, burning or electrical nature should be immediately avoided as this may signal penetration of a nerve or blood vessel.

9. DN techniques such as SDN or TrP-DN may involve static needle techniques, where the needle is left in situ for a period of time. In this case the needle may be rotated to induce mechanical stress on the fascia or myofascia. When static needling is employed, the clinician should ensure the needle is safe at rest and not in the close vicinity of vulnerable anatomical structures. Patients should be informed to stay still and not to move. They should be able to alert the clinician as needed either vocally or by the use of a call bell. Policies should be in place to avoid forgetting a patient in a treatment room (White et al., 2001).

10. It may be acceptable that an individual needle may be withdrawn and reinserted across the skin of the same patient at the same treatment session. Clinicians should follow local policies and procedures on this practice. Again, touching the needle shaft should be avoided to prevent contamination of the needle and if this occurs the needle should be disposed of and a new needle used. Needles may become blunt from piercing soft tissue and contacting bone and in this case a new needle should be employed. Of course, a used needle should never be stored or reused.

11. The clinician should actively communicate with the patient during DN and limit treatment to the patient's tolerance. The patient should be reassured throughout the procedure. This is most important for the initial treatment for a new needle-naïve patient.

12. DN technique should suit the tolerance and ability of the patient. Considerations for technique include SDN vs TrP-DN, the quantity of lancing motions, intensity and speed of the lancing motion, stimulation and quantity of local twitch responses, the length of time of active needling, static needling technique, the number of needle insertions per muscle and the number or muscles treated in one session, among others. The patient's characteristics will determine much of the approach and the patient's previous experience and response should be taken into account. The patient's perceived experience of a medical treatment is related to the intensity of the pain and the pain experience within the last 3 minutes of the procedure, therefore the treatment session should not be terminated with painful procedures (Redelmeier & Kahneman, 1996; Redelmeier et al., 2003; McEvoy & Dommerholt, 2012).

13. When needles are withdrawn, they should be immediately disposed of into a suitable certified sharps container. Sharps containers should be filled only to the fill-line mark and should be within easy reach. Sharps containers should be disposed of per local policies and procedures with a licensed medical waste removal company or agent.

Aftercare

The following are recommended for DN aftercare.

1. The muscle and treatment area needled should be compressed immediately after needle withdrawal for haemostasis for up to 30 seconds or until any bleeding has stopped. A cotton swab may be used and should be discarded as appropriate.

2. If blood is present on the skin it should be cleaned with an alcohol swab, which should be discarded as appropriate. The patient should be educated on aftercare which may include limbering exercises, gentle stretching, the use of hot packs or cold packs, activity modifications, and motor retraining, as deemed necessary.

3. Any adverse reactions should be dealt with as noted in the previous sections.

ELECTRICAL STIMULATION VIA DRY NEEDLES

Electrotherapy, such as transcutaneous electrical nerve stimulation (TENS), percutaneous electrical nerve stimulation (PENS), and neuromuscular electrical stimulation (NMES) can be delivered via solid filament needles for the treatment of pain, abnormal muscle tone or strengthening. Techniques have been described by Gunn (1997), Baldry (2005), Dommerholt and associates (2006), and White and colleagues (2008). In acupuncture, delivery of electrical currents through needles is termed electro-acupuncture (ASAP, 2007). Extra care should be noted with patients who have bleeding disorders as DN TENS or NMES related muscle contraction may lead to a greater susceptibility to bleeding. The following considerations should be taken into account (ASAP, 2007; White et al., 2008).

1. All contraindications and precautions for DN therapy and the individual electrical device used should be observed.

2. Use devices according to manufacturers' recommendations.

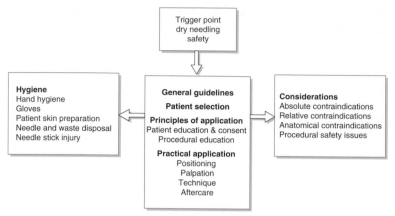

FIG. 5.1 Trigger point dry needling safety—overview.

3. Use suitable single-use, sterile, metal-handle needles, and attach the alligator clip of the electrotherapy device to the handle or directly to the shaft of a clean needle.
4. Do not connect electrical clips to contaminated needle shafts.

Contraindications and relative contraindications to electrical stimulation via DN include:

1. Patients not comfortable or phobic to either electrical stimulation or needling.
2. In the vicinity of implanted electrical devices, such as pacemakers, spinal cord stimulators (ASAP, 2007; White et al., 2008).
3. Pregnant patients in the vicinity of the mid or low back, pelvis, or abdomen.
4. In the vicinity of the anterior triangle of the neck, carotid sinus, or vagus nerve, or in the vicinity of the recurrent laryngeal nerve (White et al., 2008).
5. In areas of sensory denervation (White et al., 2008).
6. Special caution should be used with persons with epilepsy.

SUMMARY

TrP-DN is an evolving and expanding treatment (Fig. 5.1). Safety must be considered the number one priority. Clinicians should familiarise themselves with important aspects of DN safety including hygiene, contraindications, precautions, anatomical considerations, and procedural safety issues. Guidelines have been proposed to improve safe DN treatment. Patient selection and practical DN skills are required to ensure safe standardise treatment. Clinicians should encourage local jurisdictional guidelines to improve safety and standards.

ACKNOWLEDGEMENT

The author would like to acknowledge the authors and reviewers for the Irish *Guidelines for Safe Dry Needling Practice for Chartered Physiotherapists* (McEvoy et al., 2012).

REFERENCES

Aldlyami, E., Kulkarni, A., Reed, M. R., & Muller, S. D. (2010). Partington Latex-free gloves: safer for whom? *The Journal of Arthroplasty, 25,* 27–30.

APTA (2012). Physical therapists and the performance of dry needling; An educational resource paper. *American Physical Therapy Association,* 1–141.

ASAP (2007). *Guidelines for safe acupuncture and dry needling practice.* Australian Society of Acupuncture Physiotherapists Inc..

BAC (2006). *The British Acupuncture Council Code of Safe Practice.* London: BAC.

Baldry, P. (2002). Superficial versus deep dry needling. *Acupuncture in Medicine, 20,* 78–81.

Baldry, P. E. (2005). *Acupuncture, trigger points and musculoskeletal pain.* Edinburgh: Churchill Livingstone.

Barlow-Pugh, M. (2000). *Stedman's Medical dictionary.* Baltimore: Lippincott Williams & Wilkins.

Batavia, M. (2006). *Contraindications in physical rehabilitation: doing no harm.* St Louis: Saunders Elsevier.

Bond, W. W., Favero, M. S., Petersen, N. J., et al. (1981). Survival of hepatitis B virus after drying and storage for one week. *Lancet, 1,* 550–551.

Boyce, J. M., & Pittet, D. (2002). Guideline for Hand Hygiene in Health-Care Settings. Recommendations of the Healthcare Infection Control Practices Advisory Committee and the HICPAC/SHEA/APIC/IDSA Hand Hygiene Task Force. Society for Healthcare Epidemiology of America/Association for Professionals in Infection Control/Infectious Diseases Society of America. MMWR. *Recommendations and Reports, 51*(RR-16), 1–45.

Brady, S., McEvoy, J., Dommerholt, J., & Doody, C. (2014). Adverse events following trigger point dry needling: a prospective survey of chartered physiotherapists. *The Journal of Manual & Manipulative Therapy, 22*(3), 134–140.

Castelain, M., Castelain, P. R., & Ricciardi, R. (1987). Contact dermatitis to acupuncture needles. *Contact Dermatitis, 16,* 44.

Callan, A. K., Bauer, J. M., & Martus, J. E. (2016). Deep spine infection after acupuncture in the setting of spinal instrumentation. *Spine Deformity, 4,* 156–161.

Carr, D. J. (2015). The safety of obstetric acupuncture: forbidden points revisited. *Acupuncture in Medicine, 33*(5), 413–419.

CDC (1995). Centers for Disease Control and Prevention. Case-control study of HIV seroconversion in health-care workers after percutaneous exposure to HIV-infected blood–France, United Kingdom, and United States, January 1988-August 1994. *MMWR. Morbidity and Mortality Weekly Report, 44*(50), 929–933.

CDC (2011). Centers for Disease Control and Prevention. Bloodborne infectious diseases: HIV / AIDS, Hepatitis B, Hepatitis C: Emergency needle stick information. [online] Available at https://www.cdc.gov/niosh/topics/bbp/emergnedl.html (accessed 29 September 2017).

Chen, J. C., Chen, Y., Lin, S. M., Yang, H. J., Su, C. F., & Tseng, S. H. (2006). Acute spinal epidural hematoma after acupuncture. *The Journal of Trauma, 60*(2), 414–416.

Cicerone, K. D. (2005). Evidence-based practice and the limits of rational rehabilitation. *Archives of Physical Medicine and Rehabilitation, 86,* 1073–1074.

CPTA (2007). Dry needling competency profile for physical therapists. *Alberta, College of Physical Therapists of Alberta, Edmonton.,* 5.

Cummings, M., Ross-Marrs, R., & Gerwin, R. (2014). Pneumothorax complication of deep dry needling demonstration. *Acupuncture in Medicine, 32*(6), 517–519.

Dommerholt, J., 2011. Safety and hygiene in trigger point dry needling. IMT-2 Head, Neck and Shoulder Pain. Dommerholt J, Gerwin RD. Bethesda, Myopain Seminars.

Dommerholt, J., Mayoral, O., & Gröbli, C. (2006). Trigger point dry needling. *The Journal of Manual & Manipulative Therapy, 14,* E70–E87.

Ehrenkranz, N. J., & Alfonso, B. C. (1991). Failure of bland soap handwash to prevent hand transfer of patient bacteria to urethral catheters. *Infection Control and Hospital Epidemiology, 12,* 654–662.

Ernst, E., Lee, M. S., & Choi, T. Y. (2011). Acupuncture: does it alleviate pain and are there serious risks? A review of reviews. *Pain, 152,* 755–764.

Filshie, J. (2001). Safety aspects of acupuncture in palliative care. *Acupuncture in Medicine, 19,* 117–122.

Fisher, A. A. (1986). Allergic dermatitis from acupuncture needles. *Cutis, 38,* 226.

Gawande, A. (2009). *The checklist manifesto: how to get things right.* New York: Metropolitan Books.

Given. (2009). *Guidelines and standards for the clean and safe clinical practice of acupuncture.* Chaplin: National Acupuncture Foundation.

Goodman, C. C., Boissonnault, W. G., & Fuller, K. S. (2003). *Pathology: implications for the physical therapist.* Saunders, Philadelphia, London: W. B.

Gunn, C. C. (1997). *The Gunn approach to the treatment of chronic pain.* New York: Churchill Livingstone.

Hanley, J. A., & Lippman-Hand, A. (1983). If nothing goes wrong, is everything all right? Interpreting zero numerators. *JAMA, 1;* 249(13):1743–1745.

Hettiaratchy, S., Hassall, O., Watson, C., Wallis, D., & Williams, D. (1998). Glove usage and reporting of needle stick injuries by junior hospital medical staff. *Annals of the Royal College of Surgeons of England, 80,* 439–441.

Hoffman, P. (2001). Skin disinfection and acupuncture. *Acupuncture in Medicine, 19,* 112–116.

HSE (2009). Standard Precautions. *Health Service Executive. Standard Precautions version 1.0* (28th April 2009).

Huang, Y. T., Lin, S. Y., Neoh, C. A., et al. (2011). Dry needling for myofascial pain: prognostic factors. *Journal of Alternative and Complementary Medicine, 17,* 755–762.

Hutin, Y., Hauri, A., Chiarello, L., et al. (2003). Best infection control practices for intradermal, subcutaneous, and intramuscular needle injections. *Bulletin of the World Health Organization, 81,* 491–500.

Ji, G. Y., Oh, C. H., Choi, W. S., & Lee, J. B. (2015). Three cases of hemiplegia after cervical paraspinal muscle needling. *The Spine Journal, 15*(3), e9–13.

Klevens, R. M., Edwards, J. R., Richards, C. L., Jr., et al. (2007). Estimating health care-associated infections and deaths in U.S. hospitals, 2002. *Public Health Reports, 122,* 160–166.

Lee, J. H., Lee, H., & Jo, D. J. (2011). An acute cervical epidural hematoma as a complication of dry needling. *Spine, 36,* E891–E893.

Lewkonia, P., DiPaola, C., & Street, J. (2016). Incidence and risk of delayed surgical site infection following instrumented lumbar spine fusion. *Journal of Clinical Neuroscience, 23,* 76–80.

McEvoy, J., & Dommerholt, J. (2012). *Myofascial trigger points of the shoulder.* In *Physical Therapy of the Shoulder.* (pp. 351–380). R. Donatelli. St Loius: Elsevier Churchill Livingstone.

McEvoy, J., & Huijbregts, P. (2011). Reliability of myofascial trigger point palpation: a systematic review. In *Myofascial trigger Points: Pathophysiology and evidenced-informed diagnosis and management.* J. Dommerholt and P. Huijbregts.: Sudbury, Jones and Bartlett.

McEvoy, J., Dommerholt, J., Rice, D., et al., 2012. Guidelines for Safe Dry Needling Practice for Chartered Physiotherapists. http://www.iscp.ie/ Dublin.

Melchart, D., Weidenhammer, W., Streng, A., et al. (2004). Prospective investigation of adverse effects of acupuncture in 97733 patients. *Archives of Internal Medicine, 164,* 104–105.

Mockford, K., & O'Grady, H. (2017). Prevention of surgical site infections. *Surgery, 35*(9), 495–499.

Montville, R., & Schaffner, D. W. (2011). A meta-analysis of the published literature on the effectiveness of antimicrobial soaps. *Journal of Food Protection, 74,* 1875–1882.

Nelson, L. S., & Hoffman, R. S. (1998). Intrathecal injection: unusual complication of trigger-point injection therapy. *Annals of Emergency Medicine, 32,* 506–508.

O'Sullivan, P., Seoighe, D. M., Baker, J. F., et al. (2011). Hospital-based needle stick use and injuries by Dublin interns in 2010. *Irish Journal Medicine Science, 80*, 545–547.

OSHA USDOL (2011). *Occupational Safety and Health Standards, Z, Toxic and Hazardous Substances, 1910.1030, in Bloodborne pathogens. [online]*. Available at https://www.osha.gov/pls/oshaweb/owadisp.show_document?p_table=STANDARDS&p_id=10051.

Parsons, E. C. (2000). Successful reduction of sharps injuries using a structured change process. *AORN Journal, 72*, 275–279.

Paulson, D. S., Fendler, E. J., Dolan, M. J., & Williams, R. A. (1999). A close look at alcohol gel as an antimicrobial sanitizing agent. *American Journal of Infection Control, 27*, 332–338.

Peuker, E. (2004). Case report of tension pneumothorax related to acupuncture. *Acupuncture in Medicine, 22*, 40–43.

Peuker, E., & Gronemeyer, D. (2001). Rare but serious complications of acupuncture: traumatic lesions. *Acupuncture in Medicine, 19*, 103–108.

Redelmeier, D. A., & Kahneman, D. (1996). Patients' memories of painful medical treatments: real-time and retrospective evaluations of two minimally invasive procedures. *Pain, 66*, 3–8.

Redelmeier, D. A., Katz, J., & Kahneman, D. (2003). Memories of colonoscopy: a randomized trial. *Pain, 104*, 187–194.

Rodts, M. F., & Benson, D. R. (1992). HIV precautions for prevention in the workplace. *Orthopaedic Nursing, 11*, 51–57.

Romaguera, C., & Grimalt, F. (1979). Nickel dermatitis from acupuncture needles. *Contact Dermatitis, 5*, 195.

SARI (2005). Guidelines for hand hygiene in Irish healthcare settings. The Strategy for the Control of Antimicrobial Resistance in Ireland (SARI) / Health Service Executive.

Sharma, G. K., Gilson, M. M., Nathan, H., & Makary, M. A. (2009). Needle stick injuries among medical students: incidence and implications. *Academic Medicine, 84*, 1815–1821.

Siegel J, Rhinehart E, Jackson M, Chiarello L. 2007. Guideline for Isolation Precautions: Preventing Transmission of Infectious Agents in Healthcare Settings, Centre for Disease Control / Healthcare Infection Control Practices Advisory Committee.

Simons, D. G., Travell, J. G., & Simons, L. S. (1999). *Travell and Simons' Myofascial Pain and Dysfunction; the Trigger Point Manual.* Baltimore: Williams & Wilkins.

Smith, C., Crowther, C., & Beilby, J. (2002). Pregnancy outcome following women's participation in a randomised controlled trial of acupuncture to treat nausea and vomiting in early pregnancy. *Complementary Therapies in Medicine, 10*, 78–83.

Standring, S., & Gray, H. A. (2008). *Gray's anatomy: the anatomical basis of clinical practice.* Edinburgh: Churchill Livingstone.

Steentjes, K., de Vries, L. M. A., Ridwan, B. U., & Wijgman, A. J. (2016). Infectie van een heupprothese na 'dry needling'. *Nederlands Tijdschrift van de Geneeskunde, 160*, A9364.

Steinberg, B. J. (2014). Medical and dental implications of eating disorders. *Journal of Dental Hygiene, 88*(3), 156–159.

Travell, J. G., & Simons, D. G. (1983). *Myofascial pain and Dysfunction; the Trigger Point Manual.* Baltimore: Williams & Wilkins.

Travell, J. G., & Simons, D. G. (1992). *Myofascial Pain and Dysfunction: the Trigger Point manual.* Baltimore: Williams & Wilkins.

USDA (2009). USDA Policies and Procedures on Biohazardous Waste Decontamination, Management, and Quality Controls at Laboratories and Technical Facilities. In *9630-001.* USDA, Washington DC: USDA.

Vincent, C. (2001). The safety of acupuncture. *British Medical Journal, 323*, 467–468.

Vleeming, A., Albert, H. B., Ostgaard, H. C., Sturesson, B., & Stuge, B. (2008). European guidelines for the diagnosis and treatment of pelvic girdle pain. *European Spine Journal, 17*, 794–819.

White, A., Hayhoe, S., & Ernst, E. (1997). Survey of adverse events following acupuncture. *Acupuncture in Medicine, 15*, 67–70.

White, A., Hayhoe, S., Hart, A., & Ernst, E. (2001). Survey of adverse events following acupuncture (SAFA): a prospective study of 32000 consultations. *Acupuncture in Medicine, 19*, 84–92.

White, A., Cummings, M., & Filshie, J. (2008). *Evidence on the safety of acupuncture.* In *An introduction to Western medical acupuncture* (p. 122). Edinburgh: Churchill Livingstone-Elsevier.

WHO (1999). Guidelines on basic training and safety in acupuncture. *World Health Organisation, 35.*

WIP (2008). *Infectiepreventie in de acupunctuurpraktijk.* Leiden: Leids Universitair Medisch Centrum.

Witt, C. M., Pach, D., Brinkhaus, B., et al. (2009). Safety of acupuncture: results of a prospective observational study with 229,230 patients and introduction of a medical information and consent form. *Forschende Komplementärmedizin, 16*, 91–97.

World Medical Association. (2006). *Declaration of Geneva. [online].* Available at https://www.wma.net/wp-content/uploads/2017/02/WMA_DECLARATION-OF-GENEVA_A2_EN.pdf. (Accessed 18 October 2017).

Yang, L., & Mullan, B. (2011). Reducing needle stick injuries in healthcare occupations: an integrative review of the literature. *ISRN Nursing, 315432.*

Yazawa, S., Ohi, T., Sugimoto, S., Satoh, S., & Matsukura, S. (1998). Cervical spinal epidural abscess following acupuncture: successful treatment with antibiotics. *Internal Medicine, 37*, 161–165.

CHAPTER 6

Dry Needling Across Different Disciplines

JAN DOMMERHOLT

INTRODUCTION: SCOPE OF PRACTICE

Scope of practice is generally defined as the activities that an individual healthcare provider performs in the delivery of patient care. Overlap in scope of practice is recognised by many healthcare disciplines, ranging from medical radiation technologists (QSE Consulting, 2005) and nursing (Committee on Health Professions Education Summit, 2003; Association of Social Work Boards et al., 2009) to physical therapy, social work, occupational therapy (Association of Social Work Boards et al., 2009; Adrian, 2010; APTA Practice Department and APTA State Government Affairs, 2011), and medicine (Federation of State Medical Boards of the United States, 2005; Association of Social Work Boards et al., 2009). The Federation of State Medical Boards of the United States defines scope of practice as 'those health care services a physician or other health care practitioner is authorised to perform by virtue of professional license, registration, or certification' (Federation of State Medical Boards of the United States, 2005). According to the Federation, 'the concept of collaboration acknowledges that scopes of practice often overlap within the health care delivery system', which 'can be an effective means for providing safe and competent health care' (Federation of State Medical Boards of the United States, 2005). The Federation recognises that different healthcare professionals' scopes of practice may overlap and that different disciplines can collaborate based upon shared competencies.

The Pew Health Commission Taskforce on Health Care Workforce Regulation emphasised that a nearly exclusive scope of practice leads to unreasonable barriers to high quality and affordable care (Finocchio et al., 1995). In the United States, many state individual statutes also recognise the importance of overlap in scope. The Attorney General of Maryland confirmed that 'state law recognises that the scope of practice of health care professions may overlap' and confirmed that the Maryland General Assembly 'has fostered consumer choice in the selection of treatment and practitioner' by providing for overlapping scope of practice for different healthcare disciplines (Gansler & McDonald, 2010). To offer high quality, affordable, and accessible healthcare, it is crucial that all healthcare providers can practice within the full scope of their professional competencies (Safriet, 1994; Schmitt, 2001).

DRY NEEDLING BY MULTIPLE DISCIPLINES

Dry needling (DN) is a treatment technique practiced around the globe by a wide variety of healthcare disciplines, including allopathic, osteopathic, naturopathic, dental, podiatric, veterinary, acupuncture, physical therapy, occupational therapy, chiropractic medicine, myotherapy, athletic training, and massage therapy, among others, dependent on the country and local jurisdictional regulations (Dommerholt et al., 2006a). Similar to many other treatment interventions, DN is not in the exclusive scope of any discipline (APTA Practice Department and APTA State Government Affairs, 2011; Dommerholt, 2011). A chiropractor or physical therapist employing DN is practicing chiropractic or physical therapy, respectively. Uneducated patients may occasionally refer to DN as the practice of acupuncture even when performed by a nonacupuncturist, but they should be informed that only acupuncturists are practicing acupuncture. Similarly, physical therapists, chiropractors, and osteopaths administer manipulations with different names without necessarily encroaching on each other's disciplines. A physical therapist does not apply chiropractic adjustments and a chiropractor does not utilise orthopaedic manual therapy manipulations even though the techniques may appear similar. Massage therapists, physical therapists, and a variety of other professions use massage or soft tissue manipulation without claiming ownership of a technique. Irrespective of any political or philosophical disagreements, the clinical reasoning process to perform joint or soft tissue manipulations may be quite different between professions. For example, traditionally chiropractors used adjustments as a primary intervention to correct spinal subluxations for a wide range of ailments. However, more recently, the practice has evolved into targeting movement of joints rather than the position of joints, and chiropractors are increasingly adopting the term 'manipulation' (Paris, 2000). A technique does not define the scope of practice, and no profession actually owns a skill or activity in and of itself (Association of Social Work Boards et al., 2009).

Medicine

During the past centuries, several physicians have described TrPs and myofascial treatment techniques (Simons, 1975; Baldry, 2005). In 1912 physician Sir William Osler recommended inserting ladies' hatpins at tender points in the treatment of low back pain (Osler, 1912). In 1931 German physician Lange published a manual for the treatment of 'muscle hardenings' more than 50 years before Travell and Simons published their manual (Lange, 1931; Travell & Simons, 1983). When Travell developed the concepts of myofascial pain in the 1940s, she was not aware of any previous medical descriptions of TrP phenomena (Travell, 1949; Travell & Rinzler, 1952), nor was chiropractor Nimmo, who 'rediscovered' TrPs in the 1950s (Cohen & Gibbons, 1998; Schneider et al., 2001). Already in 1944, Steinbrocker suggested that the effect of TrP injections was mostly due to mechanical stimulation of TrPs irrespective of the particular type of injectate (Steinbrocker, 1944). The term 'dry needling' was first used in 1947 by Paulett in an article on low back pain published in the *Lancet* (Paulett, 1947). He emphasised that DN was most effective when the muscle would exhibit a reflex spasm, which later became known as a 'local twitch response'. Travell and Rinzler mentioned DN in a 1952 article, but they did not use DN all that much in clinical practice (Travell and Rinzler, 1952). It was not until 1979 that Lewit described needling 312 pain sites in 241 patients, including TrPs, scar tissue, ligaments, muscle spasms, tendons, entheses, periosteum, and joints (Lewit, 1979). Immediate analgesia without hypoesthesia, referred to as 'the needle effect', was noted in nearly 87% of subjects, with permanent relief of tenderness for 92 targets. In 1980 Gunn and colleagues published the first scientific study on the successful use of DN of motor points in the treatment of individuals with low back pain (Gunn et al., 1980). Since 1980, many more physicians have contributed to

the DN literature, although it appears that, at least in the North America, physicians seem to prefer using TrP injections over DN (Peng & Castano, 2005).

Veterinary Medicine

Incorporating myofascial pain constructs and DN in veterinary medicine appears to become more common (Janssens, 1991; Frank, 1999; Veenman, 2006; Haussler, 2010), especially in canine and equine medicine (Wall, 2014; Goff, 2016). MacGregor and Graf von Schweinitz (2006) studied the electromyographic activity of TrPs in equine cleidobrachialis muscles. Janssens was one of the first authors to consider TrPs in dogs (Janssens, 1991). In 2014 Wall published a comprehensive review of the importance of canine TrPs (Wall, 2014). Bowen and colleagues (2017) explored the nature and presence of TrPs in the transverse and ascending pectoral muscles of horses. Brockman (2017) described a case of a 12-year-old Akhal-Teke horse that was treated with TrP therapy, acupressure, and myofascial release. Schachinger and Klarholz (2017) recently published a book about equine DN. In the United States a growing number of veterinarians and animal physical therapists are attending canine DN courses. As is the case in human medicine, successful DN is dependent on the veterinary clinician's ability to identify TrPs or fascial adhesions and on the development of a kinesthetic awareness and visualisation of the pathway the needle takes within the body.

Dental Medicine

Although myofascial pain dysfunction syndrome was included in the 1992 research diagnostic criteria for temporomandibular disorders (Dworkin & LeResche, 1992), the guidelines did not provide much clinically useful information about how to identify and treat TrPs. More recent versions of these guidelines did not fare much better (Steenks & de Wijer, 2009). Nevertheless, early pioneering dentists recognised the importance of TrPs in dental and facial pain, occipital neuralgia, and headaches, among other areas (Jaeger, 1985, 1987, 1989; Graff-Radford et al., 1986) and they advocated including TrPs in the clinical algorithm for the treatment of patients with chronic neck and head pain (Graff-Radford et al., 1987). The same authors explored the reliability of pressure algometry (Reaves et al., 1986), TrP injections (Jaeger & Skootsky, 1987), and stretching (Jaeger & Reeves, 1986). Fricton has also contributed extensively to the dental myofascial pain literature (Fricton, 1989, 1990, 1991, 1993, 1994, 1995 1999; Fricton et al. 1985a, 1985b; Fricton & Steenks, 1996). There is no literature indicating whether DN is commonly used in dental practice.

Physical Therapy/Chiropractic/Myotherapy

All over the world DN has become a common treatment option in physical therapy. The American Physical Therapy Association has categorised DN under the umbrella of manual therapy in the most recent edition of the Guide to Physical Therapists Practice (APTA, 2014). The American Academy of Orthopaedic Manual Physical Therapists also considers DN to be within the scope of physical therapy practice. In 1984 Maryland was the first US state to approve physical therapists' use of DN. Currently DN is within the scope of physical therapy practice in most US states. National physical therapy associations in Australia, Ireland, New Zealand, Switzerland, and the United States have developed DN guidelines and educational resources. DN is also within the scope of chiropractic in a growing number of US states and in other countries. The number of DN continuing education course programs for chiropractors and physical therapists has expanded substantially not only in the United States, but also worldwide. In 2004 there were less than 10 DN courses in the US for physical therapists and chiropractors, whereas in 2018 there are nearly 30 DN course providers, each offering many DN courses. In the past decade physical therapists and chiropractors have contributed the majority of DN studies, reviews, and case reports to the scientific literature.

The Massage & Myotherapy Australia Association has issued a Myofascial Dry Needling Position Statement (https://www.massagemyotherapy.com.au/Tenant/U0000012/00000001/PDF/Polices%20and%20Procedures/Myofascial%20Dry%20Needling%20-%20Position%20Statement.pdf accessed 28 October 2017), which confirms that DN 'can be provided by trained practitioners with a minimum qualification of the Diploma of Remedial Massage'. Other healthcare providers in the US, including occupational therapists and athletic trainers, are increasingly becoming interested in DN, and a few state boards have already ruled that DN is also within their scope of practice. It remains to be seen whether this trend will expand to other countries.

Acupuncture

According to Janz and Adams, 'the relationship between the biomedical foundation of TrP-DN and clinical practice describes a variation of classical acupuncture rather than the invention of a new therapy'. From their perspective, DN constitutes a subsystem of musculoskeletal acupuncture (Janz & Adams, 2011). Many DN techniques are also described in the traditional acupuncture literature such as in *The Yellow Emperor's Inner Classic*, which was compiled 2000 years ago (Veith, 1972). Other acupuncturists maintain that DN is a kind of Western acupuncture for treating patients with myofascial pain (Zhou et al., 2015), an integral part of traditional acupuncture (Peng et al., 2016), or that it is a synonym to acupuncture or a subtype of acupuncture (Fan et al., 2017). Hobbs (2011) clarified that acupuncture is not necessarily 'limited to its historical roots and centuries' old theory, but is also a dynamic, evolving modern medical practice, which incorporates the use of neuroanatomical terminology'. In other words, acupuncture is not necessarily always based on or limited to Oriental medicine concepts, although the majority of US acupuncture state statutes define acupuncture in the context of 'Oriental medicine' or 'Oriental health concepts'. DN is clearly within the scope of acupuncture practice, even though acupuncturists tend not to use the DN terminology.

OPPOSITION TO DRY NEEDLING BY NONACUPUNCTURISTS

Initially, reputable US-based acupuncturists supported DN by physical therapists (Seem et al., 1991). However, when DN became more integrated into physical therapy practice, US acupuncture organisations increased their opposition and argued that DN would constitute the exclusive practice of acupuncture, which by definition can only be practiced by acupuncturists (Hobbs, 2007, 2011). Twenty-five years after the Maryland Board of Physical Therapy Examiners approved DN by physical therapists in 1984, the Maryland Board of Acupuncture formally opposed DN by physical therapists. Many US acupuncture organisations—such as the American Association of Acupuncture and Oriental Medicine (AAAOM), the Council of Colleges of Acupuncture and Oriental Medicine (CCAOM), the American Alliance for Professional Acupuncture Safety (AAPAS), and the National Centre for Acupuncture Safety and Integrity (NCASI), among others—have taken a firm stand and issued position papers confirming that DN is acupuncture (AAAOM, 2011a, 2011b; Hobbs, 2011). These organisations oppose DN by other disciplines such as physical therapy and chiropractic. A few medical associations and medical state boards, which in some states also regulate acupuncture practice, have also argued against DN by physical therapists and chiropractors, although the Federation of State Medical Boards copublished a statement in support of overlap of scope of practice (Association of Social Work Boards et al., 2009).

The CCAOM believes that physical therapists have recognised the benefits of acupuncture 'and its various representations such as DN due to the fact that they are attempting to use acupuncture and rename it as a physical therapy technique' (Hobbs, 2011). The AAAOM agreed that physical therapists are 'retitling' and 'repackaging' a subset of acupuncture techniques with the terms 'DN' and 'intramuscular manual therapy' (AAAOM, 2011a). Several more recent opinion papers share these sentiments (Zhou et al., 2015; Fan et al., 2016a, 2016b, 2017; Hao et al., 2016; Liu et al., 2016; Peng et al., 2016). Fan and colleagues (2017) conclude that physicians who have promoted DN have simply rebranded: (1) acupuncture as dry needling; and (2) acupuncture points as TrPs or dry needling points. Although these arguments may make some sense from a narrow acupuncture point of view, they lack a more global perspective.

Some studies conducted by Melzack suggested a 71% overlap between acupuncture points and TrP based on anatomical location (Melzack et al., 1977; Melzack, 1981); however, acupuncturist Birch concluded that Melzack erroneously had assumed that local pain indications of acupuncture points would be sufficient to establish a correlation (Birch, 2003). Instead Birch (2003) concluded that, at best, there is only an 18% to 19% overlap between acupuncture points and TrPs. Dorsher (2006) disagreed with Birch (2003) and concluded that most acupuncture points do have pain indications and can be directly compared with TrPs. He concluded that out of a total of 255 TrPs, 92% had anatomically corresponding acupuncture points and that nearly 80% of these acupuncture points had local pain indications similar to their corresponding TrPs (Dorsher, 2006). In a reply, Birch (2008) insisted that the presumed correspondence between acupoints and TrPs is based on a misunderstanding of the nature of both kinds of points. Similarly, several other acupuncturists have described similarities in between the pathways of acupuncture meridians and common referred pain patterns of TrPs (Cardinal, 2004, 2007; Dorsher & Fleckenstein, 2009).

One major flaw in comparing acupuncture points and TrP locations is that the 'TrP locations' reflect only a theoretical location as observed by Travell and Rinzler (1952). TrPs occur near motor endplates distributed widely throughout muscle bellies, which means that there are many potential TrP locations and not predetermined location of TrPs (Dommerholt et al., 2006b). Because TrPs do not have particular fixed locations, any comparison between TrPs and acupuncture points based on anatomical location is inaccurate and subject to inherent error (Dommerholt & Gerwin, 2010). As different schools of acupuncture have defined over 2500 acupuncture points worldwide, it is nearly impossible not to find topographical correspondences.

SUMMARY

Many of the controversies surrounding DN are based on a profound lack of understanding of the nature, depth of knowledge, and scope of other disciplines, turf behaviour, and perceived economic effect. Within the context of acupuncture, DN may well be similar to needling of Ashi points, but in the context of medicine, chiropractic, veterinary medicine, dentistry, and physical therapy, DN is nothing but a modification of TrP injections. Nonacupuncturists need to understand the depth of contemporary acupuncture practice; acupuncturists need to realise that DN by other disciplines does not pose any threat to acupuncture and to the public at large. Overlap in scope of practice will lead to high quality and affordable healthcare (Finocchio et al., 1995). From that perspective, DN is firmly established across many healthcare disciplines.

REFERENCES

Adrian, L. (2010). *Intramuscular manual therapy (dry needling).* Alexandria: Federation of State Boards of Physical Therapy.

American Association of Acupuncture and Oriental Medicine. (2011a). *American Association of Acupuncture and Oriental Medicine (AAAOM) Position Statement on Trigger Point Dry Needling (TDN) and Intramuscular Manual Therapy (IMT).* Washington, DC: American Association of Acupuncture and Oriental Medicine.

American Association of Acupuncture and Oriental Medicine. (2011b). *Position statement on dry needling in Illinois.* Chicago: Illinois Acupuncture Federation.

American Physical Therapy Association. (2014). *Guide to Physical Therapist Practice 3.0.* Alexandria, VA: American Physical Therapy Association.

APTA Practice Department and APTA State Government Affairs (2011). *Physical therapists & dry needling; a compendium for state policy makers.* Alexandria: American Physical Therapy Association.

Association of Social Work Boards, Federation of State Boards of Physical Therapy, Federation of State Medical Boards of the United States Inc. 2009. Changes in healthcare professions scope of practice: legislative considerations

Baldry, P. E. (2005). *Acupuncture, Trigger Points and Musculoskeletal Pain.* Edinburgh: Churchill Livingstone.

Birch, S. (2003). Trigger point: acupuncture point correlations revisited. *Journal of Alternative and Complementary Medicine, 9,* 91–103.

Birch, S. (2008). On the impossibility of trigger point-acupoint equivalence: a commentary on Peter Dorsher's analysis. *Journal of Alternative and Complementary Medicine, 14,* 343–345.

Bowen, A. G., Goff, L. M., & McGowan, C. M. (2017). Investigation of myofascial trigger points in equine pectoral muscles and girth-aversion behavior. *Journal of Equine Veterinary Science, 48,* 154–160.

Brockman, T. (2017). A case study utilizing myofascial release, acupressure and trigger point therapy to treat bilateral "Stringhalt" in a 12 year old Akhal-Teke horse. *Journal of Bodywork and Movement Therapies, 21,* 589–593.

Cardinal, S. (2004). *Points détente et acupuncture: approche neurophysiologique.* Montreal: Centre collégial de développement de matériel didactique.

Cardinal, S. (2007). *Points-détente et acupuncture: techniques de puncture.* Montreal: Centre collégial de développement de matériel didactique.

Cohen, J. H., & Gibbons, R. W. (1998). Raymond L. Nimmo and the evolution of trigger point therapy, 1929- 1986. *Journal of Manipulative and Physiological Therapeutics, 21,* 167–172.

Committee on Health Professions Education Summit. (2003). *Health Professions Education: A Bridge to Quality.* The Institute of Medicine.

Dommerholt, J., Mayoral, O., & Gröbli, C. (2006a). Trigger point dry needling. *The Journal of Manual & Manipulative Therapy, 14,* E70–E87.

Dommerholt, J., Bron, C., & Franssen, J. L. M. (2006b). Myofascial trigger points; an evidence-informed review. *The Journal of Manual & Manipulative Therapy, 14,* 203–221.

Dommerholt, J. (2011). Dry needling: peripheral and central considerations. *The Journal of Manual & Manipulative Therapy, 19,* 223–227.

Dommerholt, J., & Gerwin, R. D. (2010). Neurophysiological effects of trigger point needling therapies. In C. Fernández-de-las-Peñas, L. Arendt-Nielsen, & R. D. Gerwin (Eds.), *Diagnosis and management of tension type and cervicogenic headache.* Boston: Jones & Bartlett.

Dorsher, P. (2006). Trigger points and acupuncture points: anatomic and clinical correlations. *Medical Acupuncture, 17,* 21–25.

Dorsher, P. T., & Fleckenstein, J. (2009). Trigger points and classical acupuncture points part 3: Relationships of myofascial referred pain patterns to acupuncture meridians. *Dt Ztschr f Akup, 52,* 10–14.

Dworkin, S. F., & LeResche, L. (1992). Research diagnostic criteria for temporomandibular disorders: review, criteria, examinations and specifications, critique. *Journal of Craniomandibular Disorders, 6,* 301–355.

Fan, A. Y., & He, H. (2016a). Dry needling is acupuncture. *Acupuncture in Medicine, 34,* 241.

Fan, A. Y., Jiang, J., Faggert, S., & Xiu, J. H. (2017). Discussion about the training or education for "dry needling practice". *World Journal of Acupuncture-Moxibustion, 26,* 6–10.

Fan, A. Y., Zheng, L., & Yang, G. (2016b). Evidence that dry needling is the intent to bypass regulation to practice acupuncture in the United States. *Journal of Alternative and Complementary Medicine, 22,* 591–593.

Federation of State Medical Boards of the United States (2005). *Assessing scope of practice in health care delivery: Critical questions in assuring public access and safety.* Federation of State Medical Boards of the United States.

Finocchio, L. J., Dower, C. M., McMahon, T., & Gragnola, C. M. (1995). Taskforce on Health Care Workforce Regulation. In *Reforming Health Care Workforce Regulation: Policy Considerations for the 21st Century.* San Francisco: Pew Health Professions Commission.

Frank, E. M. (1999). Myofascial trigger point diagnostic criteria in the dog. *Journal of Musculoskeletal Pain, 7*(1-2), 231–237.

Fricton, J. R. (1989). Myofascial pain syndrome. *Neurologic Clinics, 7*(2), 413–427.

Fricton, J. R. (1990). Myofascial pain syndrome: characteristics and epidemiology. *Advances in Pain Research, 17,* 107–128.

Fricton, J. R. (1991). Clinical care for myofascial pain. *Dental Clinics of North America, 35,* 1–28.

Fricton, J. R. (1993). Clinical characteristics and diagnostic criteria. *Journal of Musculoskelet Pain, 1*(3/4), 37–47.

Fricton, J. R. (1994). Myofascial pain. *Baillière's Clinical Rheumatology, 8,* 857–880.

Fricton, J. R. (1995). Management of masticatory myofascial pain. *Seminars in Orthodontics, 1,* 229–243.

Fricton, J. R. (1999). Etiology and management of masticatory myofascial pain. *Journal of Musculoskelet Pain, 7*(1/2), 143–160.

Fricton, J. R., Auvinen, M. D., Dykstra, D., & Schiffman, E. (1985a). Myofascial pain syndrome: electromyographic changes associated with local twitch response. *Archives of Physical Medicine and Rehabilitation, 66,* 314–317.

Fricton, J. R., Kroening, R., Haley, D., & Siegert, R. (1985b). Myofascial pain syndrome of the head and neck: a review of clinical characteristics of 164 patients. *Oral Surgery, Oral Medicine, and Oral Pathology, 60,* 615–623.

Fricton, J. R., & Steenks, M. H. (1996). Diagnostiek en behandeling van myofasciale pijn. *Nederlands Tijdschrift voor Tandheelkunde, 103,* 249–253.

Gansler, D. F., & McDonald, R. N. (2010). *Opinions of the Attorney General.* Baltimore: Office of the Attorney General of Maryland.

Goff, L. (2016). Physiotherapy assessment for the equine athlete. *The Veterinary Clinics of North America Equine Practice, 32,* 31–47.

Graff-Radford, S. B., Jaeger, B., & Reeves, J. L. (1986). Myofascial pain may present clinically as occipital neuralgia. *Neurosurgery, 19,* 610–613.

Graff-Radford, S. B., Reeves, J. L., & Jaeger, B. (1987). Management of chronic head and neck pain: effectiveness of altering factors perpetuating myofascial pain. *Headache, 27,* 186–190.

Gunn, C. C., Milbrandt, W. E., Little, A. S., & Mason, K. E. (1980). Dry needling of muscle motor points for chronic low-back pain: a randomized clinical trial with long-term follow-up. *Spine, 5,* 279–291.

Hao, Y., & Liu, W. H. (2016). Traditional Chinese acupuncture manipulations and "dry needling". *World Journal of Acupuncture-Moxibustion, 26,* 15–19.

Haussler, K. K. (2010). The role of manual therapies in equine pain management. *The Veterinary Clinics of North America Equine Practice, 26,* 579–601.

Hobbs, V. (2007). *Dry needling and acupuncture emerging professional issues.* AAAOM, Sacramento: Qi Unity Report.

Hobbs, V. (2011). *Position Paper on Dry Needling*. Baltimore: Council of Colleges of Acupuncture and Oriental Medicine.

Jaeger, B. (1985). Myofascial referred pain patterns: the role of trigger points. *CDA Journal, 13*, 27–32.

Jaeger, B. (1987). Beyond TMJ: how does myofascial pain fit in? *TMJ Update, 5*, 28–32.

Jaeger, B. (1989). Are "cervicogenic" headaches due to myofascial pain and cervical spine dysfunction? *Cephalalgia, 9*, 157–164.

Jaeger, B., & Reeves, J. L. (1986). Quantification of changes in myofascial trigger point sensitivity with the pressure algometer following passive stretch. *Pain, 27*, 203–210.

Jaeger, B., & Skootsky, S. A. (1987). Double blind, controlled study of different myofascial trigger point injection techniques. *Pain, 4*, s292.

Janssens, L. A. A. (1991). Trigger points in 48 dogs with myofascial pain syndromes. *Veterinary Surgery, 20*, 274–278.

Janz, S., & Adams, J. H. (2011). Acupuncture by another name: dry needling in Australia. *Aust J Acupunct. Chinese Medicine, 6*, 3–11.

Lange, M. (1931). *Die Muskelhärten (Myogelosen)*. München: J.F. Lehmann's Verlag.

Lewit, K. (1979). The needle effect in the relief of myofascial pain. *Pain, 6*, 83–90.

Liu, L., Skinner, M. A., McDonough, S. M., & Baxter, G. D. (2016). Traditional Chinese Medicine acupuncture and myofascial trigger point needling: The same stimulation points? *Complementary Therapies in Medicine, 26*, 28–32.

MacGregor, J., & Graf von Schweinitz, D. (2006). Needle electromyographic activity of myofascial trigger points and control sites in equine cleidobrachialis muscle - an observational study. *Acupuncture in Medicine, 24*, 61–70.

Melzack, R. (1981). Myofascial trigger points: relation to acupuncture and mechanisms of pain. *Archives of Physical Medicine and Rehabilitation, 62*, 114–117.

Melzack, R., Stillwell, D. M., & Fox, E. J. (1977). Trigger points and acupuncture points for pain: correlations and implications. *Pain, 3*, 3–23.

Osler, W. (1912). *The principles and practice of medicine*. New York: Appleton.

Paris, S. V. (2000). A history of manipulative therapy through the ages and up to the current controversy in the United States. *The Journal of Manual & Manipulative Therapy, 8*, 66–77.

Paulett, J. D. (1947). Low back pain. *Lancet, 2*, 272–276.

Peng, P. W., & Castano, E. D. (2005). Survey of chronic pain practice by anesthesiologists in Canada. *Canadian Journal of Anaesthesia, 52*, 383–389.

Peng, Z. F., Nan, G., Cheng, M. N., & Zhou, K. H. (2016). The comparison of trigger point acupuncture and traditional acupuncture. *World Journal of Acupuncture-Moxibustion, 26*, 1–6.

QSE Consulting (2005). *Regulation of healthcare professionals; a report to the British Columbia Society for Laboratory Science and the British Columbia Association Of Medical Radiation Technologists*. Rose Bay: QSE Consulting.

Reeves, J. L., Jaeger, B., & Graff-Radford, S. B. (1986). Reliability of the pressure algometer as a measure of myofascial trigger point sensitivity. *Pain, 24*, 313–321.

Safriet, B. J. (1994). Impediments to progress in health care workforce policy: license and practice laws. *Inquiry, 31*, 310–317.

Schachinger, A., & Klarholz, C. (2017). *Equine Dry Needling: Guide for the Schachinger Method*. Amazon Digital Services.

Schmitt, M. H. (2001). Collaboration improves the quality of care: methodological challenges and evidence from US health care research. *Journal of Interprofessional Care, 15*, 47–66.

Schneider, M., Cohen, J., & Laws, S. (2001). *The collected writings of Nimmo & Vannerson; pioneers of chiropractic trigger point therapy*. Pittsburgh: Schneider.

Seem, M. D., Finando, S. J., & Weisberg, J. (1991). Segmental release therapy: trigger point needling for physical therapists. Empire State. *Physical Therapy*, 16–20.

Simons, D. (1975). Muscle pain syndromes-part I. *American Journal of Physical Medicine, 54*, 289–311.

Steenks, M. H., & de Wijer, A. (2009). Validity of the research diagnostic criteria for temporomandibular disorders Axis I in clinical and research settings. *Journal of Orofacial Pain, 23*, 9–16.

Steinbrocker, O. (1944). Therapeutic injections in painful musculoskeletal disorders. *JAMA, 125*, 397–401.

Travell, J. (1949). Basis for the multiple uses of local block of somatic trigger areas (procaine infiltration and ethyl chloride spray). *Miss Valley Med, 71*, 13–22.

Travell, J., & Rinzler, S. H. (1952). The myofascial genesis of pain. *Postgraduate Medicine, 11*, 425–434.

Travell, J. G., & Simons, D. G. (1983). *Myofascial pain and dysfunction; the trigger point manual*. Baltimore: Williams & Wilkins.

Veenman, P. (2006). Animal physiotherapy. *Journal of Bodywork and Movement Therapies, 10*, 317–327.

Veith, I. (1972). *Yellow Emperor's Classic of Internal Medicine. Revised paperback edition. Berkeley*. Los Angeles: University of California Press.

Wall, R. (2014). Introduction to myofascial trigger points in dogs. *Topics in Companion Animal Medicine, 9*, 43–48.

Zhou, K., Ma, Y., & Brogan, M. S. (2015). Dry needling versus acupuncture: the ongoing debate. *Acupuncture in Medicine, 33*, 485–490.

CHAPTER 7

Deep Dry Needling of the Head and Neck Muscles

CÉSAR FERNÁNDEZ-DE-LAS-PEÑAS • ANA ISABEL-DE-LA-LLAVE-RINCÓN •
RICARDO ORTEGA-SANTIAGO • BÁRBARA TORRES-CHICA •
JAN DOMMERHOLT

INTRODUCTION

Neck, head, and orofacial pain syndromes are among the most common problems seen in daily clinical practice. Headache is the most prevalent neurological pain disorder seen by physicians and experienced by almost everyone (Bendtsen & Jensen, 2010). Orofacial pain of muscular origin is as prevalent as headache (Svensson, 2007). The lifetime and point prevalence of neck pain are almost as high as low back pain. Neck pain affects 45%–54% of the general population at some time during their lives (Côte et al., 1998) and can result in severe disability (Côte et al., 2000). The lifetime prevalence of idiopathic neck pain has been estimated to be between 67% and 71%, indicating that approximately two-thirds of the general population will experience an episode of neck pain at some time during their life (Picavet et al., 2000). In a systematic review Fejer and colleagues (2006) found the 1-year prevalence for neck pain ranging from 16.7% to 75.1%. The economic burden of neck pain involves high annual compensation costs (Manchikanti et al., 2009).

Among the different primary headaches, migraine and frequent tension-type headache represent the most common forms (Bendtsen & Jensen, 2006). Globally, the percentage of adults with headache is 10% for migraine, 38% for tension-type headache, and 3% for chronic daily headache (Jensen & Stovner, 2008). Migraine is considered the sixth most disabling illness in the world (Migraine Research Foundation, 2018). In the US, about 18% of women, 6% of men, and 10% of children—equivalent to approximately 38 million people—suffer from migraine headaches (Bonafede et al., 2017). An estimated 4 million people suffer from daily chronic migraines (Migraine Research Foundation, 2018). The global prevalence of tension-type headaches

in the adult population is as high as 42% (Ferrante et al., 2013). A recent systematic review showed that the prevalence of nonspecific chronic headache after head injury in children was 39%, with a prevalence of chronic posttraumatic headache of 7.6%. Migraine and tension-type headaches were the most common headaches (Shaw et al., 2018).

In the general population, the prevalence rate of cervicogenic headache is reported as 4.1% (Sjaastad & Bakketeig, 2008). In patients with cervical spine disorders requiring surgery, the prevalence of cervicogenic headache was 21.4% (Shimohata et al., 2017). The prevalence of cervicogenic headache is, however, difficult to determine because current epidemiological studies have used different criteria for its diagnosis (Haldeman & Dagenais, 2001). Headaches cause substantial disability for patients and their families, as well as to global society (Stovner et al., 2007). In the US, the estimated total cost in 1998 was $14.4 billion for 22 million migraine sufferers (Hu et al., 1999). In Europe, the estimated cost was €13.8 billion for headaches in general (Raggi & Leonardi, 2015). According to the Global Burden of Disease Study (2015), headache, particularly tension-type headache, was the second most prevalent disorder in the world.

Clinically, orofacial pain is usually associated with headaches. Its prevalence is, however, under debate, with studies showing prevalence rates between 3% and 15% in the Western population (LeResche, 1997). Isong and colleagues (2008) determined that the prevalence of orofacial pain was 4.6% (6.3% for women; 2.8% for men). Neck, head, and facial pain are also common clinical manifestations of patients suffering from whiplash-associated disorders (Drottning et al., 2002). Neck injuries after motor-vehicle accidents comprised 28% of all injuries seen in emergency room departments in 2000 (Quinlan et al., 2004). In the US, the incidence rate was 4.2 per 1000 inhabitants (Sterner et al., 2003), whereas the prevalence rate was 1% (Richter et al., 2000). The annual costs of motor-vehicle crashes in the US from 1999 to 2001 were estimated at $346 billion, with $43 billion attributed to whiplash (Zaloshnja et al., 2006).

These pain syndromes have common clinical features and are often comorbid entities, suggesting a common nociceptive pathway with sensitisation mechanisms mediated through the trigeminal nucleus caudalis. The exact pathogenesis of the pain is not completely understood. Simons and colleagues (1999) described the referred pain elicited from trigger points (TrPs) in several muscles that can play a relevant role in the presentation of these syndromes. In this chapter we cover dry needling (DN) of TrPs in the head and neck musculature based on clinical and scientific reasoning.

CLINICAL PRESENTATION OF TRIGGER POINTS IN HEAD AND NECK PAIN SYNDROMES
Trigger Points in Headache and Orofacial Pain Populations

Since 2006, an increasing number of studies have confirmed the relevance of TrPs in head, neck, and face pain syndromes (Fernández-de-las-Peñas et al., 2007a; Fernández-de-las-Peñas, 2015). A recent systematic review and a meta-analysis support the presence of active TrPs in different spinal pain disorders, including mechanical neck pain and headaches (Lluch et al., 2015; Chiarotto et al., 2016). Clinicians should consider that differences in the pain characteristics of tension-type, cervicogenic, and migraine headaches may implicate different structures and mechanisms, which may be contributing to nociceptive irritation of the trigeminal nucleus caudalis. For instance, tension-type headache is characterised by pressing or tightening pain, pressure or bandlike tightness, and increased tenderness on palpation of the neck and shoulder muscles (ICHD-III, 2013), which resemble clinical descriptions of pain from TrPs (Simons et al., 1999; Gerwin, 2005; Fernández-de-las-Peñas, 2015). We summarise pertinent clinical and scientific evidence related to TrPs in head, neck, and face pain syndromes.

Myofascial trigger points in temporomandibular pain

There is scientific data that referred pain from masticatory muscles can be involved in orofacial pain syndromes (Svensson & Graven-Nielsen, 2001). Experimental studies reproduced motor and sensory disturbances, including hyperalgesia and referred pain, similar to those reported for temporomandibular pain patients after injecting irritating substances into the masseter muscle (Svensson et al., 2003a, 2003b, 2008). Svensson (2007) suggested that different muscles such as the masseter are involved in the pathophysiology of temporomandibular pain, whereas the upper trapezius and suboccipital muscles, for example, may be more common in tension-type headaches. Mortazavi and colleagues (2010) considered myofascial pain as one of the most common causes of chronic orofacial pain. Overall, few studies investigating the presence of TrPs in temporomandibular pain have been conducted. Wright (2000) found in a sample of 190 patients with temporomandibular pain that the upper trapezius (60%), lateral pterygoid (50%), and masseter (47%) muscles were the most common sources of referred pain into the craniofacial region. The cheek area, ear, and forehead were the most frequently reported sites of referred-pain generation. Unfortunately, this study did not include a control group, and patients were not examined in a blinded fashion.

Fernández-de-las-Peñas and colleagues (2010) conducted a blind-controlled study in which patients with myofascial temporomandibular (TMD) pain and healthy controls were examined for TrPs in the neck and head muscles. They found that active TrPs in the masticatory muscles—i.e., the superficial masseter (78%), temporalis (73%), and deep masseter (72%)—were more prevalent than TrPs within the neck and shoulder muscles, including the upper trapezius (64%), suboccipital (60%), and sternocleidomastoid (48%) muscles. This would be expected because masticatory TrPs are more likely to play a role in temporomandibular pain, whereas neck and shoulder TrPs would play a greater role in headaches. Alonso-Blanco and colleagues (2012) observed that women with temporomandibular pain exhibited more active TrPs in the temporalis and masseter muscles than women with fibromyalgia syndrome and that TrP referred pain areas were mostly located in the orofacial region in temporomandibular pain, but more pronounced in the cervical spine in subjects with fibromyalgia syndrome. DN of the masticatory muscles is effective for decreasing pain and increasing function in patients with bruxism (Blasco-Bonora & Martín-Pintado-Zugasti, 2017) and temporomandibular pain disorders (Dıraçoğlu et al., 2012; González-Pérez et al., 2015), which supports a potential myogenic role in these disorders. TrPs in the neck and shoulder muscles may be implicated in symptoms of the neck, which are commonly seen with patients suffering from temporomandibular pain (De Wijer et al., 1999). Preliminary evidence suggested that treatments targeting the cervical spine are beneficial in decreasing pain intensity and pressure pain sensitivity over the masticatory muscles and in increasing pain-free mouth opening in patients with myofascial TMD (La Touche et al., 2009). Botulinum toxin injections of the masseter and temporalis muscles reduced the pain in 77% of the subjects and reduced bruxism in 87%) (Connelly et al., 2017). In contrast, a systematic review showed only moderate short-term effects of botulinum injections (Khalifeh et al., 2016). Gerwin (2012) analysed why there are such discrepancies in the literature on botulinum toxin injections and TrPs and concluded that dosages, outcome measures, and timelines for assessment are commonly inappropriately selected.

Myofascial trigger points in tension-type headache

Tension-type headache (TTH) is a type of headache with clear scientific evidence of an aetiological role for TrPs (Fernández-de-las-Peñas & Schoenen, 2009; Fernández-de-las-Peñas, 2015). A scope review concluded that, among the musculoskeletal pain disorders associated with TTH, TrPs are proposed as the main physical outcome for assessing nociceptive pain mechanisms in this headache (Abboud et al., 2013). Marcus and colleagues (1999) reported that patients with TTH had a greater number of either active or latent TrPs than healthy controls; however, this study did not specify in which muscles TrPs most frequently were found.

In a series of blinded-controlled studies, Fernández-de-las-Peñas and colleagues found that active TrPs were extremely prevalent in individuals with chronic and episodic TTH. Patients with chronic TTH have active TrPs in: the extraocular superior oblique muscles (86%) (Fernández-de-las-Peñas et al., 2005a); the suboccipital muscles (65%) (Fernández-de-las-Peñas et al., 2006a); the upper trapezius muscle (50%–70%) (Fernández-de-las-Peñas et al., 2006b, 2007b); the temporalis muscle (60%–70%) (Fernández-de-las-Peñas et al., 2006b, 2007c); the sternocleidomastoid muscle (50%–60%) (Fernández-de-las-Peñas et al., 2006b); and the extraocular rectus lateralis muscles (60%) (Fernández-de-las-Peñas et al., 2009). Patients with chronic TTH and active TrPs in these muscles exhibited more severe headaches with greater intensity, frequency, and duration than patients with chronic TTH and latent TrPs in the same muscles (Fernández-de-las-Peñas et al., 2007e). Given that temporal summation of pain is centrally mediated (Vierck et al., 1997), a temporal integration of nociceptive signals from muscle TrPs by central nociceptive neurons is probable, leading to sen-

sitisation of central pathways in chronic TTH (Bendtsen & Schoenen, 2006). Couppe and colleagues (2007) also found a higher prevalence of TrPs in the upper trapezius muscle (85%) in patients with chronic TTH. In addition TrPs were found in children with chronic TTH. A case series of nine 13-year-old girls with TTH suggested that TrPs do play an important role in at least a subgroup of children with TTH (Von Stülpnagel et al., 2009). These girls received TrP treatments twice a week. After 6.5 sessions, the headache frequency was reduced by 67.7%, the intensity by 74.3%, and the mean duration by 77.3% (Von Stülpnagel et al., 2009). In a blinded-controlled study, Fernández-de-las-Peñas and colleagues (2011a) reported that in children with chronic TTH and a mean age of 8, the suboccipital (80%), the temporalis (54%), the ocular superior oblique (28%–30%), the upper trapezius (20%), and the sternocleidomastoid (12%–26%) muscles harbored most TrPs. Active TrPs have also been reported in episodic TTH but less frequently. The most common muscles with active TrPs included: the superior oblique muscle (15%) (Fernández-de-las-Peñas et al., 2005a); the suboccipital muscles (60%) (Fernández-de-las-Peñas et al., 2006c); the sternocleidomastoid (20%); the temporalis (45%); and the upper trapezius muscle (35%) (Fernández-de-las-Peñas et al., 2007d). Another study confirmed that active TrPs are more prevalent in chronic TTH than in episodic TTH (Sohn et al., 2010). The association of active TrPs with episodic TTH does not support the hypothesis that active TrPs are always a consequence of central sensitisation because central sensitisation is not as common in episodic TTH as in chronic TTH (Fernández-de-las-Peñas et al., 2006d). Not included in this study are TrPs located in other muscles, such as the masseter, splenius capitis, scalene, levator scapulae muscles, which may also contribute to the pain symptoms in individuals with TTH. Current evidence suggests that TrP referred pain and associated muscle hyperalgesia seem to be clinically important factors in TTH. Damping the nociceptive peripheral drive may not only reduce the number of TTH attacks but may also prevent or delay the transition from episodic into chronic TTH or both (Arendt-Nielsen et al., 2016). Recently this hypothesis has been confirmed by a study demonstrating that the number of active and latent TrPs was significantly and negatively associated with widespread pressure pain hypersensitivity in patients with frequent episodic or chronic TTH (Palacios-Ceña et al., 2016).

Finally, a few studies explored the effects of the treatment of TrP in patients with chronic TTH. Moraska and Chandler (2008) demonstrated in a pilot study that a structured massage program targeted at inactivating TrPs was effective for reducing headache pain and disability in individuals with TTH; however, this study did not include a control group. The same authors reported that a TrP massage program improved psychological measures, particularly depression and the number of events deemed as stressful (Moraska & Chandler, 2009). Moraska and colleagues (2015) found that the manual therapy treatment of TrP in cervical muscles was effective in reducing headache in a sample of TTH, but there was also a placebo effect of TrP manual therapy.

Fernández-de-las-Peñas and colleagues (2008) developed a preliminary clinical prediction rule to identify women with chronic TTH who would most likely experience short-term favourable outcomes after TrP manual therapy. Four variables were identified for immediate success and two for 1-month success (Table 7.1). If all variables (4 + LR: 5.9) were present, the chance of experiencing immediate benefit from TrP treatment improved from 54% to 87.4% (Fernández-de-las-Peñas et al., 2008). However, a limitation of this study was its relatively small sample size (n = 35). A second clinical prediction rule in which women with chronic TTH received

a multimodal therapy session identified eight variables for short-term success (Fernández-de-las-Peñas et al., 2011b). The variables are listed in Table 7.2. If five of the eight variables (5 + LR: 7.1) were present, the chance of experiencing successful treatment improved from 47% to 86.3% (Fernández-de-las-Peñas et al., 2011b). Therapeutic procedures included both joint mobilisations to the cervical and thoracic spine and soft tissue TrP therapies such as soft tissue stroking, pressure release, and muscle energy techniques applied to the neck, head, and shoulder musculature and to the temporalis, suboccipital, upper trapezius, sternocleidomastoid, and splenius capitis muscles (Fernández-de-las-Peñas et al., 2011b). These clinical prediction rules support the role of TrPs in the management of TTH; however, further studies are needed to validate the current data.

There are a small number of studies investigating the effects of DN and TTH. De Abreu Venâncio and colleagues (2008) compared the effects of TrP injections using lidocaine to TrP DN in the management of headaches of myofascial origin. They found that TrP DN was equally effective for decreasing the intensity, the frequency, and the duration of the headache and

---

TABLE 7.1

Variables Identified for Immediate Success (Top) and for 1-Month Success (Bottom), Including Accuracy Statistics With 95% Confidence Intervals for Each Variable

- Headache duration (hours per day) (< 8.5)
- Headache frequency (< 5.5)
- Body pain (< 47) from the SF-36 questionnaire
- Vitality (< 47.5) from the SF-36 questionnaire

Number of Predictor Variables Present	Sensitivity	Specificity	Positive Likelihood Ratio	Probability of Success (%)
4 +	0.37 (0.17, 0.61)	0.94 (0.68, 0.99)	5.9 (0.80, 42.9)	87.4
3 +	0.84 (0.60, 0.96)	0.75 (0.47, 0.92)	3.4 (1.4, 8.0)	80.0
2 +	0.94 (0.72, 0.99)	0.19 (0.05, 0.50)	1.2 (9.0, 1.5)	58.5
1 +	1.0 (0.79, 1.0)	0.12 (0.02, 0.41)	1.1 (0.95, 1.4)	56.4

- Headache frequency (< 5.5)
- Bodily pain (< 47) from the SF-36 questionnaire

Number of Predictor Variables Present	Sensitivity	Specificity	Positive Likelihood Ratio	Probability of Success (%)
2 +	0.58 (0.34, 0.79)	0.88 (0.60, 0.98)	4.6 (1.2, 17.9)	84.4
1 +	0.95 (0.72, 0.99)	0.56 (0.31, 0.79)	2.2 (1.2, 3.8)	72.1

The probability of success is calculated using the positive likelihood ratios and assumes a pretest probability of 54%.
From: Fernández-de-las-Peñas, C., Cleland, J.A., Cuadrado, M.L., Pareja, J. (2008). Predictor variables for identifying patients with chronic tension type headache who are likely to achieve short-term success with muscle trigger point therapy. *Cephalalgia, 28*, 264–275.

TABLE 7.2

Variables Identified for Immediate Success Including Accuracy Statistics With 95% Confidence Intervals for Each Variable Success

- Age, mean < 44.5 years
- Presence left sternocleidomastoid muscle TrP
- Presence suboccipital muscle TrPs
- Presence of left superior oblique muscle TrP
- Cervical rotation to the left > 69 degrees
- Total tenderness score < 20.5
- Neck Disability Index < 18.5
- Referred pain area of right upper trapezius muscle TrP > 42.23

Number of Predictor Variables Present	Sensitivity	Specificity	Positive Likelihood Ratio	Probability of Success (%)
8	0.1 (0.01, 0.2)	1.0 (0.89, 1.0)	∞	100
7 +	0.22 (0.10, 0.40)	1.0 (0.89, 1.0)	∞	100
6 +	0.53 (0.36, 0.69)	1.0 (0.89, 1.0)	∞	100
5 +	0.89 (0.73, 0.96)	0.88 (0.72, 0.95)	7.1 (3.1, 16.3)	86.3
4 +	0.97 (0.84, 0.99)	0.7 (0.53, 0.83)	3.2 (2.0, 5.2)	73.94
3 +	1 (0.87, 1.0)	0.23 (0.11, 0.39)	1.3 (1.1, 1.5)	53.6
2 +*				
1 +*				

The probability of success is calculated using the positive likelihood ratios and assumes a pretest probability of 47%.

*Unable to calculate as all subjects met 1 and 2 variables.

From: Fernández-de-las-Peñas, C., Cleland, J.A., Palomeque-del-Cerro, L., et al. (2011b). Development of a clinical prediction rule for identifying women with tension-type headache who are likely to achieve short-term success with joint mobilization and muscle trigger point therapy. *Headache, 51*, 246–261.

for the use of rescue medication than injections using lidocaine alone or combined with corticoids. In another study the same authors reported that TrP DN was equally effective as botulinum toxin A for decreasing the intensity, the frequency, and duration of the pain, but DN was less effective for the use of rescue medication (De Abreu Venâncio et al., 2009). These results are similar to those by Harden and associates (2009), who reported that patients who received botulinum toxin A injections over active TrPs experienced reductions in headache frequency in the short term, but the effects dissipated by week 12. Headache intensity also revealed a decrease in the botulinum toxin A group, but not in the control group (Harden et al., 2009). Therefore although TrP DN is proposed as a potential effective treatment for headaches (Kietrys et al., 2014; Fernández-de-las-Peñas & Cuadrado, 2016), there are only a small number of studies investigating this topic (France et al., 2014). It is interesting to note that the American Headache Society has recently accepted the use of TrP injections for the management of many types

of headaches (Robbins et al., 2014), supporting that myofascial TrPs seem to be relevant for headaches.

Myofascial trigger points in migraine headache

TrPs have also been found in patients with migraine headache. In unilateral migraines, active TrPs in the upper trapezius (30%), sternocleidomastoid (45%), and temporalis (40%) muscles were located only on the symptomatic side (Fernández-de-las-Peñas et al., 2006e). TrPs in the extraocular superior oblique muscle (50%) were present in the symptomatic, but not in the nonsymptomatic side (Fernández-de-las-Peñas et al., 2006f). A study of 92 patients with bilateral migraine showed that 94% exhibited TrPs in the temporalis and suboccipital muscles compared with 29% of controls (Calandre et al., 2006). The number of TrPs was related to the frequency of migraine headaches and the duration of the disease (Calandre et al., 2006). A recent study noted that the presence of TrPs was similar between women with episodic or chronic migraine supporting a role in the chronification of this headache (Ferracini et al., 2017).

Referred pain from active TrPs reproduced the pain features of migraine headache (Giamberardino et al., 2007; Fernández-de-las-Peñas et al., 2006e). Nevertheless, an association of TrPs with migraine does not necessarily constitute a causal relationship. The presence of TrPs indicates that peripheral nociceptive input from TrPs into the trigeminal nucleus may act as a migraine trigger. A link between pain generators of the neck, head, and shoulder muscles and migraine attacks may be the activation of the trigeminal nerve nucleus caudalis, and hence the activation of the trigemino-vascular system. In such instance, TrPs located in any muscle innervated by the trigeminal nerve or the upper cervical nerves may be considered as 'irritative thorns' that can precipitate, perpetuate, or aggravate migraine. Obviously, other triggers also exist for migraine.

Evidence supporting a triggering role of TrPs in migraine comes from the resolution of migraine headache by treating TrPs in neck and shoulder muscles with lidocaine or saline injections (Tfelt-Hansen et al., 1981). In addition, inactivation of active TrPs in migraine patients not only reduced the electrical pain threshold in the headache area of pain referral, but also reduced the number of headache attacks over the 60 days of the treatment period (Giamberardino et al., 2007). Garcia-Leiva and colleagues (2007) reported that TrP injection with ropivacaine (10 mg) was effective for reducing frequency and intensity of migraine attacks. The combination of TrP treatment and medication was more effective than medication alone for the management of migraine (Ghanbari et al., 2015). Sollmann and colleagues (2016) conducted a pilot study, examining the potential of peripheral magnetic stimulation of the upper treatment for the treatment of headaches, and they found a significant decrease in the number of migraine attacks, in the migraine intensity, and a reduction in analgesic medication usage when comparing the pre- and poststimulation assessments.

Myofascial trigger points in other headaches

TrPs have been also investigated in other headaches, such as cervicogenic and cluster headaches. Jaeger (1989) found in a cohort of 11 individuals with cervicogenic headache that all patients showed at least three TrPs on the symptomatic side, especially in the sternocleidomastoid and temporalis muscles. Patients who were treated reported a significant decrease in their headache frequency and intensity, which supports the role of TrPs in headache pain perception in this headache disorder (Jaeger, 1989). Roth and colleagues (2007) described a case report in which pain from TrPs in the sternocleidomastoid muscle mimicked the symptoms of cervicogenic headache. In a small clinical trial, Bodes-Pardo and colleagues (2013) found that manual therapy targeted to active TrPs in the sternocleidomastoid muscle may be effective for reducing headache and neck pain intensity and increasing motor performance in cervicogenic headache pain. Although TrPs can contribute to pain of cervicogenic headaches, it seems that referred pain from the upper cervical joints is the main source (Aprill et al., 2002). It is conceivable that the potential role of TrPs has not yet been properly studied in cervicogenic headache pain. Therefore further studies are required to elucidate the role of TrPs in this headache disorder.

Calandre and colleagues (2008) studied the presence of TrPs in 12 patients with cluster headaches. All patients showed active TrPs reproducing their headache. In this case series TrP injection was successful in about 80% of the patients. The authors suggested that, in some patients, TrPs may trigger cluster headaches (Calandre et al., 2008). In a systematic review, Ashkenazi and colleagues (2010) reported few controlled studies on the efficacy of peripheral nerve blocks and almost none on the use of TrP injections. They concluded that the technique, the type, and the doses of the anaesthetics used for nerve blockade varied greatly among studies, but, in general, the results were positive. Nevertheless this finding should be considered with caution due to the limitations of the included studies (Ashkenazi et al., 2010).

Trigger Points in Neck Pain Populations

Neck pain can have a traumatic or an insidious onset. A traumatic onset is seen, for example, after a whiplash injury (Dommerholt, 2005, 2010). An example of an insidious cause is mechanical neck pain, which is defined as generalised neck or shoulder pain with symptoms provoked by neck postures, by movement, or by palpation of the cervical muscles. Fernández-de-las-Peñas and colleagues (2007f) found that patients with mechanical insidious neck pain exhibited active TrPs in the upper trapezius (20%), the sternocleidomastoid (14%), the suboccipital (50%), and the levator scapulae (15%) muscles. A recent population-based study observed that active TrPs in the upper trapezius muscle were the most prevalent (94%), followed by TrPs in the levator scapulae (82%), multifidi (78%), and splenius cervicis (62.5%) muscles in patients with mechanical neck pain (Cerezo-Téllez et al., 2016a). The presence of TrPs in the upper trapezius muscle has been associated with the presence of cervical joint dysfunction at the levels of the C3 and C4 vertebrae in individuals suffering from neck pain (Fernández-de-las-Peñas et al., 2005b).

Therefore clinicians should include the assessment and treatment of joint mobility in the management of TrPs in individuals with mechanical neck pain (Fernández-de-las-Peñas 2009). Jung and colleagues (2016) recommended making a diagnosis of laryngeal myofascial pain when voice symptoms improve after needling of the intrinsic laryngeal muscles, combined with an unusual sensation during the needling procedure reminiscent of a local twitch response, a vocal fold movement abnormality, a history of voice abuse, and the absence of a vocal fold mucosal or neurological disorder. Researchers from Israel and the US examined the referred pain patterns of latent TrPs in the longus colli muscle in 35 healthy physicians attending a postgraduate course on DN. Although the subjects were not naïve concerning the topic, possibly introducing a bias, they found that TrP in the longus colli muscle feature mostly anterior local pain, but also included referred pain to the ipsilateral ear. A small percentage of subjects reported pain referral to the contralateral side or to the ipsilateral posterior cervical spine and occiput (Minerbi et al., 2017).

There is some evidence of the effectiveness of TrPs manual techniques in the management of mechanical neck pain. For instance, Montañez-Aguilera and colleagues (2010) reported that an ischemic compression technique was effective in the treatment of TrPs in a patient with neck pain. Bablis and colleagues (2008) found that the application of Neuro Emotional Technique, a technique incorporating central and peripheral components to alleviate the effects of distressing stimuli, may be effective for reducing pain and mechanical sensitivity over TrPs in patients with chronic neck pain. Ay and colleagues (2017) studied the effectiveness of kinesio taping on cervical myofascial pain and concluded that there was a significant improvement for pain and cervical flexion and extension, but not for cervical rotations and lateroflexion. In a comparative study of active and passive treatments of latent TrPs in the upper trapezius muscle, Kojidi and colleagues (2016) found that both approaches significantly decreased the sensitivity of myofascial TPs, increased flexibility of muscle fibres, and improved range of motion. In another study, non-thrust mobilisation techniques directed to the cervical spine and scapula were effective in pain reduction, with 3-month follow up assessments (Yildirim et al., 2016). A Spanish study showed a similar reduction of chronic neck pain using either DN and stretching, TrP compression combined with massage, or upper cervical anterior–posterior mobilisation, lateral glides to C4-C5, and a neural thoracic mobilisation (Campa-Moran et al., 2015). Ganesh and colleagues (2016) confirmed

that manual TrP therapy of the upper trapezius muscle and cervical mobilisations can be effective.

Different studies have reported that DN is effective for improving pain and related disability in individuals with nonspecific neck pain (Mejuto-Vázquez et al., 2014; Gerber et al., 2015; Cerezo-Téllez et al., 2016b), but no clear differences exist between manual therapy and DN for the management of mechanical neck pain (Llamas-Ramos et al., 2014; De Meulemeester et al., 2017). This is further supported by a few systematic reviews (Caigne et al., 2015; Liu et al., 2015). León-Hernández and colleagues (2016) established that the combination of percutaneous electrical stimulation and DN was more effective than DN alone to reduce pain in patients with chronic myofascial neck pain. Shanmugam and Mathias (2017) noted an immediate effect on pain and range of motion with DN in patients with acute facet joint lock, but they did not include a control group in their study. In another study, Ma and colleagues (2010) demonstrated that a miniscalpel-needle release was superior for reducing pain in patients with TrPs in the upper trapezius muscle compared with an acupuncture needling treatment or self-neck stretching exercises.

TrPs have been also associated with neck pain of traumatic origin, such as whiplash-associated neck pain (Dommerholt, 2005, 2010; Dommerholt et al., 2005). Schuller and associates (2000) found that 80% of 1096 individuals involved in low-velocity collisions reported muscle pain. In a review of the literature, Fernández-de-las-Peñas and colleagues found that the muscles most commonly affected by TrPs were the scalene muscles (Gerwin & Dommerholt, 1998), the splenius capitis, the upper trapezius, the posterior neck, the sternocleidomastoid (Baker, 1986), and the pectoralis minor muscles (Hong & Simons, 1993). Ettlin and colleagues (2008) reported that semispinalis capitis muscle TrPs were more frequent in patients with whiplash-associated neck pain (85%) than in patients with nontraumatic neck pain (35%) or fibromyalgia (57%). TrPs in the upper trapezius (70%–80%), the levator scapulae (60%–70%), the sternocleidomastoid (40%–50%), and the masseter (20%–30%) muscles were similar among these pain groups.

The longus colli muscles are commonly involved in whiplash injuries (Elliott, et al., 2010, 2011), as they are the farthest removed from the axis of rotation of the cervical spine and therefore prone to significant strain and deformation. Peterson and colleagues (2015) confirmed that after whiplash, deformation and deformation rates of the longus coli, sternocleidomastoid, and longus capitis muscles are altered. Whiplash injuries often result in weakness of the longus colli muscles (Prushansky et al., 2005; Pearson et al., 2009), greater rates of cervical instability, a reversal of the cervical lordosis, vertigo (Liu et al., 2017), and a loss of muscular endurance (Kumbhare et al., 2005). The longus colli muscle appears to play a key role in stabilisation of the cervical spine (Kettler et al., 2002), posture, and maintaining the cervical lordosis (Mayoux-Benhamou et al., 1994), but the exact mechanisms are not well understood (Kennedy et al., 2017).

Fernández-Pérez and colleagues (2012) observed that individuals with acute whiplash-associated neck pain exhibited a higher prevalence of active TrPs in the levator scapulae and upper trapezius muscles and that the number of active TrPs increased with higher neck pain intensity and the number of days since the accident. Additionally it seems that active TrPs are more prevalent in whiplash-associated neck pain than in mechanical neck pain (Castaldo et al., 2014). The presence of TrPs in individuals with whiplash-associated neck pain can be related to the fact that these patients usually exhibit reduced cervical stability, muscle inhibition, and hyperirritability of the cervical muscles (Headley, 2005).

Finally, a few studies have demonstrated the effects of TrP inactivation in patients with whiplash-associated neck pain. Freeman and colleagues (2009) showed that infiltrations of 1% lidocaine into TrPs in the upper trapezius were effective in the short term for increasing cervical range of motion and pressure pain thresholds in individuals with chronic whiplash-associated pain. Carroll and colleagues (2008) reported that injections of botulinum toxin type A of cervical TrPs decreased pain in patients with chronic whiplash-related neck pain. A recent randomised clinical trial reported that DN and exercise was more effective than sham DN and exercise in reducing disability at 6 and 12 months in individuals with chronic whiplash-related neck pain, although its clinical relevance was questioned (Sterling et al., 2015).

DRY NEEDLING OF HEAD MUSCLES
Corrugator Supercilii Muscle
- *Anatomy:* The corrugator supercilii muscle arises from the medial end of the superciliary arch. Its fibres pass upward and lateral between the palpebral and orbital portions of the orbicularis oculi and are inserted into the deep surface of the skin, above the middle of the orbital arch.
- *Function:* The corrugator supercilii muscle draws the eyebrow downward and medially, furrowing the forehead.

- *Innervation:* Temporal branches of the facial nerve (VII par cranial).
- *Referred pain:* TrPs in the corrugator supercilii muscle refer pain into the forehead and deep into the head, inducing frontal headaches.
- *Needling technique:* The patient lies in supine position. The muscle is needled with a pincer palpation. The needle is inserted perpendicular to the skin from either the medial or the lateral aspect of the muscle, directed towards its midportion. The needle is inserted through the skin at a shallow angle, and advanced into the muscle belly (Fig. 7.1).
- *Precautions:* The eyebrows are well vascularised, and to avoid bleeding with needling, the needle should be placed close to the skull underneath the fleshy part of the eyebrows.

Procerus Muscle
- *Anatomy:* The procerus muscle arises from the fascia overlying the surface of the nasal bones and the superior parts of the upper lateral nasal cartilages and inserts into the skin of the inferior and medial forehead.
- *Function:* The procerus muscle wrinkles the skin of the bridge of the nose.
- *Innervation:* Buccal branches of the facial nerve (VII par cranial).
- *Referred pain:* TrP in the procerus muscle refer to the forehead and possibly deep into the head, inducing frontal headaches.
- *Needling technique:* The patient lies in supine position. The muscle is needled with a pincer palpation. The needle is inserted perpendicular to the skin from superior to inferior, coming from the forehead towards the nose, or from lateral to medial. The needle is inserted through the skin at a shallow angle and advanced into the muscle belly (Fig. 7.2).
- *Precautions:* None

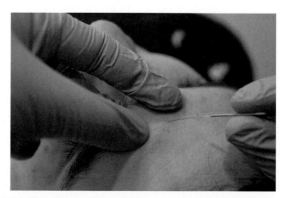

FIG. 7.1 Dry needling of the corrugator supercilii muscle.

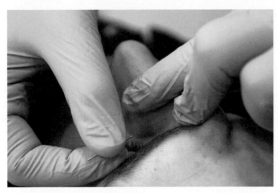

FIG. 7.2 Dry needling of the procerus muscle.

Masseter Muscle

- *Anatomy:* The masseter muscle extends from the inferior aspect of zygomatic process to the angle and lateral surface of the mandible (superficial layer); the midportion of the mandibular ramus (middle layer); and to the upper mandibular ramus and the coronoid process (deep layer).
- *Function:* The masseter muscle closes the mouth by elevating the mandible and can contribute to ipsilateral excursion of the mandible. The superficial layer also has a component of protrusion of the mandible, whereas the deep layer has a component of retraction.
- *Innervation:* Mandibular branch (V3) of the trigeminal nerve (V par cranial).
- *Referred pain:* The superficial layer refers pain to the eyebrow and retroorbital area, the maxilla, the anterior aspect of the mandible, and the upper or lower molar teeth. TrPs in the deep layer spread pain deep into the ear and to the temporomandibular joint area.

- *Needling technique:* The patient lies in supine position. The muscle is usually needled with a flat palpation, although it is also possible to treat the masseter muscle with an intraoral pincer palpation, whereby the palpating finger is placed inside the mouth against the buccal mucosa with two fingers on the external surface of the skin bracing the TrP. The needle is inserted perpendicular to the skin towards the TrP (Fig. 7.3).
- *Precautions:* None

Temporalis Muscle

- *Anatomy:* The temporalis muscle extends from the temporal fossa (except that portion of it which is formed by the zygomatic bone) to the anterior border of the mandibular coronoid process and to the anterior border of the ramus of the mandible.
- *Function:* The temporalis muscle closes the mouth by elevating the mandible. The temporalis muscle also helps lateral deviation of the mandible to the same side and is instrumental in the details of mouth closing.
- *Innervation:* Mandibular branch (V3) of the trigeminal nerve (V par cranial).
- *Referred pain:* TrPs in the temporalis muscle refer deep in the temporoparietal region and inside the head, contributing to temporal headache and maxillary toothache.
- *Needling technique:* The patient is in supine position. The muscle is needled with a flat palpation. The needle is fixed with the index and middle fingers of the nonneedling hand and then inserted perpendicular to the skin towards the TrP (Fig. 7.4).
- *Precautions:* The superficial temporal artery should be identified and avoided.

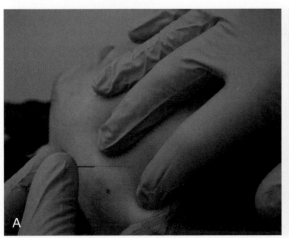
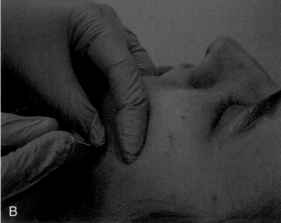

FIG. 7.3 Dry needling of the masseter muscle.

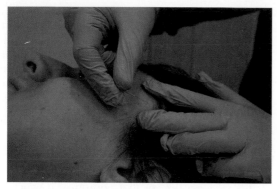

FIG. 7.4 Dry needling of the temporalis muscle.

Zygomatic Muscle

- *Anatomy:* The zygomatic major and minor muscles extend from the zygomatic bone and insert into the muscles of the mouth, including the orbicularis oris, the levator, and the depressor anguli oris.
- *Function:* The zygomatic muscles elevate the angle of the mouth as in smiling.
- *Innervation:* Facial nerve (VII par cranial).
- *Referred pain:* TrPs in the zygomatic muscles refer to the nose and forehead, and pain is perceived in an arc close to the side of the nose up to the forehead.
- *Needling technique:* The patient is in supine position. The zygomatic muscle can be needled with flat palpation or with an intraoral pincer palpation. The needle is inserted perpendicular to the skin towards the zygomatic bone using flat palpation. It is also possible to treat the zygomatic muscles with an intraoral pincer palpation, whereby the palpating finger is placed inside the mouth against the buccal

mucosa with two fingers on the external surface of the skin bracing the TrP (Fig. 7.5).
- *Precautions:* None

Buccinator and Risorius Muscles

- *Anatomy:* The buccinator muscle forms the lateral wall of the oral cavity and attaches laterally to a pterygomandibular raphe, a tendinous inscription connecting the buccinator muscle with the more posterior superior pharyngeal constrictor muscle. Some fibres may attach to the maxilla and the mandible. The risorius muscle attaches to the parotid fascia over the fascia. Kim and colleagues (2015) identified three distinct variations of the risorius muscle, including the zygomaticus risorius, platysma risorius, and triangularis risorius muscles; the platysma risorius muscle was the most common variation. Anteriorly the buccinator and risorius muscles merge into the fibres of the orbicularis oris muscle. According to Kim and colleagues (2015), the risorius muscle attaches closely to the depressor anguli oris muscle in three distinct layers.
- *Function:* The buccinator muscle is one of the first muscles a baby can more or less control as the muscle is responsible for the sucking reflex. The risorius muscle is primarily a muscle of facial expression, especially smiling. Both muscles are involved in speech, vocalisations, chewing, whistling, and playing a wind instrument. For wind instrumentalists, these muscles are of prime importance and considered to be part of what is referred to as the embouchure, or the coordinated control of the facial muscles required to play the instrument.
- *Innervation:* Buccal branch of facial nerve (N. VII).

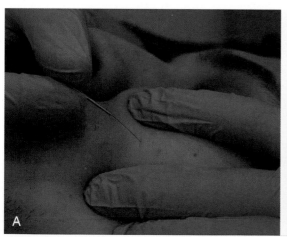
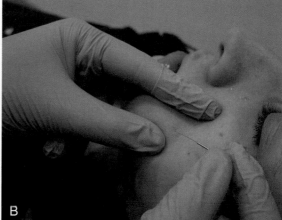

FIG. 7.5 Dry needling of the zygomatic muscle.

- *Referred pain:* TrPs in the buccinator muscle refer pain deep to the cheek experienced as an aching sensation underneath the zygomatic arch. The referred pain pattern of TrPs in the risorius muscle has not been described.
- *Needling technique:* The patient is in supine position. The buccinator and risorius muscle can be needled with flat palpation or with an intraoral pincer palpation. The needle is inserted perpendicular to the skin using flat palpation (Fig. 7.6). It is also possible to treat the muscles with an intraoral pincer palpation, whereby the palpating finger is placed inside the mouth against the buccal mucosa with two fingers on the external surface of the skin bracing the TrP similarly to the zygomaticus approach.
- *Precautions:* None

Superior Pharyngeal Constrictor Muscle

- *Anatomy:* The superior pharyngeal constrictor muscle originates anteriorly from the pterygoid hamulus, with occasional attachments to the posterior margin of the medial pterygoid plate, the pterygomandibular raphe, the mylohyoid line of the mandible, and the side of the tongue and it attaches to the pharyngeal tubercle of basilar part of the occiput. The posterior and lateral walls of the oropharynx are enclosed by the superior pharyngeal constrictor muscle.
- *Function:* The superior pharyngeal constrictor muscle constricts the upper part of the pharynx and assists in moving a bolus of food into the oesophagus, but it can also exert force on the mandible via its connections to the buccinator muscle.
- *Innervation:* The cranial part of the accessory nerve from the pharyngeal plexus.

- *Referred pain:* Rocabado (1983) described a 'buccinator aponeurosis pharyngeal syndrome' characterised by retrusion of the mandible and posterior cranial rotation, with three primary areas of pain, including ipsilateral posterior condylar pain, suboccipital pain, and pain in the buccinator pharyngeal aponeurosis pain. Ernest (2006) reported pain at the superior lateral pharynx, pain at the medial edge of the temporomandibular joint, ear aches, temporal pain, soreness and pain on swallowing, and dyscoordination of the swallowing reflex. Referred pain patterns of TrPs in the superior pharyngeal constrictor muscle have not yet been described.
- *Needling technique:* The superior pharyngeal constrictor muscle can be needled immediately posterior to the pterygomandibular raphe and the buccinator muscle underneath the anterior aspect of the superficial masseter muscle (Fig. 7.7).
- *Precautions:* None

Medial Pterygoid Muscle

- *Anatomy:* The medial pterygoid muscle originates on the medial surface of the lateral pterygoid plate of the sphenoid bone, the maxillary tuberosity, and the pyramidal process of the palatine bone and inserts into the lower back part of the medial surface of the ramus and angle of the mandible.
- *Function:* The medial pterygoid muscle closes the mouth by elevating the mandible. It has a component of retraction of the mandible.
- *Innervation:* Medial pterygoid nerve, via the mandibular branch (V3) of the trigeminal nerve (V par cranial).
- *Referred pain:* TrPs in the medial pterygoid muscle refer to poorly circumscribed areas in the mouth, including the tongue, hard palate, and pharynx, but also deep into the ear and the throat.

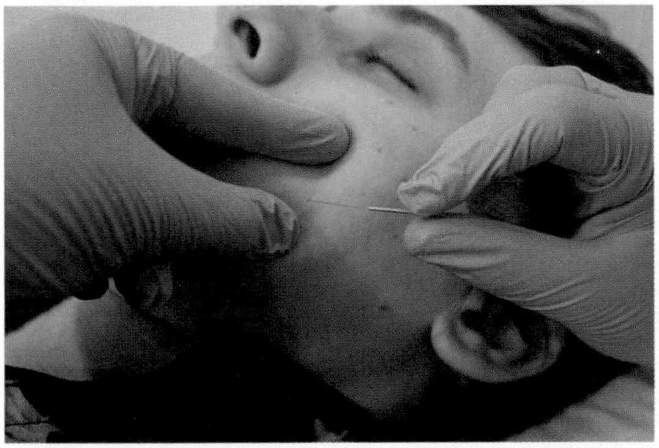

FIG. 7.6 Dry needling of the buccinator and risorius muscles.

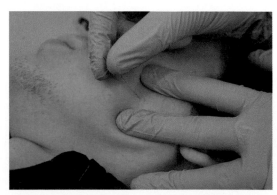

FIG. 7.7 Dry needling of the superior pharyngeal constrictor muscle.

- *Needling technique:* The patient is in supine position. The muscle can be needled in its superior–medial or inferior–lateral part. The superior–medial part of the muscle is needled through the mandibular fossa, similar to needling the inferior lateral pterygoid muscle (Fig. 7.8). With a flat palpation, the needle is fixed between the index and middle fingers of the nonneedling hand and inserted through the skin at a shallow angle towards the medial surface of the ramus and angle of the mandible (Fig. 7.9). This approach is similar to needling TrPs in the supraspinatus and the iliacus muscles.
- *Precautions:* Avoid needling the lingual nerve with the superior–medial approach and the alveolar nerve with the inferior–lateral approach.

Lateral Pterygoid Muscle

- *Anatomy:* The superior lateral pterygoid muscle arises from the infratemporal surface of the greater wing of the sphenoid bone, and the inferior lateral pterygoid muscle arises from the lateral surface of the lateral pterygoid plate. The inferior head attaches to the neck of the mandible. Two types of attachments have been identified for the superior head (Omami & Lurie, 2012). With the Type 1 insertion, the superior head attaches only to the intraarticular disc, whereas with the Type 2 insertion, it attaches to the disc and condyle (Omami & Lurie, 2012). The lateral pterygoid muscle also attaches to the intraarticular cartilage of the temporomandibular joint.
- *Function:* The superior division of the lateral pterygoid muscle may play a role in the positioning of the intraarticular disc. Both heads contribute to protrusion and contralateral deviation of the mandible. The inferior head may initiate mouth opening even before the digastric muscles are activated (Moyers, 1950).
- *Innervation:* Lateral pterygoid nerve, via the mandibular branch (V3) of the trigeminal nerve (V par cranial).
- *Referred pain:* TrPs in the lateral pterygoid muscle project to the maxilla and the temporomandibular joint.
- *Needling technique:* The patient is in supine position. For the superior division, the needle is inserted perpendicular to the skin through the mandibular fossa, which is located anterior to the temporomandibular joint and posterior to the coronoid process. The needle is directed superior–medial-forward direction underneath the zygomatic arch towards the sphenoid bone (Fig. 7.10). Using an alternate approach, the needle is inserted above the zygomatic arch just behind the eye socket and directed in an inferior direction (Fig. 7.11). For the inferior division, the patient needs to open the mouth slightly. The needle is inserted perpendicular to the skin through the mandibular fossa and directed towards in a medial-forward direction towards the sphenoid bone (Fig. 7.12).

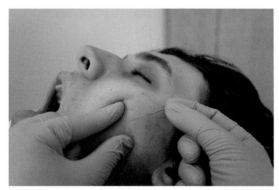

FIG. 7.8 Dry needling of the medial pterygoid muscle through the mandibular fossa.

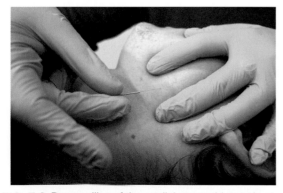

FIG. 7.9 Dry needling of the medial pterygoid muscle at the mandible.

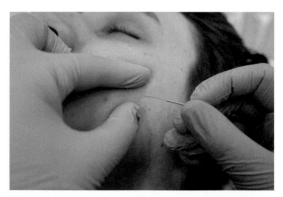

FIG. 7.10 Dry needling of the superior division of the lateral pterygoid muscle through the mandibular fossa.

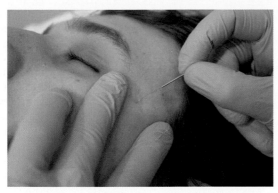

FIG. 7.11 Dry needling of the superior division of the lateral pterygoid muscle behind the zygomatic bone.

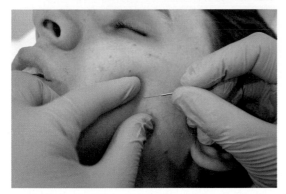

FIG. 7.12 Dry needling of the inferior division of the lateral pterygoid muscle.

- *Precautions:* The maxillary artery overlies the lateral pterygoid muscle and should be avoided by needling close to the coronoid process. In patients taking anticoagulants, extra caution is warranted as it is not possible to apply hemostasis after the needling procedure. Use of sonography in Doppler mode can accurately locate the maxillary artery. Needling the temporomandibular joint can easily be avoided by accurately locating the mandibular fossa and needling slightly posterior to the coronoid process.

Digastric Muscles

- *Anatomy:* The posterior digastric muscle arises from the mastoid notch at the mastoid process of the temporal bone at the digastric groove, whereas the anterior digastric muscle arises from the inferior border of the mandible, close to its symphysis. The two muscles are joined together by a common tendon that is indirectly anchored to the hyoid bone through a fibrous loop.

- *Function:* The digastric muscles protrude and open the mouth by descending the mandible.
- *Innervation:* Digastric branch, via the facial nerve (VII par cranial) for the posterior digastric muscle; and mylohyoid nerve, via the mandibular branch (V3) of the trigeminal nerve (V par cranial) for the anterior digastric muscle.
- *Referred pain:* TrPs in the posterior digastric muscle refer pain to the upper part of the sternocleidomastoid muscle, whereas TrPs in the anterior digastric muscle project pain to the four lower incisor teeth.
- *Needling technique:* The patient is in supine. For the posterior digastric muscle, the needle is directed towards the mastoid process using a flat palpation technique (Fig. 7.13). For the anterior belly the head and neck of the patient are slightly extended. The muscle is then needled with a flat palpation technique. The TrP is fixed between the index and middle fingers of the nonneedling hand, and the needle is inserted perpendicular to the skin (Fig. 7.14).

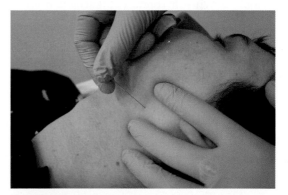

FIG. 7.13 Dry needling of the posterior belly of the digastric muscle.

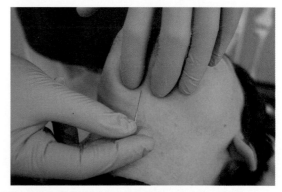

FIG. 7.14 Dry needling of the anterior belly of the digastric muscle.

- *Precautions:* When needling the posterior digastric muscle, avoid the external jugular vein. To avoid needling through the very thin muscles, a superficial to slowly deeper needling technique is recommended.

DRY NEEDLING OF NECK–SHOULDER MUSCLES

Several of the shoulder muscles are reviewed in Chapters 8 and 10.

Trapezius Muscle: Upper Portion

- *Anatomy:* The superior region (descending part) of the trapezius muscle arises from the external occipital protuberance, the medial third of the superior nuchal line of the occipital bone, the ligamentum nuchae, and the spinous process of C7 and inserts into the posterior border of the lateral third of the clavicle.
- *Function:* When the upper trapezius contracts unilaterally, it induces ipsilateral sidebending and contralateral rotation of the head and elevation of the shoulder. When it contracts bilaterally, it extends the neck.
- *Innervation:* Accessory nerve (XI par cranial) and cervical spinal nerves C3-C4.
- *Referred pain:* TrPs in the upper trapezius muscle refer pain ipsilaterally from the posterior–lateral region of the neck, behind the ear, and to the temporal region.
- *Needling technique:* The patient is in sidelying, prone, or supine position. The muscle is needled with a pincer palpation. The needle is inserted perpendicular to the skin and directed towards the practitioner's finger. The needle is kept between the fingers in the shoulder. The needle can be inserted from anterior to posterior (Fig. 7.15) or posterior to anterior

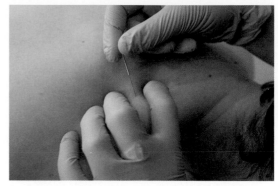

FIG. 7.16 Dry needling of the upper portion of the trapezius muscle in prone position.

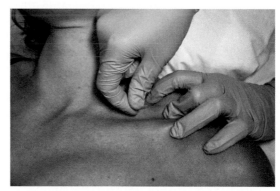

FIG. 7.17 Dry needling of the upper portion of the trapezius muscle in supine position.

(Fig. 7.16). Needling the muscle in supine position is indicated to reach the anterior fibres of the upper trapezius muscle (Fig. 7.17).

- *Precautions:* The most common serious adverse event is penetrating the lung and producing a pneumothorax. This is minimised by needling strictly between the fingers holding the muscle in a pincer grasp and needling directed towards the practitioner's finger.

Levator Scapulae Muscle

- *Anatomy:* The levator scapulae muscle originates from the dorsal tubercles of the transverse processes of C1 to C4 vertebrae and inserts on the superior medial angle and adjacent medial border of the scapula.
- *Function:* The levator scapulae muscle extends and sidebends the neck. When the head is turned to the opposite side and forward flexed, it rotates the head towards the midline. The muscle rotates the scapula glenoid fossa downward when the neck is fixed.

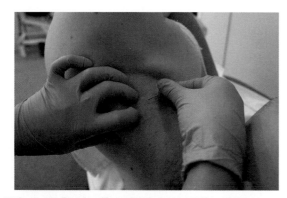

FIG. 7.15 Dry needling of the upper portion of the trapezius muscle in sidelying position.

- *Innervation:* Cervical spinal nerves C3-C5 via the dorsal scapular nerve.
- *Referred pain:* TrPs in the levator scapulae muscle refer to the angle of the neck and along the vertebral border of the scapula.
- *Needling technique:* The patient is in the lateral decubitus position. The muscle is needled via a pincer palpation. For the superior (cervical) portion, the muscle is felt as a ropy muscle band. The needle is inserted perpendicular to the skin and directed towards the practitioner's thumb (Fig. 7.18). For the lower (shoulder) portion, the muscle is identified over the superior medial border of scapula. The needle is inserted through the skin at a shallow angle and directed towards the upper, medial border of the scapula (Fig. 7.19). Placing the arm in a hammerlock position (hand on the lower back with the arm in internal rotation and support under the shoulder) makes it easier to palpate the muscle.
- *Precautions:* Do not needle towards the rib cage to avoid creating a pneumothorax.

Sternocleidomastoid Muscle

- *Anatomy:* The two heads of the sternocleidomastoid muscle (sternal and clavicular) originate in the mastoid process of the temporal bone. The sternal head attaches to the anterior surface of the manubrium sterni and the clavicular head attaches to the superior border and anterior surface of the medial third of the clavicle.

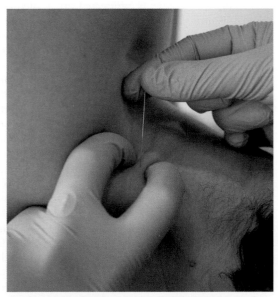

FIG. 7.18 Dry needling of the superior portion of the levator scapulae muscle.

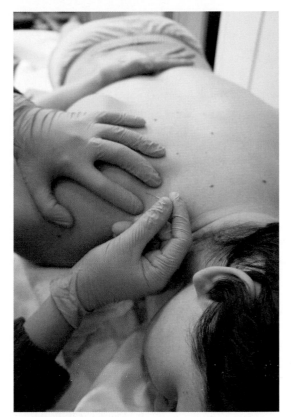

FIG. 7.19 Dry needling of the inferior portion of the levator scapulae muscle.

- *Function:* When the sternocleidomastoid muscle contracts unilaterally, it sidebends the head to the same side, rotates it to the opposite side, and tilts the chin upward. When the sternocleidomastoid muscle contracts bilaterally, it flexes the neck against gravity.
- *Innervation:* Accessory nerve (XI par cranial) and cervical spinal nerves C2-C3.
- *Referred pain:* TrPs in the sternal division may refer pain to the vertex, to the occiput, across the cheek, over the eye, to the throat, and to the sternum, whereas TrPs in the clavicular division refer pain to the forehead and deep into the ear, inducing frontal headache and earache.
- *Needling technique:* The patient is in supine position. Both heads, clavicular and sternal, are needled by pincer palpation. The needle is inserted perpendicular to the skin and directed towards the practitioner's thumb (Fig. 7.20). The more proximal part of the muscle can also be treated in sidelying position using a flat palpation. The needle is placed perpendicular to the skin about 1 cm caudal of the TrP.

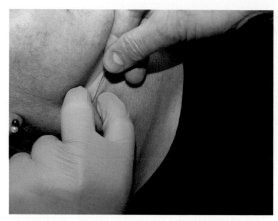

FIG. 7.20 Dry needling of the sternocleidomastoid muscle.

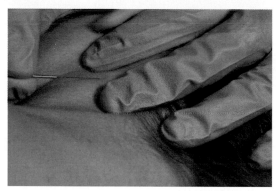

FIG. 7.21 Dry needling of the sternocleidomastoid muscle proximal part.

Next, the needle is redirected initially in a very shallow manner towards the TrP in the direction of the mastoid process. The needle can be directed deeper until the TrP has been reached (Fig. 7.21).

- *Precautions:* There are several structures clinicians need to be aware of, including the apex of the lung above the clavicle, the carotid artery and internal jugular vein medial to the sternocleidomastoid muscle, the external jugular vein that crosses the muscle, and the vertebral artery. By needling the sternocleidomastoid mastoid in a pincer palpation, most of these structures can be avoided except the external jugular vein. To avoid needling the external jugular vein, the vein needs to be identified if possible. If the vein is not visible, the patient may perform a Valsalva maneuver to accentuate the vein. If the vein remains invisible, dry needling can still be performed, realising that the vein may get punctured.

Splenius Capitis Muscle

- *Anatomy:* The splenius capitis muscle arises from the lower half of the ligamentum nuchae and from the spinous process of C7 to T3-T4 vertebrae and insets, under cover of the sternocleidomastoid, into the mastoid process of the temporal bone and into the rough surface of the occipital bone, below the lateral third of the superior nuchal line.
- *Function:* The splenius capitis muscle extends, side-bends, and rotates the neck to the same side.
- *Innervation:* Dorsal rami of the cervical spinal nerves.
- *Referred pain:* TrPs in the splenius capitis muscle project to the vertex of the head.
- *Needling technique:* The needling approach is basically the same for all posterior cervical muscles. It is very difficult, if not impossible, to distinguish the various posterior cervical muscles with manual palpation and, for the purpose of DN, we can safely consider the posterior cervical muscles as 'one muscle'. The patient is in the prone or sidelying position. For less experienced clinicians, it is recommended to exclusively use the prone position. Pertinent anatomical landmarks are the spinous processes of C2 and C6 and the transverse processes. All needling is performed between C2 and C6 and posterior to the transverse processes. Once the TrP is located, the needle is placed perpendicular to the skin slightly lateral and cranial from the TrP location. Generally, the needle is placed about 1 to 2 cm lateral to the spinous processes. After the needle has punctured the skin, the needle is redirected in a medial–caudal–ventral direction towards the lamina. The needle depth is dependent on the location of the TrP and the targeted muscle. For the splenius capitis muscle, needle depth is much less than for the cervical multifidus muscles, but the needle direction is basically the same (Fig. 7.22). Recently this approach has been validated for the cervical multifidi muscles with cadaver and sonography verification (Fernández-de-las-Peñas et al., 2017). For some posterior cervical muscles, a pincer palpation may also be possible. In this case the needle is directed towards the thumb similar to the levator scapulae (see Fig. 7.18). Because the lower fibres of the splenius capitis muscle are located in the upper thoracic spine region, needling procedures must follow the same approach and consider the same precautions as described in Chapter 10 for the thoracic multifidi and longissimus thoracis muscles.
- *Precautions:* Needling above C2 is not recommended except for the oblique capitis inferior muscle (see later in this chapter). When needling close to the

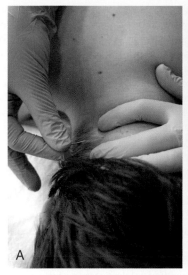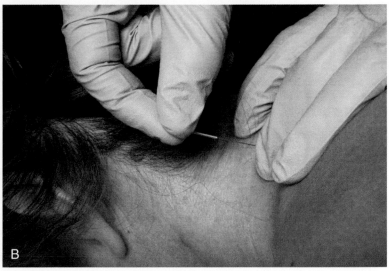

FIG. 7.22 Dry needling of the posterior cervical muscles.

spine, needling strictly in a medial-caudal-ventral direction is important as needling in a cranial-medial or even lateral-medial direction may cause an epidural hematoma with possible paralysis and loss of bladder control (Chen et al., 2006; Lee et al., 2011).

Splenius Cervicis Muscle

- *Anatomy:* The splenius cervicis muscle extends from the spinous processes of the T2-T6 vertebrae to the posterior tubercles of the transverse processes of C1-C3 vertebrae.
- *Function:* The splenius cervicis muscle extends the neck and rotates the head to the same side.
- *Innervation:* Dorsal rami of the cervical spinal nerves.
- *Referred pain:* TrPs in the splenius cervicis muscle refers upwards to the occiput, diffusely through the cranium, and to the back of the orbit. Sometimes it is projected to the angle of the neck.
- *Needling technique:* Because the lower fibres of the splenius cervicis muscle are located in the upper thoracic spine region, needling procedures must follow the same approach and consider the same precautions as described in Chapter 10 for the thoracic multifidi and longissimus thoracis muscles. For the upper fibres of the splenius cervicis muscle, the muscle can be palpated and needled either with a flat or pincer palpation as described previously for the splenius capitis muscle.
- *Precautions:* When needling close to the spine, needling strictly in a medial–caudal–ventral direction is

important, as needling in a cranial–medial or even lateral–medial direction may cause an epidural hematoma with possible paralysis and loss of bladder control (Chen et al., 2006; Lee et al., 2011).

Semispinalis Capitis and Cervicis Muscles

- *Anatomy:* The semispinalis capitis muscle arises from the tips of the transverse processes of C7 and T1-T6 vertebrae and the articular processes of C4-C6 and inserts between the superior and inferior nuchal lines of the occipital bone. The semispinalis cervicis muscle arises from the transverse processes of T2-T6 vertebrae and inserts into the posterior spinous processes of C2 to C5.
- *Function:* The semispinalis capitis extends, sidebends, and rotates the neck to the same side; the semispinalis cervicis extends and rotates the neck to the opposite side.
- *Innervation:* Dorsal rami of the cervical spinal nerves.
- *Referred pain:* TrPs in the semispinalis capitis and cervicis muscles refer pain over the posterior occiput and above the orbit.
- *Needling technique:* Because the lower fibres of the semispinalis capitis and cervicis muscles are located in the upper thoracic spine region, needling procedures must follow the same approach and consider the same precautions as described in Chapter 10 for the thoracic multifidi and longissimus thoracis muscles. For the upper fibres of the semispinalis capitis and cervicis muscles, the muscle can be palpated

and needled either with a flat or pincer palpation, as described previously for the splenius capitis muscle.

- *Precautions:* When needling close to the spine, needling strictly in a medial–caudal–ventral direction is important as needling in a cranial–medial or even lateral–medial direction may cause an epidural hematoma with possible paralysis and loss of bladder control (Chen et al., 2006; Lee et al., 2011).

Cervical Multifidi Muscles

- *Anatomy:* The cervical multifidi muscles cross two to four vertebral levels. The superior attachments are the posterior processes of C2 to C5, whereas the inferior attachments include the articular processes of the C2 to C7 vertebrae.
- *Function:* The main function of the cervical multifidi muscles is stabilisation of the cervical spine. They may assist in extension and rotation of the cervical spine to the opposite side.
- *Innervation:* Posterior primary rami of the cervical nerves at each level.
- *Referred pain:* TrPs in the cervical multifidi muscles spread to the suboccipital region and downward over the neck and upper part of the shoulder. Pain is perceived deep into the cervical zygapophyseal joint.
- *Needling technique:* The patient is in the prone position. Cervical multifidi muscles are not directly palpable; but clinicians can suspect the presence of relevant TrPs when patients report deep pain. The cervical multifidi muscles are palpated and needled with a flat palpation as described previously for the splenius capitis muscle.
- *Precautions:* When needling close to the spine, needling strictly in a medial–caudal–ventral direction is important as needling in a cranial–medial or even lateral–medial direction may cause an epidural hematoma with possible paralysis and loss of bladder control (Chen et al., 2006; Lee et al., 2011).

Suboccipital Muscles

- *Anatomy:* The rectus capitis posterior minor muscle extends from the posterior tubercle of the atlas (C1) to the medial aspect of the nuchal line on the occiput. The rectus capitis posterior major muscle originates from the spinous process of axis (C2) and inserts into the lateral part of the inferior nuchal line of the occiput. The oblique capitis superior muscle originates at the transverse process of the atlas (C1) and inserts into the occiput between the superior and inferior nuchal lines. The oblique capitis inferior muscle begins at the spinous process of the axis (C2) and attaches to the transverse process of the

atlas (C1). It is important to realise that the suboccipital triangle, shaped by the rectus capitis posterior major muscle and the oblique capitis muscle, lies practically in the horizontal plane when the head is kept in the anatomical position.

- *Function:* The rectus capitis posterior major and minor and the oblique capitis superior muscles extend the head on the neck; however, they are primarily postural muscles. The oblique capitis superior also assists in ipsilateral sidebending. The oblique capitis inferior is an ipsilateral rotator of the head and atlas on the axis.
- *Innervation:* Dorsal ramus of the first cervical spinal nerve.
- *Referred pain:* Referred pain from TrPs in the suboccipital muscles is perceived as deep pain spreading from the occiput towards the region of the orbit, mimicking a bilateral tension-type headache.
- *Needling technique:* Only the oblique capitis inferior muscle can be needled safely because of the proximity of the vertebral artery above the arch of the atlas and the foramen magnum. The patient is in prone position. The muscle is needled only in its medial half between the transverse process of C1 and the spinous process of C2. The needle is inserted perpendicular to the skin directly in the medial half of the muscle towards the posterior arch of C1. This equates to directing the needle towards the patient's opposite eye in a cranial–medial direction. To assist in directing the needle properly, it is helpful to have the patient point to the contralateral eye with the index finger (Fig. 7.23).
- *Precautions:* Avoid directing the needle strictly cranially or too laterally to prevent inadvertent penetration of the vertebral artery (Hong et al., 2018) or foramen magnum (Miyamoto et al., 2010).

Scalene Muscles

- *Anatomy:* The anterior scalene muscle extends from the anterior aspect of the transverse processes of the C3 to C6 vertebrae and inserts on the first rib anterior to the neurovascular bundle. The middle scalene muscle arises from the posterior aspects of transverse processes of C3 to C7 and attaches to the first rib posterior to the neurovascular bundle. The posterior scalene muscle originates for the posterior tubercles of the transverse processes of C4 to C6 and attaches to the second rib.
- *Function:* The scalene muscles sidebend the neck to the same side. The anterior scalene assists in rotating the head to the opposite side. The scalene muscles are accessory respiratory muscles and can assist in elevating the first and second rib.

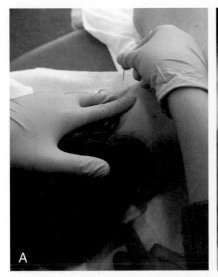
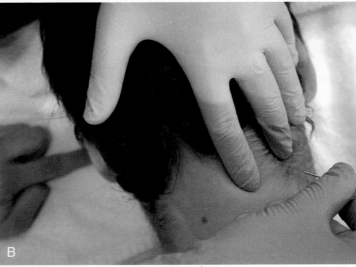

FIG. 7.23 Dry needling of the oblique capitis inferior muscle.

- *Innervation:* The anterior scalene is innervated by cervical spinal nerves from C4-C6. The middle scalene is innervated by cervical spinal nerves from C3-C8, and the posterior scalene is innervated by cervical spinal nerves from C5-C8.
- *Referred pain:* TrPs in the scalene muscles refer pain to the upper and medial vertebral borders of the scapula, to the pectoral region and down the front and back of the arm, on the radial forearm, and to the thumb and index finger.
- *Needling technique:* For needling the anterior scalene muscle, the patient is in the supine position. The anterior scalene muscle can be identified by having

the patient sniff sharply, which activates the respiratory component of the muscle function (Katagiri et al., 2003). The anterior scalene is palpated in the triangle formed by the jugular vein, the lateral edge of the clavicular head of the sternocleidomastoid muscle, and the clavicle as the base, whereas the middle scalene is palpated in the triangle formed by the brachial plexus, the posterior scalene, and the clavicle as the base. For the anterior scalene the needle is inserted perpendicular to the skin at least 2 cm above the clavicle, parallel to the table (Fig. 7.24). Considering the thickness of the muscle, the needle should not be inserted more than 1 to 1.5 cm. TrPs

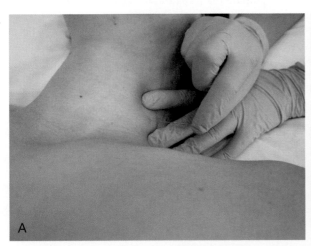
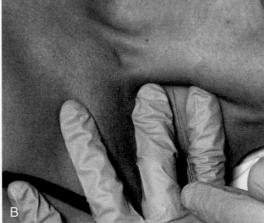

FIG. 7.24 Dry needling of the scalene muscles.

in the medial scalene can also be needled in the supine position. The needle is inserted perpendicular to the skin behind the brachial plexus and directed towards the posterior tubercle transverse processes of the cervical spine. For novices it is, however, easier to needle TrPs in the medial scalene with the patient in the sidelying position. The medial scalene is located in the midline of the neck just behind the sternocleidomastoid muscle overlying the transverse processes. To needle a TrP in the middle scalene, the needle is placed perpendicular to the skin about 1 cm caudal of the TrP. Next, the needle is redirected initially in a very shallow manner towards the TrP in the direction of the mastoid process. The needle can be directed deeper until the TrP has been reached. This approach is similar to the approach for the proximal part of the sternocleidomastoid muscle (see Fig. 7.21). Although it is possible to needle TrPs in the posterior scalene muscle, ultrasound-guided needling is preferred due to the close proximity to the lungs.

- *Precautions:* To avoid needling the apex of the lung, the scalene muscles can only be needled at least 2 cm above the clavicle.

Longus Colli Muscle

- *Anatomy:* The longus colli muscle is located anterior to the spine between the atlas and the third thoracic vertebra. The muscle consists of three parts: the superior oblique part originates from the transverse process of the third, fourth, and fifth cervical vertebrae and inserts at the anterior arch of the atlas; the inferior oblique part arises from the anterior surface of the bodies of the first two or three thoracic vertebrae and inserts at the transverse process of the fifth and sixth cervical vertebrae; and the vertical part comes from the anterior surfaces of the bodies of the upper three thoracic and lower three cervical vertebrae with attachments at the anterior surfaces of the second, third, and fourth cervical vertebrae.
- *Function:* The longus colli muscle flexes the neck and may assist in sidebending (superior and inferior obliques) and rotation (inferior oblique).
- *Innervation:* Branches of the ventral rami of the C2-C6 spinal nerves.
- *Referred pain:* According to Minerbi and colleagues (2017), TrPs in the longus colli muscles may refer to the ipsilateral ear, contralateral neck, posterior neck, and occiput, although local pain was the most common finding.
- *Needling technique:* The patient is in supine position. After locating the carotid artery, place the

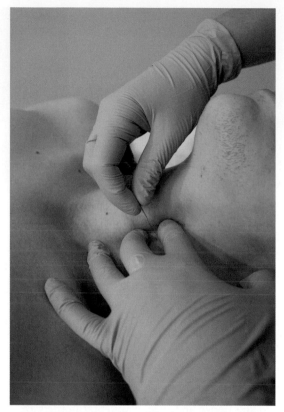

FIG. 7.25 Dry needling of the longus colli muscle.

palpating fingers in between the carotid artery and the trachea at the level of C4-C6. Move the trachea to the contralateral side and drop the finger tips towards the ventral surface of the cervical spine to palpate the longus colli muscle. Before placing the needle, verify that the carotid artery is lateral to the palpating fingers. Next, insert the needle perpendicular to the skin into the longus colli muscle (Fig. 7.25).

- *Precautions:* Avoid the carotid artery.

REFERENCES

Abboud, J., Marchand, A. A., Sorra, K., & Descarreaux, M. (2013). Musculoskeletal physical outcome measures in individuals with tension-type headache: a scoping review. *Cephalalgia, 33,* 1319–1336.

Alonso-Blanco, C., Fernández-de-las-Peñas, C., de-la-Llave-Rincón, A. I., Zarco-Moreno, P., Galán-del-Río, F., & Svensson, P. (2012). Characteristics of referred muscle pain to the head from active trigger points in women with myofascial temporomandibular pain and fibromyalgia syndrome. *Journal of Headache and Pain, 13,* 625–637.

Aprill, C., Axinn, M. J., & Bogduk, N. (2002). Occipital headaches stemming from the lateral atlanto-axial (C1-C2) joint. *Cephalalgia, 22*, 15–22.

Arendt-Nielsen, L., Castaldo, M., Mechelli, F., & Fernández-de-las-Peñas, C. (2016). Muscle triggers as a possible source of pain in a subgroup of tension-type headache patients? *The Clinical Journal of Pain, 32*, 711–718.

Ashkenazi, A., Blumenfeld, A., Napchan, U., Grosberg, B., Nett, R., DePalma, T., et al. Interventional Procedures Special Interest Section of the American. (2010). Peripheral nerve blocks and trigger point injections in headache management - a systematic review and suggestions for future research. *Headache, 50*, 943–952.

Ay, S., Konak, H. E., Evcik, D., & Kibar, S. (2017). The effectiveness of Kinesio Taping on pain and disability in cervical myofascial pain syndrome. *Revista Brasileira de Reumatologia English Edition, 57*, 93–99.

Baker, B. A. (1986). The muscle trigger point: evidence of overload injury. *Journal of Neurological and Orthopaedic Medicine and Surgery, 7*, 35–44.

Bablis, P., Pollard, H., & Bonello, R. (2008). Neuro-emotional technique for the treatment of trigger point sensitivity in chronic neck pain sufferers: a controlled clinical trial. *Chiropractic & Osteopathy, 16*, 4.

Bendtsen, L., & Jensen, R. (2006). Tension type headache: the most common, but also the most neglected headache disorder. *Current Opinion in Neurology, 19*, 305–309.

Bendtsen, L., & Jensen, R. (2010). Epidemiology of tension-type headache, migraine and cervicogenic headache. In C. Fernández de las Peñas, L. Arendt-Nielsen, & R. Gerwin (Eds.), *Tension type and cervicogenic headache: pathophysiology, diagnosis and treatment* (pp. 7–13). Baltimore: Jones & Bartlett.

Bendtsen, L., & Schoenen, J. (2006). Synthesis of tension type headache mechanisms. In J. Olesen, P. Goasdby, N. M. Ramdan, et al. (Eds.), *The headaches.* (3rd ed.). Philadelphia: Lippincott Williams & Wilkins.

Blasco-Bonora, P. M., & Martín-Pintado-Zugasti, A. (2017). Effects of myofascial trigger point dry needling in patients with sleep bruxism and temporomandibular disorders: a prospective case series. *Acupuncture in Medicine, 35*(1), 69–74.

Bodes-Pardo, G., Pecos-Martín, D., Gallego-Izquierdo, T., Salom-Moreno, J., Fernández-de-las-Peñas, C., & Ortega-Santiago, R. (2013). Manual treatment for cervicogenic headache and active trigger point in the sternocleidomastoid muscle: a pilot randomized clinical trial. *Journal of manipulative and physiological therapeutics, 36*, 403–411.

Bonafede, M., Cai, Q., Cappell, K., Kim, G., Sapra, S. J., Shah, N., et al. (2017). Factors associated with direct health care costs among patients with migraine. *Journal of Managed Care & Specialty Pharmacy, 23*(11), 1169–1176.

Cagnie, B., Castelein, B., Pollie, F., Steelant, L., Verhoeyen, H., & Cools, A. (2015). Evidence for the use of ischemic compression and dry needling in the management of trigger points of the upper trapezius in patients with neck pain: a systematic review. *American Journal of Physical Medicine & Rehabilitation, 94*, 573–583.

Calandre, E. P., Hidalgo, J., García-Leiva, J. M., & Rico-Villademoros, F. (2006). Trigger point evaluation in migraine patients: an indication of peripheral sensitization linked to migraine predisposition? *European Journal of Neurology, 13*, 244–249.

Calandre, E. P., Hidalgo, J., García-Leiva, J. M., Rico-Villademoros, F., & Delgado-Rodriguez, A. (2008). Myofascial trigger points in cluster headache patients: a case series. *Head & Face Medicine, 4*, 32.

Campa-Moran, I., Rey-Gudin, E., Fernandez-Carnero, J., Paris-Alemany, A., Gil-Martinez, A., Lerma Lara, S., et al. (2015). Comparison of dry needling versus orthopedic manual therapy in patients with myofascial chronic neck pain: a single-blind, randomized pilot study. *Pain Research and Treatment.* Article ID 327307.

Carroll, A., Barnes, M., & Comiskey, C. (2008). A prospective randomized controlled study of role of botulinum toxin in whiplash-associated disorder. *Clinical Rehabilitation, 22*, 513–519.

Castaldo, M., Ge, H. Y., Chiarotto, A., Villafane, J. H., & Arendt-Nielsen, L. (2014). Myofascial trigger points in patients with whiplash-associated disorders and mechanical neck pain. *Pain Medicine, 15*, 842–849.

Cerezo-Téllez, E., Torres-Lacomba, M., Mayoral-del Moral, O., Sánchez-Sánchez, B., Dommerholt, J., & Gutiérrez-Ortega, C. (2016a). Prevalence of myofascial pain syndrome in chronic non-specific neck pain: a population-based cross-sectional descriptive study. *Pain Medicine, 17*, 2369–2377.

Cerezo-Téllez, E., Torres-Lacomba, M., Fuentes-Gallardo, I., Perez-Muñoz, M., Mayoral-del-Moral, O., Lluch-Girbés, E., et al. (2016b). Effectiveness of dry needling for chronic nonspecific neck pain: a randomized, single-blinded, clinical trial. *Pain, 157*, 1905–1917.

Chen, J. C., Chen, Y., Lin, S. M., Yang, H. J., Su, C. F., & Tseng, S. H. (2006). Acute spinal epidural hematoma after acupuncture. *The Journal of Trauma, 60*, 414–416.

Chiarotto, A., Clijsen, R., Fernández-de-las-Peñas, C., & Barbero, M. (2016). Prevalence of myofascial trigger points in spinal disorders: a systematic review and meta-analysis. *Archives of Physical Medicine and Rehabilitation, 97*, 316–337.

Connelly, S. T., Myung, J., Gupta, R., Tartaglia, G. M., Gizdulich, A., Yang, J., et al. (2017). Clinical outcomes of Botox injections for chronic temporomandibular disorders: do we understand how Botox works on muscle, pain, and the brain? *International Journal of Oral and Maxillofacial Surgery, 46*, 322–327.

Côte, P., Cassidy, J. D., & Carroll, L. (1998). The Saskatchewan Health and Back Pain Survey: the prevalence of neck pain and related disability in Saskatchewan adults. *Spine, 23*, 1689–1698.

Côte, P., Cassidy, J. D., & Carroll, L. (2000). The factors associated with neck pain and its related disability in the Saskatchewan population. *Spine, 25*, 1109–1117.

Couppé, C., Torelli, P., Fuglsang-Frederiksen, A., Andersen, K. V., & Jensen, R. (2007). Myofascial trigger points are very prevalent in patients with chronic tension-type headache: a double-blinded controlled study. *The Clinical Journal of Pain, 23*, 23–27.

De Abreu Venâncio, R., Alencar, F. G., & Zamperini, C. (2008). Different substances and dry-needling injections in patients with myofascial pain and headaches. *Cranio, 26,* 96–103.

De Abreu Venâncio, R., Alencar, F. G., & Zamperini, C. (2009). Botulinum toxin, lidocaine, and dry-needling injections in patients with myofascial pain and headaches. *Cranio, 27,* 46–53.

De Meulemeester, K. E., Castelein, B., Coppieters, I., Barbe, T., Cools, A., & Cagnie, B. (2017). Comparing trigger point dry needling and manual pressure technique for the management of myofascial neck/shoulder pain: a randomized clinical trial. *Journal of Manipulative and Physiological Therapeutics, 40,* 11–20.

De Wijer, A., De Leeuw, J. R., Steenks, M., & Bosman, F. (1999). Temporomandibular and cervical spine disorders. Self-reported signs and symptoms. *Spine, 21,* 1638–1646.

Dıraçoğlu, D., Vural, M., Karan, A., & Aksoy, C. (2012). Effectiveness of dry needling for the treatment of temporomandibular myofascial pain: a double-blind, randomized, placebo controlled study. *Journal of Back and Musculoskeletal Rehabilitation, 25,* 285–290.

Drottning, M., Staff, P., & Sjaastad, O. (2002). Cervicogenic headache after whiplash injury. *Cephalalgia, 22,* 165–171.

Dommerholt, J. (2005). Persistent myalgia following whiplash. *Current Pain and Headache Reports, 9,* 326–330.

Dommerholt, J. (2010). Whiplash injury, muscle pain and motor dysfunction. In S. Mense & R. D. Gerwin (Eds.), *Muscle pain - an update: mechanisms, diagnosis and treatment* (pp. 247–288). Heidelberg: Springer.

Dommerholt, J., Royson, M. W., & Whyte-Ferguson, L. (2005). Neck pain and dysfunction following whiplash. In L. Ferguson & R. Gerwin (Eds.), *Clinical mastery in the treatment of myofascial pain* (pp. 57–89). Philadelphia: Lippincott Williams & Wilkins.

Elliott, J. M., O'Leary, S., Sterling, M., Hendrikz, J., Pedler, A., & Jull, G. (2010). Magnetic resonance imaging findings of fatty infiltrate in the cervical flexors in chronic whiplash. *Spine (Phila Pa 1976), 35*(9), 948–954.

Elliott, J., Pedler, A., Kenardy, J., Galloway, G., Jull, G., & Sterling, M. (2011). The temporal development of fatty infiltrates in the neck muscles following whiplash injury: an association with pain and posttraumatic stress. *PLoS One, 6*(6), e21194.

Ernest, E. (2006). Superior pharyngeal constrictor muscle. Practical. *Pain Management, 6*(6), 52–53.

Ettlin, T., Schuster, C., Stoffel, R., Brüderlin, A., & Kischka, U. (2008). A distinct pattern of myofascial findings in patients after whiplash injury. *Archives of Physical Medicine and Rehabilitation, 89,* 1290–1293.

Fejer, R., Ohm-Kyvik, K., & Hartvigsen, J. (2006). The prevalence of neck pain in the world population: a systematic critical review of the literature. *European Spine Journal, 15,* 834–848.

Fernández-de-las-Peñas, C. (2009). Interaction between trigger points and joint hypo-mobility: a clinical perspective. *The Journal of Manual & Manipulative Therapy, 17,* 74–77.

Fernández-de-las-Peñas, C., & Schoenen, J. (2009). Chronic tension type headache: what's new? *Current Opinion in Neurology, 22,* 254–261.

Fernández-de-las-Peñas, C., Cuadrado, M. L., Gerwin, R. D., & Pareja, J. A. (2005a). Referred pain from the trochlear region in tension-type headache: myofascial trigger point from the superior oblique muscle. *Headache, 45,* 731–737.

Fernández-de-las-Peñas, C., Fernández, J., & Miangolarra, J. C. (2005b). Musculoskeletal disorders in mechanical neck pain: myofascial trigger points versus cervical joint dysfunctions: a clinical study. *Journal of Musculoskeletal Pain, 13*(1), 27–35.

Fernández-de-las-Peñas, C., Alonso-Blanco, C., Cuadrado, M. L., Gerwin, R. D., & Pareja, J. A. (2006a). Trigger points in the suboccipital muscles and forward head posture in tension type headache. *Headache, 46,* 454–460.

Fernández-de-las-Peñas, C., Alonso-Blanco, C., Cuadrado, M. L., Gerwin, R. D., & Pareja, J. A. (2006b). Myofascial trigger points and their relationship to headache clinical parameters in chronic tension type headache. *Headache, 46,* 1264–1272.

Fernández-de-las-Peñas, C., Alonso-Blanco, C., Cuadrado, M. L., & Pareja, J. A. (2006c). Myofascial trigger points in the suboccipital muscles in episodic tension type headache. *Manual Therapy, 11,* 225–230.

Fernández-de-las-Peñas, C., Arendt-Nielsen, L., & Simons, D. (2006d). Contributions of myofascial trigger points to chronic tension type headache. *The Journal of Manual & Manipulative Therapy, 14,* 222–231.

Fernández-de-las-Peñas, C., Cuadrado, M. L., & Pareja, J. (2006e). Myofascial trigger points, neck mobility and forward head posture in unilateral migraine. *Cephalalgia, 26,* 1061–1070.

Fernández-de-las-Peñas, C., Cuadrado, M. L., Gerwin, R. D., & Pareja, J. A. (2006f). Myofascial disorders in the trochlear region in unilateral migraine: a possible initiating or perpetuating factor. *The Clinical Journal of Pain, 22,* 548–553.

Fernández-de-las-Peñas, C., Simons, D. G., Cuadrado, M. L., & Pareja, J. A. (2007a). The roles of myofascial trigger points in musculoskeletal pain syndromes of the head and neck. *Current Pain and Headache Reports, 11,* 365–372.

Fernández-de-las-Peñas, C., Ge, H., Arendt-Nielsen, L., Cuadrado, M. L., & Pareja, J. A. (2007b). Referred pain from trapezius muscle trigger point shares similar characteristics with chronic tension type headache. *European Journal of Pain, 11,* 475–482.

Fernández-de-las-Peñas, C., Ge, H., Arendt-Nielsen, L., Cuadrado, M. L., & Pareja, J. A. (2007c). The local and referred pain from myofascial trigger points in the temporalis muscle contributes to pain profile in chronic tension-type headache. *The Clinical Journal of Pain, 23,* 786–792.

Fernández-de-las-Peñas, C., Cuadrado, M. L., & Pareja, J. A. (2007d). Myofascial trigger points, neck mobility and forward head posture in episodic tension type headache. *Headache, 47,* 662–672.

Fernández-de-las-Peñas, C., Cuadrado, M. L., Arendt-Nielsen, L., Simons, D. G., & Pareja, J. A. (2007e). Myofascial trigger points and sensitisation: an updated pain model for tension type headache. *Cephalalgia, 27,* 383–393.

Fernández-de-las-Peñas, C., Alonso-Blanco, C., & Miangolarra, J. C. (2007f). Myofascial trigger points in subjects presenting with mechanical neck pain: a blinded, controlled study. *Manual Therapy, 12,* 29–33.

Fernández-de-las-Peñas, C., Cleland, J. A., Cuadrado, M. L., & Pareja, J. (2008). Predictor variables for identifying patients with chronic tension type headache who are likely to achieve short-term success with muscle trigger point therapy. *Cephalalgia, 28,* 264–275.

Fernández-de-las-Peñas, C., Cuadrado, M. L., Gerwin, R., & Pareja, J. (2009). Referred pain from the lateral rectus muscle in subjects with chronic tension type headache. *Pain Medicine, 10,* 43–48.

Fernández-de-las-Peñas, C., Galán-del-Río, F., Alonso-Blanco, C., Jiménez-García, R., Arendt-Nielsen, L., & Svensson, P. (2010). Referred pain from muscle trigger points in the masticatory and neck-shoulder musculature in women with temporomandibular disorders. *The Journal of Pain, 11,* 1295–1304.

Fernández-de-las-Peñas, C., Fernández-Mayoralas, D. M., Ortega-Santiago, R., Ambite-Quesada, S., Palacios-Ceña, D., & Pareja, J. A. (2011a). Referred pain from myofascial trigger points in head and neck-shoulder muscles reproduces head pain features in children with chronic tension type headache. *The Journal of Headache and Pain, 12,* 35–43.

Fernández-de-las-Peñas, C., Cleland, J. A., Palomeque-del-Cerro, L., Caminero, A. B., Guillem-Mesado, A., & Jiménez-García, R. (2011b). Development of a clinical prediction rule for identifying women with tension-type headache who are likely to achieve short-term success with joint mobilization and muscle trigger point therapy. *Headache, 51,* 246–261.

Fernández-de-las-Peñas, C. (2015). Myofascial head pain. *Current Pain and Headache Reports, 19*(7), 28.

Fernández-de-las-Peñas, C., & Cuadrado, M. L. (2016). Dry needling for headaches presenting active trigger points. *Expert Review of Neurotherapeutics, 16,* 365–366.

Fernández-de-las-Peñas, C., Mesa-Jiménez, J. A., Paredes-Mancilla, J. A., Koppenhaver, S. L., & Fernández-Carnero, S. (2017). Cadaveric and ultrasonographic validation of needling placement in the cervical multifidus muscle. *Journal of Manipulative and Physiological Therapeutics, 40,* 365–370.

Ferracini, G. N., Florencio, L. L., Dach, F., Chaves, T. C., Palacios-Ceña, M., Fernández-de-las-Peñas, C., et al. (2017). Myofascial trigger points and migraine-related disability in women with episodic and chronic migraine. *The Clinical Journal of Pain, 33,* 109–115.

Fernández-Pérez, A. M., Villaverde-Gutiérrez, C., Mora-Sánchez, A., Alonso-Blanco, C., Sterling, M., & Fernández-de-las-Peñas, C. (2012). Muscle trigger points, pressure pain threshold, and cervical range of motion in patients with high level of disability related to acute whiplash injury. *The Journal of Orthopaedic and Sports Physical Therapy, 42,* 634–641.

Ferrante, T., Manzoni, G. C., Russo, M., Camarda, C., Taga, A., Veronesi, L., et al. (2013). Prevalence of tension-type headache in adult general population: the PACE study and review of the literature. *Neurological Sciences, 34,* S137–138.

France, S., Bown, J., Nowosilskyj, M., Mott, M., Rand, S., & Walters, J. (2014). Evidence for the use of dry needling and physiotherapy in the management of cervicogenic or tension-type headache: a systematic review. *Cephalalgia, 34,* 994–1003.

Freeman, M.D., Nystrom, A., Centeno, C. 2009. Chronic whiplash and central sensitization; an evaluation of the role of a myofascial trigger points in pain modulation. *Journal of Brachial Plexus and Peripheral Nerve Injury,* 23;4:2.

Ganesh, G. S., Singh, H., Mushtaq, S., Mohanty, P., & Pattnaik, M. (2016). Effect of cervical mobilization and ischemic compression therapy on contralateral cervical side flexion and pressure pain threshold in latent upper trapezius trigger points. *Journal of Bodywork and Movement Therapies, 20,* 477–483.

García-Leiva, J. M., Hidalgo, J., Rico-Villademoros, F., Moreno, V., & Calandre, E. P. (2007). Effectiveness of ropivacaine trigger points inactivation in the prophylactic management of patients with severe migraine. *Pain Medicine, 8,* 65–70.

Gerber, L. H., Shah, J., Rosenberger, W., Armstrong, K., Turo, D., Otto, P., et al. (2015). Dry needling alters trigger points in the upper trapezius muscle and reduces pain in subjects with chronic myofascial pain. *PMR, 7,* 711–718.

Gerwin, R. (2005). Headache. In L. Ferguson & R. Gerwin (Eds.), *Clinical mastery in the treatment of myofascial pain* (pp. 1–24). Philadelphia: Lippincott Williams & Wilkins.

Gerwin, R. D., & Dommerholt, J. (1998). Myofascial trigger points in chronic cervical whiplash syndrome [abstract]. *Journal of Musculoskeletal Pain, 6,* 28.

Gerwin, R. (2012). Botulinum toxin treatment of myofascial pain: a critical review of the literature. *Current Pain and Headache Reports, 16*(5), 413–422.

Ghanbari, A., Askarzadeh, S., Petramfar, P., & Mohamadi, M. (2015). Migraine responds better to a combination of medical therapy and trigger point management than routine medical therapy alone. *NeuroRehabilitation, 37,* 157–163.

Giamberardino, M. A., Tafuri, E., Savini, A., et al. (2007). Contribution of myofascial trigger points to migraine symptoms. *The Journal of Pain, 8,* 869–878.

Global Burden of Disease Study 2013 Collaborators. (2015). Global, regional, and national incidence, prevalence, and years lived with disability for 301 acute and chronic diseases and injuries in 188 countries, 1990–2013: a systematic analysis for the Global Burden of Disease Study 2013. *Lancet, 386,* 743–800.

Gonzalez-Perez, L. M., Infante-Cossio, P., Granados-Nunez, M., Urresti-Lopez, F. J., Lopez-Martos, R., & Ruiz-Canela-Mendez, P. (2015). Dry needling of trigger points located in the lateral pterygoid muscle: efficacy and safety of treatment for management of myofascial pain and temporomandibular dysfunction. *Medicina Oral, Patología Oral y Cirugía Bucal, 20,* e326–333.

Haldeman, S., & Dagenais, S. (2001). Cervicogenic headaches. a critical review. *Spine Journal, 1,* 31–46.

Harden, R. N., Cottrill, J., Gagnon, C. M., Smitherman, T. A., Weinland, S. R., Tann, B., et al. (2009). Botulinum toxin A in the treatment of chronic tension-type headache with cervical myofascial trigger points: a randomized, double-blind, placebo-controlled pilot study. *Headache, 49,* 732–743.

Headley, B. J. (2005). A surface electromyography assessment of patients subsequent to motor vehicle crash (MVC) and controls to establish presence of soft-tissue injury: a pilot study. *Journal of Whiplash & Related Disorders, 4,* 57–71.

Hong, S., Park, Y., & Lee, C.-N. (2018). Lateral medullary infarction caused by Oriental acupuncture. *European Neurology, 79,* 63.

Hong, C. Z., & Simons, D. G. (1993). Response to treatment for pectoralis minor: myofascial pain syndrome after whiplash. *Journal of Musculoskeletal Pain, 1,* 89–132.

Hu, X. H., Markson, L. E., Lipton, R. B., Stewart, W. F., & Berger, M. L. (1999). Burden of migraine in the USA: disability and economic costs. *Archives of Internal Medicine, 159,* 813–818.

ICHD-III. (2013). International Classification of Headache Disorders: Headache Classification Subcommittee of the International Headache Society, 3nd edition. *Cephalalgia, 33,* 629–808.

Isong, U., Gansky, S. A., & Plesh, O. (2008). Temporomandibular joint and muscle disorder-type pain in US adults: the National Health Interview Survey. *Journal of Orofacial Pain, 22,* 317–322.

Jaeger, B. (1989). Are cervicogenic headache due to myofascial pain and cervical spine dysfunction? *Cephalalgia, 9,* 157–164.

Jensen, R., & Stovner, L. J. (2008). Epidemiology and comorbidity of headache. *Lancet Neurology, 7,* 354–361.

Jung, S. Y., Park, H. S., Bae, H., Yoo, J. H., Park, H. J., Park, K. D., et al. (2016). Laryngeal myofascial pain syndrome as a new diagnostic entity of dysphonia. *Auris, Nasus, Larynx, 44*(2), 182–187.

Katagiri, M., Abe, T., Yokoba, M., Dobashi, Y., Tomita, T., & Easton, P. A. (2003). Neck and abdominal muscle activity during a sniff. *Respiratory Medicine, 97*(9), 1027–1035.

Kennedy, E., Albert, M., & Nicholson, H. (2017). Do longus capitis and colli really stabilise the cervical spine? A study of their fascicular anatomy and peak force capabilities. *Musculoskelet Sci Pract., 32,* 104–113.

Kettler, A., Hartwig, E., Schultheiss, M., Claes, L., & Wilke, H. J. (2002). Mechanically simulated muscle forces strongly stabilize intact and injured upper cervical spine specimens. *Journal of Biomechanics, 35*(3), 339–346.

Khalifeh, M., Mehta, K., Varguise, N., Suarez-Dural, P., & Enciso, R. (2016). Botulinum toxin type A for the treatment of head and neck chronic myofascial pain syndrome. A systematic review and meta- analysis. *J American Dental Assoc, 147*(12), 959–973.

Kietrys, D. M., Palombaro, K. M., & Mannheimer, J. S. (2014). Dry needling for management of pain in the upper quarter and craniofacial region. *Current Pain and Headache Reports, 18*(8), 437.

Kim, H. S., Pae, C., Bae, J. H., Hu, K. S., Chang, B. M., Tansatit, T., et al. (2015). An anatomical study of the risorius in Asians and its insertion at the modiolus. *Surgical and Radiologic Anatomy, 37,* 147–151.

Kojidi, M. M., Okhovatian, F., Rahimi, A., Baghban, A. A., & Azimi, H. (2016). Comparison between the effects of passive and active soft tissue therapies on latent trigger points of the upper trapezius muscle in women: a single-blind, randomized clinical trial. *Journal of chiropractic medicine, 15*(4), 235–242.

Kumbhare, D. A., Balsor, B., Parkinson, W. L., Harding Bsckin, P., Bedard, M., Papaioannou, A., et al. (2005). Measurement of cervical flexor endurance following whiplash. *Disability and Rehabilitation, 27*(14), 801–807.

La Touche, R., Fernández de las Peñas, C., Fernández-Carnero, J., Escalante, K., Angulo-Díaz-Parreño, S., Paris-Alemany, A., et al. (2009). The effects of manual therapy and exercise directed at the cervical spine on pain and pressure pain sensitivity in patients with myofascial temporomandibular disorders. *Journal of Oral Rehabilitation, 36,* 644–652.

Lee, J. H., Lee, H., & Jo, D. J. (2011). An acute cervical epidural hematoma as a complication of dry needling. *Spine (Phila Pa 1976), 36,* E891–893.

León-Hernández, J.V., Martín-Pintado-Zugasti, A., Frutos, L.G., Alguacil-Diego, I.M., de la Llave-Rincón, A.I., Fernandez-Carnero, J. 2016. Immediate and short-term effects of the combination of dry needling and percutaneous TENS on post-needling soreness in patients with chronic myofascial neck pain. *Brazilian Journal of Physical Therapy, 20*(5), 422–431.

LeResche, L. (1997). Epidemiology of temporomandibular disorders: implications for the investigation of etiologic factors. *Critical Reviews in Oral Biology and Medicine, 8,* 291–305.

Liu, L., Huang, Q. M., Liu, Q. G., Ye, G., Bo, C. Z., Chen, M. J., et al. (2015). Effectiveness of dry needling for myofascial trigger points associated with neck and shoulder pain: a systematic review and meta-analysis. *Archives of Physical Medicine and Rehabilitation, 96,* 944–955.

Liu, X. M., Pan, F. M., Yong, Z. Y., Ba, Z. Y., Wang, S. J., Liu, Z., et al. (2017). Does the longus colli have an effect on cervical vertigo? A retrospective study of 116 patients. *Medicine (Baltimore), 96*(12), e6365.

Llamas-Ramos, R., Pecos-Martín, D., Gallego-Izquierdo, T., Llamas-Ramos, I., Plaza-Manzano, G., Ortega-Santiago, R., et al. (2014). Comparison of the short-term outcomes between trigger point dry needling and trigger point manual therapy for the management of chronic mechanical neck pain: a randomized clinical trial. *The Journal of Orthopaedic and Sports Physical Therapy, 44,* 852–861.

Lluch, E., Nijs, J., De Kooning, M., Van Dyck, D., Vanderstraeten, R., Struyf, F., et al. (2015). Prevalence, incidence, localization, and pathophysiology of myofascial trigger points in patients with spinal pain: a systematic literature review. *Journal of Manipulative and Physiological Therapeutics, 38,* 587–600.

Ma, C., Wu, S., Li, G., Xiao, X., Mai, M., & Yan, T. (2010). Comparison of miniscalpel-needle release, acupuncture needling, and stretching exercise to trigger point in myofascial pain syndrome. *The Clinical Journal of Pain, 26,* 251–257.

Manchikanti, L., Singh, V., Datta, S., Cohen, S. P., Hirsch, J. A., & American Society of Interventional Pain Physicians. (2009). Comprehensive review of epidemiology, scope, and impact of spinal pain. *Pain Physician, 12,* E35–E70.

Marcus, D., Scharff, L., Mercer, S., & Turk, D. (1999). Musculoskeletal abnormalities in chronic headache: a controlled comparison of headache diagnostic groups. *Headache, 39,* 21–27.

Mayoux-Benhamou, M. A., Revel, M., Vallée, C., Roudier, R., Barbet, J. P., & Bargy, F. (1994). Longus colli has a postural function on cervical curvature. *Surgical and Radiologic Anatomy, 16*(4), 367–371.

Mejuto-Vázquez, M. J., Salom-Moreno, J., Ortega-Santiago, R., Truyols-Domínguez, S., & Fernández-de-las-Peñas, C. (2014). Short-term changes in neck pain, widespread pressure pain sensitivity, and cervical range of motion after the application of trigger point dry needling in patients with acute mechanical neck pain: a randomized clinical trial. *The Journal of Orthopaedic and Sports Physical Therapy, 44,* 252–256.

Migraine Research Foundation. https://migraineresearchfoundation.org/about-migraine/migraine-facts. Accessed 22 January, 2018.

Minerbi, A., Ratmansky, M., Finestone, A., Gerwin, R., & Vulfsons, S. (2017). The local and referred pain patterns of the longus colli muscle. *Journal of Bodywork and Movement Therapies, 21*(2), 267–273.

Montañez-Aguilera, F. J., Valtueña-Gimeno, N., Pecos-Martín, D., Arnau-Masanet, R., Barrios-Pitarque, C., & Bosch-Morell, F. (2010). Changes in a patient with neck pain after application of ischemic compression as a trigger point therapy. *Journal of Back and Musculoskeletal Rehabilitation, 23,* 101–104.

Moraska, A., & Chandler, C. (2008). Changes in clinical parameters in patients with tension-type headache following massage therapy: a pilot study. *The Journal of Manual & Manipulative Therapy, 16,* 106–112.

Moraska, A., & Chandler, C. (2009). Changes in psychological parameters in patients with tension-type headache following massage therapy: a pilot study. *The Journal of Manual & Manipulative Therapy, 17,* 86–94.

Moraska, A. F., Stenerson, L., Butryn, N., Krutsch, J. P., Schmiege, S. J., & Mann, J. D. (2015). Myofascial trigger point-focused head and neck massage for recurrent tension-type headache: a randomized, placebo-controlled clinical trial. *The Clinical Journal of Pain, 31,* 159–168.

Mortazavi, H., Javadzadeh, A., Delavarian, Z., & Mahmoodabadi, R. Z. (2010). Myofascial pain dysfunction syndrome (MPDS). *Iranian Journal of Otorhinolaryngology, 4,* 131–136.

Moyers, R. E. (1950). An electromyographic analysis of certain muscles involved in temporomandibular movement. *American Journal of Orthodontics, 36,* 481–515.

Miyamoto, S., Ide, T., & Takemura, N. (2010). Risks and causes of cervical cord and medulla oblongata injuries due to acupuncture. *World Neurosurgery, 73*(6), 735–741.

Omami, G., & Lurie, A. (2012). Magnetic resonance imaging evaluation of discal attachment of superior head of lateral pterygoid muscle in individuals with symptomatic temporomandibular joint. *Oral Surgery, Oral Medicine, Oral Pathology, Oral Radiology, 114*(5), 650–657.

Palacios-Ceña, M., Wang, K., Castaldo, M., Guillem-Mesado, A., Ordás-Bandera, C., Arendt-Nielsen, L., et al. (2016). Trigger points are associated with widespread pressure pain sensitivity in people with tension-type headache. *Cephalalgia.* [Epub ahead of print].

Pearson, I., Reichert, A., De Serres, S. J., Dumas, J. P., & Côté, J. N. (2009). Maximal voluntary isometric neck strength deficits in adults with whiplash-associated disorders and association with pain and fear of movement. *The Journal of Orthopaedic and Sports Physical Therapy, 39*(3), 179–187.

Peterson, G., Dedering, Å., Andersson, E., Nilsson, D., Trygg, J., Peolsson, M., et al. (2015). Altered ventral neck muscle deformation for individuals with whiplash associated disorder compared to healthy controls: a case-control ultrasound study. *Manual Therapy, 20*(2), 319–327.

Picavet, H.S.J., Van Gils, H.W.V., Schouten, J.S.A.G. 2000. Musculoskeletal complaints in the Dutch population. RIVM (National Institute of Public Health and the Environment), The Netherlands. [In Dutch: Klachten aan het bewegingsapparaat in de Nederlandse bevolking prevalenties, consequenties en risicogroepen].

Prushansky, T., Gepstein, R., Gordon, C., & Dvir, Z. (2005). Cervical muscles weakness in chronic whiplash patients. *Clinical Biomechanics (Bristol, Avon), 20*(8), 794–798.

Quinlan, K. P., Annest, J. L., Myers, B., Ryan, G., & Hill, H. (2004). Neck strains and sprains among motor vehicle occupants—USA, 2000. *Accident; Analysis and Prevention, 36,* 21–27.

Raggi, A., & Leonardi, M. (2015). Burden and cost of neurological diseases: a European North-South comparison. *Acta Neurologica Scandinavica, 132,* 16–22.

Richter, M., Otte, D., Pohlemann, T., Krettek, C., & Blauth, M. (2000). Whiplash-type neck distortion in restrained car drivers: frequency, causes and long-term results. *European Spine Journal, 9,* 109–117.

Robbins, M. S., Kuruvilla, D., Blumenfeld, A., Charleston, L., 4th, Sorrell, M., Robertson, C. E., et al. Peripheral Nerve Blocks and Other Interventional Procedures Special Interest Section of the American Headache Society. (2014). Trigger point injections for headache disorders: expert consensus methodology and narrative review. *Headache, 54,* 1441–1459.

Rocabado, M. (1983). Biomechanical relationship of the cranial, cervical, and hyoid regions. *The Journal of Cranio-Mandibular Practice, 1,* 61–66.

Roth, R., Roth, J., & Simons, D. (2007). Cervicogenic headache caused by myofascial trigger points in the sternocleidomastoid: a case report. *Cephalalgia, 27,* 375–380.

Schuller, E., Eisenmenger, W., & Beier, G. (2000). Whiplash injury in low speed car accidents. *Journal of Musculoskeletal Pain, 8,* 55–67.

Shanmugam, S., & Mathias, L. (2017). Immediate effects of paraspinal dry needling in patients with acute facet joint lock induced wry neck. *Journal of Clinical and Diagnostic Research, 11*(6), YM01–YM03.

Shaw, L., Morozova, M., & Abu-Arafeh, I. (2018). Chronic post-traumatic headache in children and adolescents: systematic review of prevalence and headache features. *Pain Manag., 8*(1), 57–64.

Shimohata, K., Hasegawa, K., Onodera, O., Nishizawa, M., & Shimohata, T. (2017). The clinical features, risk factors, and surgical treatment of cervicogenic headache in patients with cervical spine disorders requiring surgery. *Headache, 57*(7), 1109–1117.

Simons, D. G., Travell, J., & Simons, L. S. (1999). *Travell & Simons' Myofascial pain and dysfunction: the trigger point manual: vol. 1* (2nd ed.). Baltimore: Williams & Wilkins.

Sjaastad, O., & Bakketeig, I. S. (2008). Prevalence of cervicogenic headache: Vaga study of headache epidemiology. *Acta Neurologica Scandinavica, 117*, 173–180.

Sohn, J. H., Choi, H., Lee, S., & Jun, A. (2010). Differences in cervical musculoskeletal impairment between episodic and chronic tension-type headache. *Cephalalgia, 30*, 1514–1523.

Sollmann, N., Trepte-Freisleder, F., Albers, L., Jung, N. H., Mall, V., Meyer, B., et al. (2016). Magnetic stimulation of the upper trapezius muscles in patients with migraine - A pilot study. *European Journal of Paediatric Neurology, 20*, 888–897.

Sterling, M., Vicenzino, B., Souvlis, T., & Connelly, L. B. (2015). Dry-needling and exercise for chronic whiplash-associated disorders: a randomized single-blind placebo-controlled trial. *Pain, 156*, 635–643.

Sterner, Y., Toolanen, G., Gerdle, B., & Hildingsson, C. (2003). The incidence of whiplash trauma and the effects of different factors on recovery. *Journal of Spinal Disorders & Techniques, 16*, 195–199.

Stovner, L., Hagen, K., Jensen, R., Katsarava, Z., Lipton, R., Scher, A., et al. (2007). The global burden of headache: a documentation of headache prevalence and disability worldwide. *Cephalalgia, 27*, 193–210.

Svensson, P. (2007). Muscle pain in the head: overlap between temporomandibular disorders and tension-type headaches. *Current Opinion in Neurology, 20*, 320–325.

Svensson, P., & Graven-Nielsen, T. (2001). Craniofacial muscle pain: review of mechanisms and clinical manifestations. *Journal of Orofacial Pain, 15*, 117–145.

Svensson, P., Bak, J., & Troest, T. (2003a). Spread and referral of experimental pain in different jaw muscles. *Journal of Orofacial Pain, 17*, 214–223.

Svensson, P., Cairns, B. E., Wang, K., Hu, J. W., Graven-Nielsen, T., Arendt-Nielsen, L., et al. (2003b). Glutamate-evoked pain and mechanical allodynia in the human masseter muscle. *Pain, 101*, 221–227.

Svensson, P., Castrillon, E., & Cairns, B. E. (2008). Nerve growth factor-evoked masseter muscle sensitization and perturbation of jaw motor function in healthy women. *Journal of Orofacial Pain, 22*, 340–348.

Tfelt-Hansen, P., Lous, I., & Olesen, J. (1981). Prevalence and significance of muscle tenderness during common migraine attacks. *Headache, 21*, 49–54.

Vierck, C. J., Jr., Cannon, R. L., Fry, G., Maixner, W., & Whitsel, B. (1997). Characteristics of temporal summation of second pain sensations elicited by brief contact of glabrous skin by a preheated thermode. *Journal of Neurophysiology, 78*, 992–1002.

Von Stülpnagel, C., Reilich, P., Straube, A., Schäfer, J., Blaschek, A., Lee, S. H., et al. (2009). Myofascial trigger points in children with tension-type headache: a new diagnostic and therapeutic option. *Journal of Child Neurology, 24*, 406–409.

Wright, E. (2000). Referred craniofacial pain patterns in patients with temporomandibular disorder. *Journal of the American Dental Association (1939), 131*, 1307–1315.

Yildirim, A., Akbaş, A., Sürücü, G. D., Karabiber, M., Gedik, D. E., & Aktürk, S. (2016). The effectiveness of mobilization practices for patients with neck pain due to myofascial pain syndrome: a randomized clinical trial. *Turkish J Phys Med Rehabil, 62*(4), 337–345.

Zaloshnja, E., Miller, T., Council, F., & Persaud, B. (2006). Crash costs in the USA by crash geometry. *Accident; Analysis and Prevention, 38*, 644–651.

CHAPTER 8

Deep Dry Needling of the Shoulder Muscles

CAREL BRON • JO L.M. FRANSSEN • BETTY T.M. BEERSMA • JAN DOMMERHOLT

INTRODUCTION

Shoulder pain, shoulder complaints, and shoulder disorders are common terms that frequently are used interchangeably as there is some overlap between these concepts. In this chapter we will use the term shoulder pain, which is a very common musculoskeletal disorder. In primary care the yearly incidence of shoulder pain is estimated to be 14.2 per 1000 people. The 1-year prevalence in the general population is estimated to be 20% to 50%. The estimates are strongly influenced by the definition of shoulder disorders, as well as by inclusion and exclusion criteria such as limited motion, age, gender, and anatomical areas. Thus shoulder pain is widespread and imposes a considerable burden on the affected person and on society. Women are slightly more affected than men, and the frequency of shoulder pain peaks between 46 and 64 years of age (van der Windt et al., 1995). Shoulder pain tends to be persistent or recurrent despite medical treatment (Ginn & Cohen, 2004). The pathophysiological mechanisms are poorly understood, in spite of a growing body of knowledge of shoulder kinematics, injury mechanisms, and the technical advances of medical imaging, including sonography, magnetic resonance imaging, and more conventional techniques such as x-rays.

Most shoulder pains are caused by a small number of relatively common conditions. Although subacromial impingement is often suggested to be the most common potential source of shoulder pain (Neer, 1972; Hawkins & Hobeika, 1983), solid evidence is lacking (Bron, 2008). Moreover, in 2011 Papadonikolakis and colleagues (2011) reported in a systematic review that there was no published evidence to support the diagnosis of subacromial impingement. This syndrome includes tendonitis or tendinopathy of the rotator cuff and the long head of the biceps brachii muscle, or subacromial or subdeltoid bursitis. In fact, calcifications, acromion spurs, subacromial fluid, or signs of tendon degeneration are equally prevalent in healthy subjects and in individuals with shoulder pain (Milgrom et al., 1995). Furthermore, physical examination tests of subacromial impingement are not reliable (Hegedus et al., 2008), and the results of imaging diagnostics do not correlate well with pain (Bradley et al., 2005). In addition, interventions targeting subacromial problems are, at best, only moderately effective at treating patients with shoulder complaints (Coghlan et al., 2008; Buchbinder et al., 2009; Dorrestijn et al., 2009). Other less common causes of shoulder pain are tumours, infections, and nerve-related injuries.

Histological studies have determined that the rotator cuff is made of multiple confluent tissue layers functioning in concert. The tendons of the supraspinatus and the infraspinatus merge together at the level of the greater tuberosity, whereas the infraspinatus and teres minor merge near their musculotendinous junctions. The subscapularis tendon and the supraspinatus tendon join as a sheath around the biceps tendon at the entrance of the bicipital groove (Matava et al., 2005).

CLINICAL RELEVANCE OF MYOFASCIAL TRIGGER POINTS IN SHOULDER PAIN SYNDROMES

Myofascial trigger points (TrPs) in patients with shoulder pain are most prevalent in the infraspinatus, upper trapezius, and deltoid muscles; most of the time, multiple TrPs in more than one muscle are involved. Ingber (2000) successfully treated the subscapularis muscle, which he considered to be the main cause of shoulder pain in three overhead athletes. Hidalgo-Lozano and colleagues (2010) found that the muscles most affected by active TrPs were the supraspinatus, infraspinatus, and subscapularis in patients with shoulder pain with a medical diagnosis of shoulder impingement. Elite swimmers with shoulder pain presented with similar findings (Hidalgo-Lozano et al., 2013).

In an older study, Sola and Kuitert (1955) concluded that the supraspinatus muscle was one of the least frequently involved shoulder girdle muscles, both in patients and in young healthy adults. The supraspinatus muscle is rarely involved by itself but usually appears in association with the infraspinatus or upper trapezius muscles (Bron et al., 2011b) or the subscapularis muscle (Hidalgo-Lozano et al., 2010), which very commonly harbor TrPs in patients with shoulder pain and dysfunction. In addition, other muscles such as the levator scapulae, biceps brachii, deltoid, pectoralis minor, pectoralis major, scalene, latissimus dorsi, and teres major and minor muscles may also be involved in shoulder pain. Additionally, it should be mentioned that not only are multiple muscles involved in patients with shoulder pain, but that each and every muscle can harbor multiple TrPs, both active and latent (Ge et al., 2008). In fact, two studies demonstrated that TrPs in the latissimus dorsi and pectoralis major muscles reproduced axillary arm pain in women with breast cancer who had undergone mastectomies (Fernandez-Lao et al., 2010).

Two randomised controlled trials showed promising results of manual TrP therapy in patients with shoulder pain (Hains et al., 2010; Bron et al., 2011a). Furthermore, an increasing number of studies report the effects of dry needling (DN) on pain and function with varying results. Arias-Buria and colleagues (2017) found that the inclusion of two sessions of TrP DN had significant positive effects on function but not on pain, which lasted for at least 12 months. In another study, patients aged 65 years and older were needled once in the infraspinatus muscle. Needling of an active TrP with or without needling of a latent TrP in the infraspinatus muscle had a significant effect on pain, pressure pain thresholds, and grip strength. Unfortunately, no comparison is made with a control group that received no treatment or sham treatment (Calvo-Lobo et al., 2017). In a study comparing a single session of DN of the infraspinatus on the symptomatic shoulder with the asymptomatic shoulder, researchers found that pain sensitivity and range of motion (ROM) increased after 3 to 4 days posttreatment in the symptomatic shoulder, whereas the muscle function was unchanged (Koppenhaver et al., 2016). Lane and colleagues (2017) described a case report of a 60-year-old woman with complaints of shoulder pain and upper extremity numbness and tingling elicited by compression of TrPs in the infraspinatus and teres minor muscles; DN resolved her symptoms in just two sessions.

Even patients suffering from spasticity after stroke may benefit from DN of shoulder muscles (Mendigutia-Gomez et al., 2016) as discussed in detail in Chapter 4.

One study investigated the effects of TrP DN in patients with poststroke shoulder pain and reported that patients in the intervention group reduced their analgesic medication use, improved their sleep and mood, and more effectively prepared them for their rehabilitation program than those in the control group (DiLorenzo et al., 2004). Others concluded that DN was not a valuable adjunct to an individual physical therapy protocol in the treatment of shoulder pain (Perez-Palomares et al., 2017). Finally, a research group from Taiwan reported that one single session of DN of myofascial TrPs in the extensor group of the forearm had an immediate small but significant effect on pain and pressure pain threshold in the ipsilateral trapezius muscle with an increase of the cervical ROM in contralateral sidebending (Tsai et al., 2010).

Shoulder Pain and Movement Dysfunction

Shoulder pain and disturbed movement patterns are closely related. A disturbed movement pattern of the scapular musculature such as the upper or lower trapezius and the anterior serratus muscles may cause mechanical dysfunction and deep shoulder pain (Cools et al., 2003; Kibler, 2006). On the other hand, there is evidence that muscle pain can create a different motor activation pattern. Falla and colleagues (2007) demonstrated that an injection with hypertonic saline reduced the electromyographic (EMG) activity in the painful (injected) muscle and led to hyperactivity of the muscles in the ipsilateral and contralateral shoulder. Another study found that latent TrPs in the posterior deltoid muscles were associated with reduced efficiency of reciprocal inhibition, which may lead to unbalanced muscle activation (Ibarra et al., 2011).

These findings appear consistent with the pain adaptation model of Lund and colleagues (1991), which maintains that muscle pain causes a decrease of EMG activity in the agonist muscle but causes an increase of EMG activity in the antagonists, finally leading to motor control changes. Martin and colleagues (2008) showed, however, that muscle nociception may result in excitation of both elbow flexor and extensor muscles; other researchers noted that the activity of motor neurons is not necessarily uniformly decreased (Farina et al., 2004, 2005; Tucker et al., 2009). As active TrPs cause muscle pain, they may also cause muscle inhibition and disturbances of motor activation patterns. In fact several researchers demonstrated that latent TrPs can disturb motor activation patterns (Lucas et al., 2010; Ibarra et al., 2011; Bohlooli et al., 2016).

Trigger Points and Range of Motion Restrictions

Adhesive capsulitis, also referred to as primary frozen shoulder, is the most common cause of severely restricted shoulder joint mobility. Of interest is that thickening of the shoulder capsule was identified as a primary shoulder motion restriction independent of adhesions (Texeira et al., 2012). Although the natural history of a frozen shoulder is usually described as consisting of episodes with stiffness and recovery phases eventually progressing to full recovery, there is no scientific evidence in support of this notion (Wong et al., 2017). Based on clinical experience of the authors of this chapter, inactivation of TrP in shoulder muscles, particularly the subscapularis muscle, frequently reduces patients' symptoms—including pain and restricted mobility—which may lead to an early and proper recovery within weeks. Again, there is no scientific evidence from the literature to support this clinical experience. In a multiple case study of five patients with primary frozen shoulders, all patients improved after a subscapular nerve block and subscapularis muscle injections (Jankovic & van Zundert, 2006). Recently another case report described the clinical reasoning behind the use of TrP DN in the treatment of a patient with adhesive capsulitis in which the rapid improvement seen after DN may suggest that muscles may indeed be a significant source of pain in this condition (Clewley et al., 2014).

Trigger Points and Stability

Another enigmatic shoulder disorder is referred to as minor, subtle, occult, or functional instability, which is often associated with shoulder pain and diagnosed as secondary shoulder impingement. Patients with this disorder complain of a feeling of instability in the absence of true instability, confirmed by physical examination tests such as the apprehension test. Although not mentioned in the literature, these patients often respond well to DN of the adductor muscles of the shoulder, including the teres major, latissimus dorsi, and subscapularis muscles. Unfortunately, until now there are no studies that have reported the clinical effects of DN on subtle shoulder instability, although the study by Ibarra and colleagues (2011) found evidence of fine movement control disturbances due to shoulder muscle TrPs.

DRY NEEDLING OF THE SHOULDER MUSCLES

Some of the shoulder muscles are covered in other chapters. The coracobrachialis, biceps, and triceps muscles are described in Chapter 9; the rhomboid and latissimus dorsi muscles are included in Chapter 10.

Supraspinatus Muscle

- *Anatomy:* The supraspinatus muscle originates from the supraspinous fossa of the scapula and inserts at the superior facet of the greater tubercle of the humerus.
- *Function:* The supraspinatus muscle assists in abduction and stabilises the humeral head together with the other rotator cuff muscles during all movements of the shoulder. The muscle prevents caudal dislocation during carrying of heavy loads such as bags and suitcases.
- *Innervation:* Suprascapular nerve, from the C5 and C6 nerve roots.
- *Referred pain:* TrP may refer to the middeltoid region, often extending down the lateral aspect of the arm and forearm, sometimes focusing strongly over the lateral epicondyle of the elbow.
- *Needling technique:* The patient lies prone (Fig. 8.1) or on the uninvolved side with the arm close to the body and relaxed (in sidelying position supported by a pillow) (Fig. 8.2). The supraspinatus muscle is only accessible through the upper trapezius muscle and is identified by flat palpation with sufficient pressure. After localisation of the TrP, the needle is inserted and directed longitudinal to the frontal plane or slightly posterior towards the base of the supraspinous fossa.
- *Precautions:* The apex of the lung is in front of the scapula, and clinicians should avoid needling in a ventral direction.

Infraspinatus Muscle

- *Anatomy:* The infraspinatus muscle originates from the infraspinous fossa of the scapula and inserts at the dorsosuperior facet of the greater tubercle of the humerus.

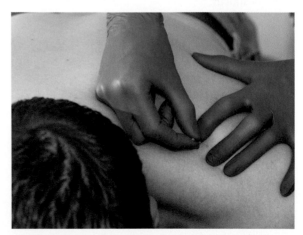

FIG. 8.1 Dry needling of the supraspinatus muscle in prone position.

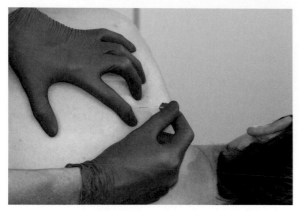

FIG. 8.2 Dry needling of the supraspinatus muscle in sidelying position.

- *Function:* The infraspinatus muscle assists in external rotation and stabilises the humeral head together with the other rotator cuff muscles and prevents upwards migration of the humeral head during all movements.
- *Innervation:* Suprascapular nerve, from the C5 and C6 nerve roots.
- *Referred pain:* TrP may refer to the front of the shoulder (intraarticular pain) and the middeltiod region, extending downwards the arm to the ventrolateral aspect of the arm and forearm and the radial aspect of the hand. The referred pain from this muscle can mimic the symptoms of carpal tunnel syndrome (Qerama et al., 2009).
- *Needling technique:* The patient lies prone (Fig. 8.3) or on the uninvolved side with the arm supported by a pillow (Fig. 8.4). The needle is directed towards the scapula.

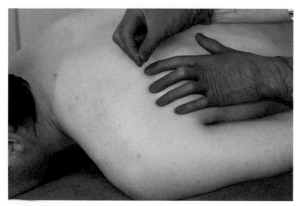

FIG. 8.3 Dry needling of the infraspinatus muscle in prone position.

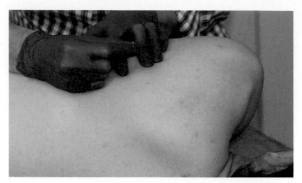

FIG. 8.4 Dry needling of the infraspinatus muscle in sidelying position.

- *Precautions:* In osteoporotic patients, fenestration of the scapula has been reported, which would imply that clinicians should avoid needling through the scapula. Pate and colleagues (1985) confirmed that scapular fenestration is indeed quite rare; in clinical practice, fenestration has not been an issue.

Teres Minor Muscle

- *Anatomy:* The teres minor muscle originates from the upper one-third of the lateral border of the dorsal surface of the scapula and inserts on the dorsal facet of the greater tubercle below the insertion of the infraspinatus muscle.
- *Function:* The teres minor muscle has the same function as the infraspinatus muscle but can also adduct the upper arm.
- *Innervation:* Axillary nerve, from the C5 and C6 nerve roots.
- *Referred pain:* TrPs refer to the dorsal aspect of the shoulder and may cause numbness and tingling in the ulnar aspect of the forearm and hand.
- *Needling technique:* The patient lies prone or in sidelying position with the arm supported by a pillow. TrPs in the teres minor muscle are palpated with a pincer palpation with the thumb of the clinician placed underneath the bulk of the muscle deep into the axilla and the fingers on either side of the TrP over the palpable taut band. The needle is directed to the thumb (Fig. 8.5).
- *Precautions:* When needling in front of the scapula, clinician can easily pass through the intercostal space and enter the pleura and lung.

Subscapularis Muscle

- *Anatomy:* The subscapularis muscle originates from the subscapular fossa and inserts to the lesser tubercle and reinforces the transverse ligament that overlies the bicipital sulcus.

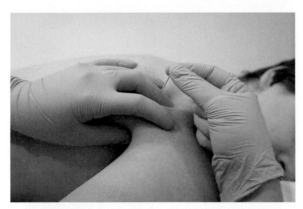

FIG. 8.5 Dry needling of the teres minor muscle in prone position.

- *Function:* The subscapularis muscle is an internal rotator assisted by the pectoral major muscle. It stabilises the humeral head together with the other rotator cuff muscles and prevents upward migration of the humeral head during all movements.
- *Innervation:* Subscapular nerve from the C5, C6, and C7 nerve roots.
- *Referred pain:* TrPs may refer to the dorsal aspect of the shoulder extending to the dorsal aspect of the upper arm and around the wrist.
- *Needling technique:*
  1. Axillary approach: The patient lies supine with the arm 90 degrees abducted and 90 degrees externally rotated. Bringing the scapula more laterally will optimise access to the muscle. The needle is directed parallel to the ribcage perpendicular to the scapula (Fig. 8.6).
  2. Medial approach: The patient lies prone with the arm in internal rotation and the forearm resting on the back at the lumbar level (hammerlock position). The needle is inserted from medial to lateral under the scapula (Fig. 8.7). The muscle can be also needled when the patient lies on the involved shoulder (Fig. 8.8).
- *Precautions:* As the subscapularis muscle is located between the ventral surface of the scapula and the ribcage, the needle has to be directed away from the ribcage to avoid entering the intercostal space.

Deltoid Muscle

- *Anatomy:* The deltoid muscle originates from the lateral third of the clavicle (ventral part), the entire lateral border of the acromion (middle part), and the lateral half of the spine of the scapula (posterior part). The entire muscle inserts on the deltoid

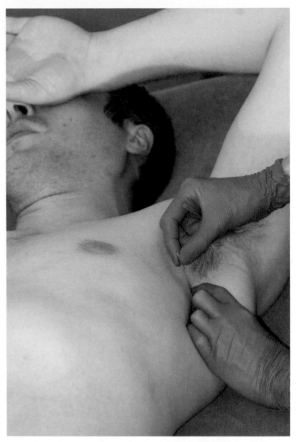

FIG. 8.6 Dry needling of the subscapularis muscle in supine position (axillary approach).

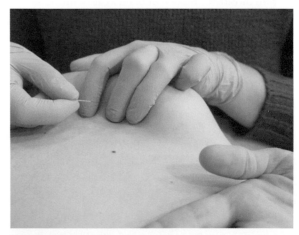

FIG. 8.7 Dry needling of the subscapularis muscle in prone position (medial approach).

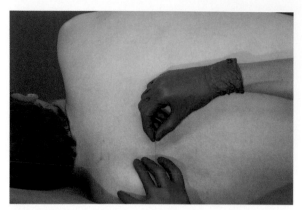

FIG. 8.8 Dry needling of the subscapularis muscle in sidelying position (medial approach).

tuberosity, which is a rough triangular area midway the anterolateral border of the humerus.

- *Function:* This thick, multipennate muscle is a prime mover for abduction of the upper arm and assists in flexion and internal rotation (ventral fibres) or extension and external rotation (dorsal fibres).
- *Innervation:* Axillary nerve from the C5 and C6 nerve roots.
- *Referred pain:* TrPs may refer to the region of the affected part (anterior, middle, or posterior) of the muscle.
- *Needle technique:* The anterior part can be needled in the supine position (Fig. 8.9), the posterior part in prone position (Fig. 8.10), and the middle part can be treated in the prone, supine, or sidelying position (Fig. 8.11). In all positions the upper arm is slightly abducted and supported by a pillow if necessary. The needle is inserted perpendicularly through the skin directly into the taut band against the humerus.
- *Precautions:* No special precautions.

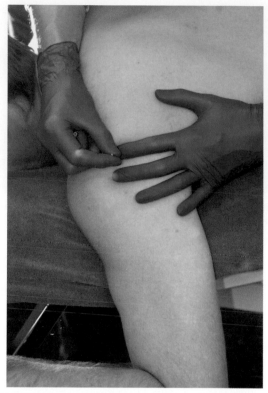

FIG. 8.10 Dry needling of the posterior deltoid muscle in prone position.

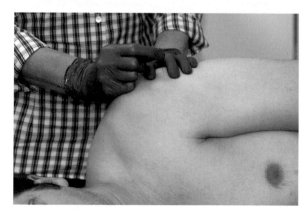

FIG. 8.11 Dry needling of the middle deltoid muscle in sidelying position.

Teres Major Muscle

- *Anatomy:* The teres major muscle originates from the posterior surface of the inferior angle of the scapula. The tendon of the teres major muscle fuses with the tendon of the latissimus dorsi muscle and inserts to the medial lip of the bicipital groove.

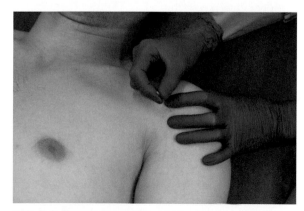

FIG. 8.9 Dry needling of the anterior deltoid muscle in supine position.

- *Function:* The teres major muscle assists the latissimus dorsi muscle in extension, internal rotation, and adduction of the arm.
- *Innervation:* Lower subscapularis nerve from the C6 and C7 nerve roots.
- *Referred pain:* TrPs may refer to the posterior deltoid, the posterior glenohumeral joint, over the long head of the triceps brachii, and occasionally to the dorsal forearm.
- *Needling technique:* The patient lies prone with the arm slightly abducted (Fig. 8.12). The muscle is grasped between the thumb and the second and third fingers, and the needle is directed ventral and lateral. It is also possible to needle this muscle in sidelying position, when a pillow in front of the patient supports the arm (Fig. 8.13). The treatment is the same for the axillar part of the latissimus dorsi muscle.
- *Precautions:* There is no danger for injury of the neurovascular bundle or entering the ribcage as long as the needle is directed ventrally and slightly laterally.

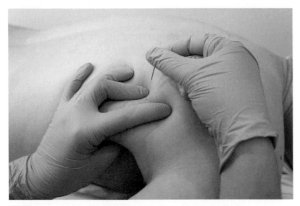

FIG. 8.12 Dry needling of the teres major muscle in prone.

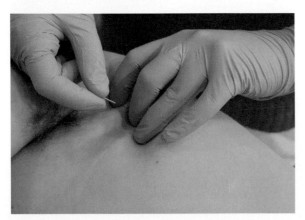

FIG. 8.13 Dry needling of the teres major muscle in sidelying position.

Pectoralis Minor Muscle

- *Anatomy:* The pectoralis minor muscle originates from the third, fourth, and fifth ribs near their costal cartilages and inserts at the coracoid process of the scapula together with the coracobrachialis muscle and the biceps brachii brevis.
- *Function:* The pectoralis minor muscle protracts and draws the scapula forward, downward, and inward. It also depresses the shoulder girdle and stabilises it against forceful upward pressure of the arm. Downward force of the pectoralis minor causes winging of the scapula. When the scapula is fixed by the trapezius and levator scapulae muscles, the pectoralis minor is an accessory respiratory muscle.
- *Innervation:* Medial pectoral nerve from the C8 and T1 nerve roots.
- *Referred pain:* TrPs may refer to the ventral aspect of the shoulder extending to the anterior chest region and the ulnar side of the arm to the third, fourth, and fifth finger. The referred pain is almost the same as from the referred pain area of the pectoralis major. The pain may mimic angina pectoris, pain of the tendon of the biceps brachii muscle, and a golfer's elbow.
- *Needling technique:* The patient lies in the supine position with the arm in approximately 80 degrees of abduction. A woman with ample breasts should be asked to cover her breast with the opposite hand. The coracoid process is identified, and the taut bands of the pectoralis minor muscle are subsequently palpated beneath the pectoralis major muscle. The thumb is moved over the ribcage underneath the pectoralis major muscle until the pectoralis minor muscle is palpated. The muscle is held between the thumb and the fingers in a pincer grip with the tips of the fingers and thumb slightly above the ribcage. The needle is now directed towards the thumb, preventing the needle to enter the thorax or the neurovascular bundle (Fig. 8.14).
- *Precautions:* As the pectoralis minor muscle is located over the ventral surface of the ribcage, clinicians have to be certain to avoid entering the intercostal space and penetrating the lung. The neurovascular bundle to the arm lies under the pectoralis minor muscle close to the coracoid process.

Pectoralis Major Muscle

- *Anatomy:* The pectoralis major muscle crosses three joints: the sternoclavicular, acromioclavicular, and glenohumeral joint. The pectoralis major muscle is a thick, fan-shaped muscle. Medially, it originates from four separate attachments: the clavicular fibres, which attach to the anterior surface of the

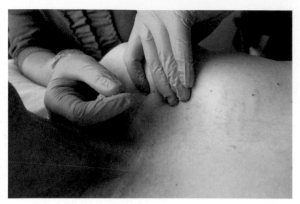

FIG. 8.14 Dry needling of the pectoralis minor muscle in supine position.

manubrium and along the medial half of the clavicle; the sternal fibres, which attach along the entire length of the sternum; the costal fibres, which attach to the first through seventh costal cartilages (sometimes the first and seventh are omitted); and the abdominal fibres, which attach to the aponeurosis of the external oblique. Laterally, all fibres converge to a flat, bilaminar tendon, which attaches to the crest of the greater tubercle of the humerus, along the lateral lip of the bicipital groove. The ventral layer, which is formed by fibres from the manubrium, clavicle, sternum, and second to fifth costal cartilages, is laminated like playing cards. The dorsal layer, which is formed by fibres from the sixth and often seventh costal cartilages, sixth rib, sternum, and aponeurosis of the external oblique, is folded, reversing the order of attachment of the fibres with the inferior fibres becoming superior fibres at the attachment site, where it blends with the capsular ligament of the shoulder joint. This arrangement should be kept in mind when palpating TrPs and eliciting local twitch responses.

- *Function:* The pectoralis major muscle protracts the shoulder girdle with the subclavius muscle and depresses the shoulder girdle with the sternal, costal, and abdominal fibres. It gives internal rotation and adduction of the arm and medial flexion across the chest and oblique upward and forward movement of the arm with the clavicular fibres. The pectoralis muscle is active in forceful inhalation.
- *Innervation:* The lateral pectoral nerve from the C5-C7 nerve roots and medial pectoral nerve from the C8 and T1 nerve roots.
- *Referred pain:* TrPs in the clavicular section refer pain over the anterior deltoid muscle. TrPs in the

intermediate sternal fibres refer pain to the anterior chest, down the inner aspect of the arm, and, possibly, to the volar aspect of the arm and ulnar side of the hand. TrPs in the medial sternal section refer to the sternum; TrPs in the costal and abdominal fibres cause breast tenderness and nipple hypersensitivity. Left pectoralis major TrPs may mimic angina, whereas a point on the right side in the intercostal space between the fifth and sixth ribs just lateral to the xyphoid process may be linked to cardiac arrhythmias (Simons et al., 1999).

- *Needling technique:* Position the patient in the supine position with the arm slightly abducted. Women, particularly those with ample breast tissue, may be asked to place their hand over their breast and move the breast out of the way. Stand or sit adjacent to the patient on the same or opposite side to be needled.
  1. Axillary portion: The axillar portion of the pectoralis major muscle is grasped with a pincer palpation. The needle is directed towards the thumb (Fig. 8.15).
  2. When needling the clavicular portion of the pectoralis major muscle, the needle is placed slightly medial to the TrP and directed in a shallow manner towards the TrP in the direction of the humerus (medial to lateral) (Fig. 8.16).
  3. TrPs near the costochondral junctions can be needled perpendicular to the direction of the ribs with a shallow to deeper approach using a 5 cm needle. The needle is always directed in a 'downhill' direction that can either be cranially or caudally, depending on the shape of the chest (Fig. 8.17).

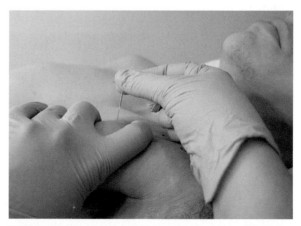

FIG. 8.15 Dry needling of the pectoralis major muscle (axillar portion).

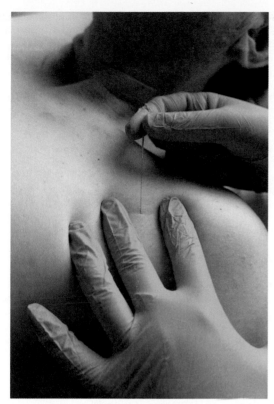

FIG. 8.16 Dry needling of the pectoralis major muscle (clavicular part).

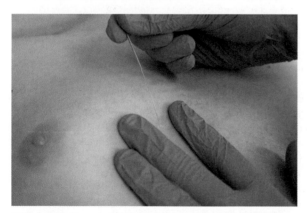

FIG. 8.17 Dry needling of the pectoralis major muscle (sternal part).

4. TrPs on the chest wall can only be needled safely over a rib with the index and long fingers placed over the intercostal spaces on either side of the rib. The needle should be inserted at a shallow angle, tangential to the chest wall, between the distal phalangeal joints of the fingers right above

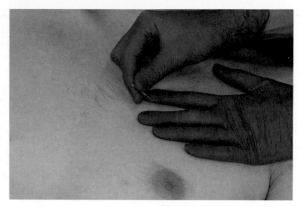

FIG. 8.18 Dry needling of the pectoralis major muscle (chest).

the rib with the TrP located between the proximal phalangeal joints (Fig. 8.18).
- *Precautions:* Care must be taken to prevent penetration into the lung, creating a pneumothorax. A special precaution to consider is the presence of breast or pectoral implants. DN is contraindicated in the presence of implants.

Subclavius Muscle
- *Anatomy:* The subclavius muscle lies beneath the clavicle over the first rib and attaches medially by a short thick tendon to the junction of the first rib with its cartilage. The muscle attaches laterally in a groove on the caudal aspect of the middle third of the clavicle.
- *Function:* The subclavius muscle indirectly assists in protraction of the shoulder by approximating the clavicle and the first rib.
- *Innervation:* Subclavius nerve from the C5 and C6 nerve roots.
- *Referred pain:* The pain travels across the front of the shoulder and down the front of the arm and along the radial side of the forearm and hand, skipping the elbow and wrist. In addition, the dorsal and volar aspects of the thumb, the index finger, and the middle finger also may hurt.
- *Needling technique:* The patient lies in the supine position. The needle is inserted and directed towards the point of maximum tenderness beneath the clavicle, usually in the middle of the muscle towards the junction of its medial and middle thirds. Strong referred pain patterns are likely to be elicited by needle penetration of TrPs (Fig. 8.19). To avoid needling the subclavian artery and vein, needling towards the sternum may be preferred.

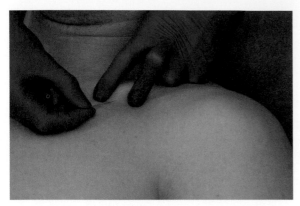

FIG. 8.19 Dry needling of subclavius muscle in supine position.

- *Precautions:* As the subclavius muscle is located over the ventral surface of the ribcage one has to be certain to avoid entering the intercostal space and penetrating the lung. The neurovascular bundle to the arm lies under the pectoralis minor muscle close to the coracoid process. The subclavian artery and vein are in very close proximity to the muscle and must be avoided.

REFERENCES

Arias-Buria, J. L., Fernandez-de-Las-Penas, C., Palacios-Cena, M., Koppenhaver, S. L., & Salom-Moreno, J. (2017). Exercises and dry needling for subacromial pain syndrome: a randomized parallel-group trial. *The Journal of Pain*, 18(1), 11–18.

Bohlooli, N., Ahmadi, A., Maroufi, N., Sarrafzadeh, J., & Jaberzadeh, S. (2016). Differential activation of scapular muscles, during arm elevation, with and without trigger points. *Journal of Bodywork and Movement Therapies*, 20, 26–34.

Bradley, M. P., Tung, G., & Green, A. (2005). Overutilization of shoulder magnetic resonance imaging as a diagnostic screening tool in patients with chronic shoulder pain. *Journal of Shoulder and Elbow Surgery*, 14, 233–237.

Bron, C. (2008). The subacromial impingement syndrome. *Tijdschrift Man Ther IFOMT Special*, 12–18.

Bron, C., De Gast, A., Dommerholt, J., Stegenga, B., Wensing, M., & Oostendorp, R. A. (2011a). Treatment of myofascial trigger points in patients with chronic shoulder pain: a randomized, controlled trial. *BMC Medicine*, 9, 8.

Bron, C., Dommerholt, J., Stegenga, B., Wensing, M., & Oostendorp, R. A. (2011b). High prevalence of shoulder girdle muscles with myofascial trigger points in patients with shoulder pain. *BMC Musculoskeletal Disorders*, 12, 139.

Buchbinder, R., Green, S., & Youd, J. M. (2009). Corticosteroid injections for shoulder pain. *Cochrane Database of Systematic Reviews*, CD004016.

Calvo-Lobo, C., Pacheco-Da-Costa, S., & Hita-Herranz, E. (2017). Efficacy of deep dry needling on latent myofascial trigger points in older adults with nonspecific shoulder pain: a randomized, controlled clinical trial pilot study. *Journal of Geriatric Physical Therapy (2001)*, 40(2), 63–73.

Clewley, D., Flynn, T. W., & Koppenhaver, S. (2014). Trigger point dry needling as an adjunct treatment for a patient with adhesive capsulitis of the shoulder. *The Journal of Orthopaedic and Sports Physical Therapy*, 44, 92–101.

Coghlan, J. A., Buchbinder, R., Green, S., Johnston, R. V., & Bell, S. N. (2008). Surgery for rotator cuff disease. *Cochrane Database of Systematic Reviews*, CD005619.

Cools, A. M., Witvrouw, E. E., Declercq, G. A., Danneels, L. A., & Cambier, D. C. (2003). Scapular muscle recruitment patterns: trapezius muscle latency with and without impingement symptoms. *The American Journal of Sports Medicine*, 31, 542–549.

Dilorenzo, L., Traballesi, M., Morelli, D., Pompa, A., Brunelli, S., Buzzi, M. G., & Formisano, R. (2004). Hemiparetic shoulder pain syndrome treated with deep dry needling during early rehabilitation: a prospective, open-label, randomized investigation. *Journal of Musculoskeletal Pain*, 12(2), 25–34.

Dorrestijn, O., Stevens, M., Winters, J. C., Van Der Meer, K., & Diercks, R. L. (2009). Conservative or surgical treatment for subacromial impingement syndrome? A systematic review. *Journal of Shoulder and Elbow Surgery*, 18, 652–660.

Falla, D., Farina, D., & Graven-Nielsen, T. (2007). Experimental muscle pain results in reorganization of coordination among trapezius muscle subdivisions during repetitive shoulder flexion. *Experimental Brain Research*, 178, 385–393.

Farina, D., Arendt-Nielsen, L., Merletti, R., & Graven-Nielsen, T. (2004). Effect of experimental muscle pain on motor unit firing rate and conduction velocity. *Journal of Neurophysiology*, 91, 1250–1259.

Farina, D., Arendt-Nielsen, L., & Graven-Nielsen, T. (2005). Spike triggered average torque and muscle fiber conduction velocity of low-threshold motor units following submaximal endurance contractions. *Journal of Applied Physiology*, 98, 1495–1502.

Fernandez-Lao, C., Cantarero-Villanueva, I., Fernandez-De-Las-Penas, C., Del-Moral L-Avila, R., Arendt-Nielsen, L., & Arroyo-Morales, M. (2010). Myofascial trigger points in neck and shoulder muscles and widespread pressure pain hypersensitivtiy in patients with postmastectomy pain: evidence of peripheral and central sensitization. *The Clinical Journal of Pain*, 26, 798–806.

Ge, H. Y., Fernandez-De-Las-Penas, C., Madeleine, P., & Arendt-Nielsen, L. (2008). Topographical mapping and mechanical pain sensitivity of myofascial trigger points in the infraspinatus muscle. *European Journal of Pain*, 12, 859–865.

Ginn, K. A., & Cohen, M. L. (2004). Conservative treatment for shoulder pain: prognostic indicators of outcome. *Archives of Physical Medicine and Rehabilitation*, 85, 1231–1235.

Hains, G., Descarreaux, M., & Hains, F. (2010). Chronic shoulder pain of myofascial origin: a randomized clinical trial using ischemic compression therapy. *Journal of Manipulative and Physiological Therapeutics*, 33, 362–369.

Hawkins, R. J., & Hobeika, P. E. (1983). Impingement syndrome in the athletic shoulder. *Clinics in Sports Medicine*, 2, 391–405.

Hegedus, E. J., Goode, A., Campbell, S., Morin, A., Tamaddoni, M., Moorman, C. T., 3rd, & Cook, C. (2008). Physical examination tests of the shoulder: a systematic review with meta-analysis of individual tests. *British Journal of Sports Medicine*, 42(2), 80–92.

Hidalgo-Lozano, A., Fernández-de-las-Peñas, C., Alonso-Blanco, C., Ge, H.-Y., Arendt-Nielsen, L., & Arroyo-Morales, M. (2010). Muscle trigger points and pressure pain hyperalgesia in the shoulder muscles in patients with unilateral shoulder impingement: a blinded, controlled study. *Experimental Brain Research*, 202(4), 915–925.

Hidalgo-Lozano, A., Fernandez-de-Las-Penas, C., Calderon-Soto, C., Domingo-Camara, A., Madeleine, P., & Arroyo-Morales, M. (2013). Elite swimmers with and without unilateral shoulder pain: mechanical hyperalgesia and active/latent muscle trigger points in neck-shoulder muscles. *Scandinavian Journal of Medicine & Science in Sports*, 23(1), 66–73.

Ibarra, J. M., Ge, H. Y., Wang, C., Martinez Vizcaino, V., Graven-Nielsen, T., & Arendt-Nielsen, L. (2011). Latent myofascial trigger points are associated with an increased antagonistic muscle activity during agonist muscle contraction. *The Journal of Pain*, 12(12), 1282–1288.

Ingber, R. S. (2000). Shoulder impingement in tennis/racquetball players treated with subscapularis myofascial treatments. *Archives of Physical Medicine and Rehabilitation*, 81(5), 679–682.

Jankovic, D., & Van Zundert, A. (2006). The frozen shoulder syndrome. Description of a new technique and five case reports using the subscapular nerve block and subscapularis trigger point infiltration. *Acta Anaesthesiologica Belgica*, 57, 137–143.

Kibler, W. B. (2006). Scapular involvement in impingement: signs and symptoms. *Instructional Course Lectures*, 55, 35–43.

Koppenhaver, S., Embry, R., Ciccarello, J., Waltrip, J., Pike, R., Walker, M., … Flynn, T. (2016). Effects of dry needling to the symptomatic versus control shoulder in patients with unilateral subacromial pain syndrome. *Manual therapy*, 26, 62–69.

Lane, E., Clewley, D., & Koppenhaver, S. (2017). Complaints of upper extremity numbness and tingling relieved with dry needling of the teres minor and infraspinatous: a case report. *The Journal of Orthopaedic and Sports Physical Therapy*, 47(4), 287–292.

Lucas, K. R., Rich, P. A., & Polus, B. I. (2010). Muscle activation patterns in the scapular positioning muscles during loaded scapular plane elevation: the effects of latent myofascial trigger points. *Clinical Biomechanics*, 25(8), 765–770.

Lund, J., Donga, R., Widmer, C., & Stohler, C. (1991). The pain-adaptation model: a discussion of the relationship between chronic musculoskeletal pain and motor activity. *Canadian Journal of Physiology and Pharmacology*, 69(5), 683–694.

Martin, P. G., Weerakkody, N., Gandevia, S. C., & Taylor, J. L. (2008). Group III and IV muscle afferents differentially affect the motor cortex and motoneurones in humans. *The Journal of Physiology*, 586, 1277–1289.

Matava, M. J., Purcell, D. B., & Rudzki, J. R. (2005). Partial-thickness rotator cuff tears. *The American Journal of Sports Medicine*, 33, 1405–1417.

Mendigutia-Gomez, A., Martin-Hernandez, C., Salom-Moreno, J., & Fernandez-de-las-Penas, C. (2016). Effect of dry needling on spasticity, shoulder range of motion, and pressure pain sensitivity in patients with stroke: a crossover study. *Journal of Manipulative and Physiological Therapeutics*, 39, 348–358.

Milgrom, C., Schaffler, M., Gilbert, S., & Van Holsbeeck, M. (1995). Rotator-cuff changes in asymptomatic adults. The effect of age, hand dominance and gender. *Journal of Bone and Joint Surgery. British Volume (London)*, 77(2), 296–298.

Neer, C. S. (1972). Anterior acromioplasty for the chronic impingement syndrome in the shoulder: a preliminary report. *The Journal of Bone and Joint Surgery. American Volume*, 54, 41–50.

Papadonikolakis, A., McKenna, M., Warme, W., Martin, B. I., & Matsen, F. A. (2011). Published evidence relevant to the diagnosis of impingement syndrome of the shoulder. *The Journal of Bone and Joint Surgery. American Volume*, 93(19), 1827–1832.

Pate, D., Kursunoglu, S., Resnick, D., & Resnik, C. S. (1985). Scapular foramina. *Skeletal Radiology*, 14(4), 270–275.

Perez-Palomares, S., Olivan-Blazquez, B., Perez-Palomares, A., Gaspar-Calvo, E., Perez-Benito, M., Lopez-Lapena, E., … Magallon-Botaya, R. (2017). Contribution of dry needling to individualized physical therapy treatment of shoulder pain: a randomized clinical trial. *J Orthop Sports Phys Ther*, 47(1), 11–20.

Qerama, E., Kasch, H., & Fuglsang-Frederiksen, A. (2009). Occurrence of myofascial pain in patients with possible carpal tunnel syndrome - a single-blinded study. *European Journal of Pain*, 13, 588–591.

Simons, D. G., Travell, J. G., & Simons, L. S. (1999). *Travell and Simons' myofascial pain and dysfunction; the trigger point manual*, Vol 1, 2nd ed. Baltimore: Williams & Wilkins.

Sola, A. E., & Kuitert, J. H. (1955). Myofascial trigger point pain in the neck and shoulder girdle; report of 100 cases treated by injection of normal saline. *Northwest Medicine*, 54, 980–984.

Teixeira, P., Balaj, C., Chanson, A., Lecocq, S., Louis, M., & Blum, A. (2012). Adhesive capsulitis of the shoulder: value of inferior glenohumeral ligament signal changes on T2-weighted fat saturated images. *American Journal of Roentgram*, 198, W589–596.

Tsai, C. T., Hsieh, L. F., Kuan, T. S., Kao, M. J., Chou, L. W., & Hong, C. Z. (2010). Remote effects of dry needling on the irritability of the myofascial trigger point in the upper trapezius muscle. *American Journal of Physical Medicine & Rehabilitation, 89*(2), 133–140.

Tucker, K., Butler, J., Graven-Nielsen, T., Riek, S., & Hodges, P. (2009). Motor unit recruitment strategies are altered during deep tissue pain. *The Journal of Neuroscience, 29,* 10820–10826.

Van Der Windt, D. A., Koes, B. W., De Jong, B. A., & Bouter, L. M. (1995). Shoulder disorders in general practice: incidence, patient characteristics, and management. *Annals of the Rheumatic Diseases, 54,* 959–964.

Wong, C. K., Levine, W. N., Deo, K., Kesting, R. S., Mercer, E. A., Schram, G. A., & Strang, B. L. (2017). Natural history of frozen shoulder: fact or fiction? A systematic review. *Physiotherapy, 103*(1), 40–47.

CHAPTER 9

Deep Dry Needling of the Arm and Hand Muscles

CÉSAR FERNÁNDEZ-DE-LAS-PEÑAS • JAVIER GONZÁLEZ IGLESIAS •
CHRISTIAN GRÖBLI • MARÍA PALACIOS-CEÑA • JOSÉ L. ARIAS-BURÍA

INTRODUCTION

Arm pain syndromes constitute a complex entity which can arise from a wide range of different conditions. Symptoms in the upper quadrant, including the neck, shoulder, arm, forearm, or hand not related to an acute trauma or underlying systemic diseases, can be provoked by trigger points (TrPs). In fact, there are several neck and shoulder muscles with referred pain pattern perceived throughout the upper extremity, for example, the scalenes, subclavius, pectoralis minor, supraspinatus, infraspinatus, subscapularis, pectoralis major, latissimus dorsi, serratus posterior superior, and serratus anterior muscles (Simons et al., 1999). A combination of referred pain patterns from TrPs in multiple neck, shoulder, and forearm muscles can create a complex clinical pattern of nonspecific arm pain (Fernández-de-las Peñas et al., 2012). Furthermore, TrP referred pain in some muscles can mimic some neuropathic pain conditions. Qerama and colleagues (2009) demonstrated that 49% of individuals with normal electrophysiological findings in the median nerve, but with symptoms mimicking carpal tunnel syndrome, presented with active TrPs in the infraspinatus muscle with paresthesia and referred pain to the arm and fingers. In the same study, patients with mild electrophysiological signs of carpal tunnel syndrome exhibited a significantly higher occurrence of infraspinatus muscle TrPs in the symptomatic arm compared with patients with moderate to severe electrophysiological signs (33% versus 20%). Dry needling (DN) of the shoulder musculature can improve pain, sensitivity, and grip power of individuals presenting with lateral epicondylalgia (Kheradmandi et al., 2015). DN of the neck and shoulder muscles is covered in Chapter 7 (neck) and Chapter 8 (shoulders).

TrP taut bands in the musculature of the upper quadrant can be related to neural or articular dysfunctions. For instance, because the brachial plexus runs anatomically between the anterior and the medial scalene muscles, taut bands and TrPs in the scalene muscles may be related to entrapment of the brachial plexus. Similarly, shortening of the scalene muscles induced by TrP taut bands may be related to first rib dysfunctions (Ferguson & Gerwin, 2005), which means that clinicians should integrate TrP DN within the overall clinical reasoning process and management. In the current chapter we will cover deep DN of TrPs in the arm and hand muscles.

CLINICAL RELEVANCE OF TRIGGER POINTS IN ARM AND HAND PAIN SYNDROMES

There are only a few studies demonstrating the relevance of TrPs in the aetiology of different arm pain syndromes. The most commonly described muscle pain syndrome in the arm is probably lateral epicondylalgia (Slater et al., 2003). Fernández-Carnero and colleagues (2007) found that active TrPs in the extensor wrist musculature reproduced the pain symptoms in subjects with lateral epicondylalgia (65% extensor carpi radialis brevis; 55% extensor carpi radialis longus; 50% brachioradialis; 25% extensor digitorum communis muscle). In a subsequent study, Fernández-Carnero and colleagues (2008) reported that subjects with unilateral lateral epicondylalgia also exhibited latent TrPs in muscles of the unaffected elbow (88% extensor carpi radialis brevis; 80% extensor carpi radialis longus), which may be related to the development of bilateral symptoms in this patient population. Active TrPs in the extensor carpi radialis brevis were very prevalent (68% right side; 57% left side) in women with fibromyalgia syndrome (Alonso-Blanco et al., 2011). Although these studies support the role of TrPs in arm pain syndromes, particularly in lateral epicondylalgia, further studies are needed (Shmushkevich & Kalichman, 2013). A recent study reported almost excellent agreement on TrP location and classification in the extensor carpi radialis brevis and extensor digitorum communis muscles (Mora-Relucio, et al., 2016). It is also important to consider that when TrPs are present in the brachioradialis (Mekhail et al., 1999) or extensor carpi radialis brevis muscles (Clavert et al., 2009), entrapment of the radial nerve is feasible. The only randomised clinical trial investigating the effectiveness of DN in lateral epicondylalgia observed that TrP DN was more effective than medical drug treatment at 6 months (Uygur et al., 2017).

In clinical practice an association between TrPs in the wrist flexor muscles and medial epicondylalgia is commonly seen, particularly in individuals with high muscular demands in the forearm (i.e., climbers) (González-Iglesias et al., 2011), or with low but repetitive loading (i.e., manual or office workers) (Fernández-de-las Peñas et al., 2012). Again, TrPs in the wrist flexor musculature can be also related to different nerve entrapments. For instance, as the pronator teres muscle is a common place for median nerve entrapment, commonly referred to as pronator syndrome (Lee & LaStayo, 2004), tension induced by TrP taut bands may be relevant for symptoms associated with median nerve compression (Simons et al., 1999). Similarly, the median nerve can be entrapped by TrPs in the flexor digitorum profundus and superficialis muscles, whereas the ulnar nerve can be entrapped by TrPs in the flexor carpi ulnaris and flexor digitorum profundus (Chaitow & Delany, 2008). Therefore clinicians should consider muscle–nerve interrelations in their daily practice even though no scientific study has confirmed the clinical observations.

Finally, TrPs within the intrinsic muscles of the hand, that is, the interossei and lumbricals, can also be clinically relevant for unspecific wrist–hand pain. For instance, manual laborers or boxers who have suffered a traumatic event over the wrist or the hand frequently develop TrPs in these muscles. There is clinical evidence that TrP DN of the intrinsic hand muscles such as the dorsal interossei is highly effective in these patients. TrPs in the thenar muscles are commonly seen in complaints of presumed arthritic changes in the joints of the thumb. DN of TrPs in the abductor pollicis brevis may relieve the pain associated with these joint problems (Villafañe & Herrero, 2016). Again, no scientific study has been published confirming these clinical observations.

It is important for clinicians to combine scientific and empirical evidence, as often there is no scientific evidence yet for several approaches that clinically are found to be effective. In this chapter we cover DN of TrPs in the arm and hand musculature based on clinical and scientific reasoning.

DRY NEEDLING OF THE ARM AND HAND MUSCLES
Coracobrachialis Muscle

- *Anatomy:* The coracobrachialis muscle originates from the coracoid process and inserts to the mid-portion of the humerus bone.
- *Function:* The coracobrachialis muscle assists in flexion and adduction of the arm at the glenohumeral joint.
- *Innervation:* Musculocutaneous nerve via the lateral cord from the C5 and C6 roots. It should be noted that the musculocutaneous nerve crosses the muscle belly of the coracobrachialis underneath the pectoralis major muscle.
- *Referred pain:* TrPs in the coracobrachialis muscle refer to the anterior aspect of the shoulder and also down the back of the arm and dorsum of the forearm to the back of the hand. The pain may mimic bicipital tendinopathy of the short head of the biceps.
- *Needling technique:* The patient lies supine with slight external rotation and abduction of the humerus. The muscle is needled with flat palpation. For the proximal part of the muscle between the coracoid process and the pectoralis major muscle, the tendon of the short head of the biceps brachii is palpated first. By gliding medially of the biceps tendon, the coracobrachialis muscle can be palpated. The location of the coracobrachialis muscle can be verified by flexion of the arm with the biceps in passive flexion at the elbow. The needle is inserted medial from the TrP in the coracobrachialis muscle and directed in a shallow manner towards the TrP (Fig. 9.1). Below the

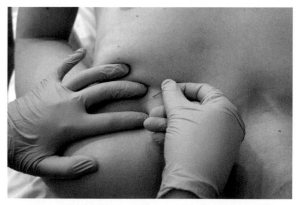

FIG. 9.1 Dry needling of the coracobrachialis muscle (proximal).

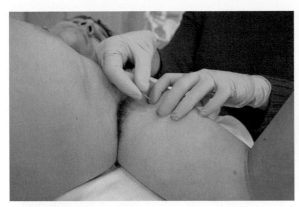

FIG. 9.2 Dry needling of the coracobrachialis muscle (distal).

pectoralis major muscle the needle is inserted perpendicular to the skin from the medial to lateral side towards the humerus (Fig. 9.2).

- *Precautions:* In the proximal part of the coracobrachialis muscle, the neurovascular bundle, which includes the median nerve, the musculocutaneous nerve, the ulnar nerve, and the brachial artery, is located underneath the muscle. In the distal part, it is dorsal and medial to the muscle. The musculocutaneous nerve passes through the muscle underneath the pectoralis muscle.

Biceps Brachii Muscle

- *Anatomy:* The long head of the biceps brachii muscle attaches to the upper margin of the glenoid fossa. The tendon passes through the glenohumeral joint over the head of the humerus. The short head attaches to the coracoid process of the scapula. Both heads join in a common tendon to insert at the radial tuberosity, facing the ulna in the supinated forearm.
- *Function:* The long head of the biceps brachii seats the humerus in the glenoid fossa when the arm is extended and loaded. Both heads assist in flexion of the arm at the shoulder and abduction of the arm at the shoulder in the externally rotated (and supinated) arm. The muscle is one of the three flexors at the elbow (together with the brachialis and the brachioradialis muscles) and acts most strongly when the hand is supinated. It also supinates the forearm when the arm is not fully extended.
- *Innervation:* Musculocutaneous nerve, via the lateral cord from the C5 and C6 roots. It should be noted that, anatomically, the median nerve runs medial to the muscle belly of the biceps brachii (Maeda et al., 2009).

- *Referred pain:* TrPs in the biceps brachii refer pain upward over the muscle and over the anterior deltoid region of the shoulder and occasionally to the suprascapular region; they can mimic symptoms of long head bicipital tendonitis. TrPs also may initiate another additional pattern of milder pain downward in the antecubital space.
- *Needling technique:* The patient lies supine with the arm slightly flexed. The muscle is grasped between the thumb and index and long fingers. Taut bands are identified. The muscle is commonly needled from a lateral approach to avoid needling the neurovascular bundle at the medial side, but with careful palpation it is quite easy to needle the muscle wherever clinically relevant trigger points are found. The needle is directed into the taut bands to elicit local twitch responses. The two heads of the biceps are palpated and treated separately (Fig. 9.3).

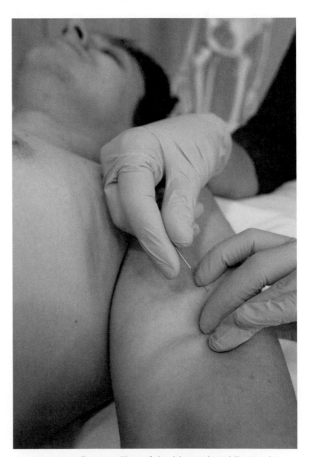

FIG. 9.3 Dry needling of the biceps brachii muscle.

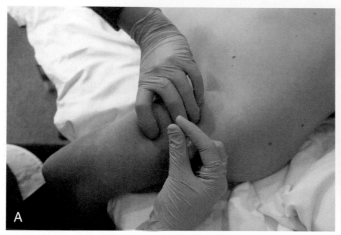
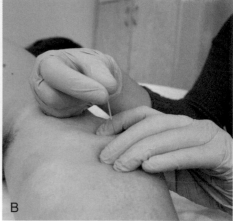

FIG. 9.4 Dry needling of the triceps brachii muscle.

- *Precautions:* The neurovascular bundle, which includes the median nerve, the musculocutaneous nerve, the ulnar nerve, and the brachial artery, is located medially to the biceps brachii muscle and must be avoided. In addition, avoid the radial nerve that lies along the lateral border of the distal biceps and the brachialis muscles.

Triceps Brachii Muscle

- *Anatomy:* The long head of the triceps brachii muscle originates from the scapula inferior to the glenoid fossa and is the only head that crosses the shoulder joint. The medial head originates from the medial portion of the humerus and the lateral head originates from the lateral side of the humerus. All three heads insert to the olecranon process on the ulna via a common tendon.
- *Function:* This triceps brachii muscle extends the forearm at the elbow and is an antagonist of the biceps brachii muscle. The main function of the long head of the triceps brachii muscle is adduction of the arm at the shoulder and rotation of the scapula to elevate the humeral head towards the acromion.
- *Innervation:* Radial nerve, via the posterior cord of the brachial plexus from spinal roots C7 and C8.
- *Referred pain:* TrP in the triceps brachii muscle refer up and down the posterior aspect of the shoulder, spreading potentially to the upper trapezius region, the posterior part of the arm, the dorsum of the forearm, the fourth and fifth digits (lateral head), and the lateral and sometimes the medial epicondyle (medial head).

- *Needling technique:* The triceps brachii can be treated with the patient in supine, sidelying, or prone position. The prone position is the preferred position as the entire triceps muscle can be treated. The muscle is palpated with a pincer palpation and the needle is directed to the underlying thumb (Fig. 9.4). The muscle can also be needled with a flat palpation, but it is harder to avoid needling into the radial nerve.
- *Precautions:* The radial nerve runs deep to the lateral head of the triceps muscle (Rezzouk et al., 2002) and must be avoided. A recent case report showed that needling the radial nerve could cause major complications (McManus & Cleary, 2018).

Anconeus Muscle

- *Anatomy:* The anconeus muscle originates from the side of the olecranon process and to the dorsal surface of the ulna and inserts to the lateral epicondyle.
- *Function:* The anconeus muscle assists the extension movement of the forearm at the elbow and is an agonist of the triceps brachii muscle.
- *Innervation:* Radial nerve, via the posterior cord of the brachial plexus from spinal roots C7 and C8.
- *Referred pain:* TrPs in the anconeus muscle induce pain and tenderness locally to the lateral epicondyle.
- *Needling technique:* The patient lies in the prone position with the forearm flexed about 45 degrees at the elbow. The muscle is needled with flat palpation. As the anconeus muscle is often a thin muscle, the needle is inserted slightly proximal to the TrP and redirected towards the TrP (Fig. 9.5).
- *Precautions:* None

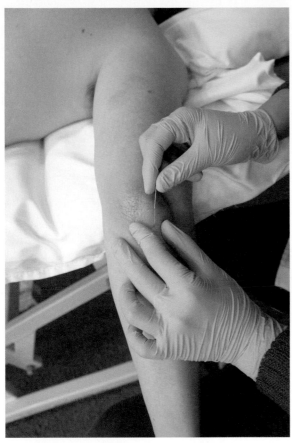

FIG. 9.5 Dry needling of the anconeus muscle.

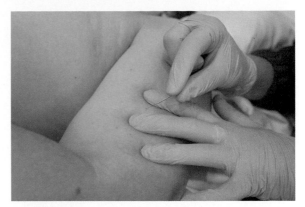

FIG. 9.6 Dry needling of the brachialis muscle.

the medial aspect is indicated, the neurovascular bundle and especially the median nerve must be avoided.

- *Precautions:* The neurovascular bundle should be avoided over the medial head of the muscle.

Brachioradialis Muscle

- *Anatomy:* The brachioradialis muscle starts from the upper two-thirds of the supracondylar ridge of the humerus and attaches over the distal radius at the styloid process.
- *Function:* In the neutral position of the forearm, the brachioradialis muscle flexes the forearm at the elbow.
- *Innervation:* Radial nerve, via the posterior cord of the brachial plexus from spinal roots C7 and C8.
- *Referred pain:* TrPs in the brachioradialis muscle refer to the lateral epicondyle, the radial aspect of the forearm, the wrist, and the base of the thumb.
- *Needling technique:* The patient lies in the supine position. The brachioradialis muscle is needled with pincer palpation. The needle is inserted from either the medial or the lateral aspect of the forearm and directed towards the practitioner's finger (Fig. 9.7). In patients with a very thin brachioradialis muscle, needling in between the fingers may be a safer option for the clinician to avoid needling the opposing finger.
- *Precautions:* The brachioradialis muscle is the most superficial muscle over the lateral elbow. The radial nerve passes close to it (Mekhail et al., 1999) and must be avoided. Clinicians should be aware of needling their opposing finger in patients with a very thin brachioradialis muscle when they used the pincer procedure.

Brachialis Muscle

- *Anatomy:* The brachialis muscle originates from the distal two-thirds of the humerus and inserts at the coronoid process of the ulnar tuberosity. This muscle extends into the anterior part of the joint capsule of the elbow.
- *Function:* The brachialis muscle flexes the forearm at the elbow.
- *Innervation:* Musculocutaneous nerve, via the lateral cord and by spinal roots C5 and C6.
- *Referred pain:* TrPs in the brachialis muscle refer to the base of the thumb and often to the antecubital region of the elbow.
- *Needling technique:* The patient lies supine with the elbow relaxed and slightly flexed. The muscle is needled with a flat palpation towards the humerus. The muscle is needled primarily from the lateral aspect of the arm to avoid hitting the neurovascular bundle (Fig. 9.6). When needling TrPs in

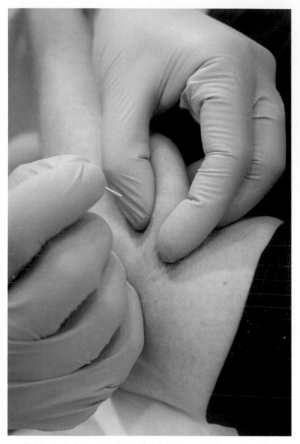

FIG. 9.7 Dry needling of the brachioradialis muscle.

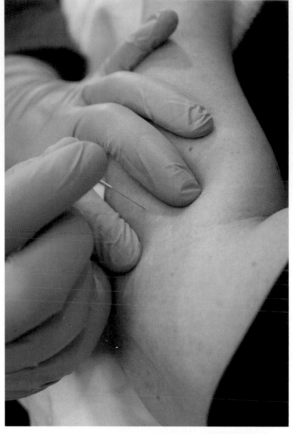

FIG. 9.8 Dry needling of the supinator muscle.

Supinator Muscle

- *Anatomy:* The supinator muscle originates from the lateral humeral epicondyle, the radial collateral ligament, the annular ligament, and the supinator crest of the ulna. The muscle inserts over the radial tuberosity and upper third of the radial shaft.
- *Function:* The supinator muscle supinates the forearm and may assist flexion at the elbow.
- *Innervation:* Radial nerve, via the posterior cord of the brachial plexus from spinal roots C7 and C8. In fact, the radial nerve crosses the fibrous arch of the supinator muscle, called the arcade of Frohse. Muscle tension induced by TrPs taut bands in this muscle can entrap the radial nerve, particularly the posterior interosseous muscle, which is the motor branch (Schneider, 2005; Tatar et al., 2009).
- *Referred pain:* TrPs in the supinator muscle refer mainly to the lateral epicondyle, the lateral area of

the elbow, and sometimes can project spillover pain to the dorsal aspect of the web of the thumb.
- *Needling technique:* The patient is in the supine position. The muscle is needled with flat palpation. The needle is inserted perpendicular to the skin at the dorsal aspect of the forearm at the level of upper third of the radial bone (Fig. 9.8). Trps at the ventral part of the muscles can be needled in a similar fashion.
- *Precautions:* There is a risk of hitting the superficial branch of the radial nerve over the muscle or the posterior interosseous nerve between the two heads of the muscle.

Wrist and Finger Extensor Muscles

- *Anatomy:* The wrist–finger extensor muscles, including the extensor carpi radialis longus, extensor carpi radialis brevis, extensor digitorum communis, and extensor carpi ulnaris muscles, originate from the lateral supracondylar ridge of the humerus, the lateral epicondyle, the radial ligament of the elbow, and the intermuscular septa through a common tendon. The attachments are at the base of the second metacarpal bone for the extensor carpi radialis longus muscle, the base of the third metacarpal bone for the extensor carpi radialis brevis muscle, the ulnar aspect of the base of the fifth metacarpal bone for the extensor carpi ulnaris muscle, and the distal phalanx of the second to fourth fingers for the extensor digitorum communis muscle.

- *Function:* The wrist–finger extensor muscles extend the wrist. The extensor carpi radialis longus muscle provides radial abduction of the hand, and the extensor carpi ulnaris muscle provides ulnar abduction. The extensor digitorum communis extends the phalanges.
- *Innervation:* Deep branch of the radial nerve (posterior interosseous nerve), via the posterior cord of the brachial plexus from spinal roots C7 and C8. The radial nerve may get entrapped in the superior-lateral aspect of the extensor carpi radialis brevis muscle (Clavert et al., 2009).
- *Referred pain:* TrPs in the extensor carpi radialis longus muscle refer pain to the lateral epicondyle and to the dorsum of the hand next to the thumb. TrPs in the extensor carpi radialis brevis muscle project pain to the radial and posterior aspects of the hand and the wrist. TrPs in the extensor digitorum communis muscle refer pain downward to the forearm, reaching the same digit that the fibres activate; TrPs in the extensor carpi ulnaris muscle refer pain to the ulnar side of the back of the wrist.
- *Needling technique:* The patient lies in supine position with the forearm pronated. The extensor carpi radialis longus is usually needled with a pincer palpation (Fig. 9.9). The extensor carpi radialis brevis, located medial to the extensor digitorum muscles, can be needled with a pincer (similar to the extensor carpi radialis longus) or flat palpation depending upon the size of the muscle. The extensor digitorum muscles are needled with flat palpation. The needle is inserted perpendicular to the skin and directed towards the radius bone (Fig. 9.10). For the extensor carpi ulnaris the needle is inserted perpendicular to the skin and directed towards the ulnar bone (Fig. 9.11). Because these are relatively flat muscles, needling directly over a TrP may not be as accurate as inserting the needle 1 cm or so away

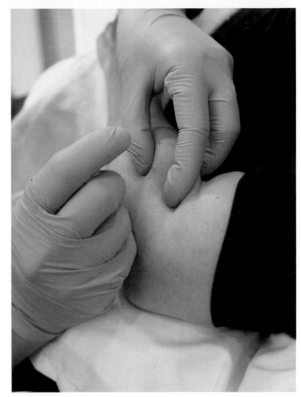

FIG. 9.9 Dry needling of the extensor carpi radialis longus muscle.

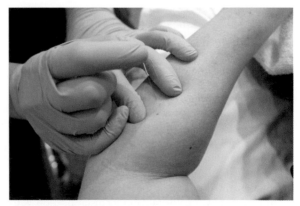

FIG. 9.10 Dry needling of the extensor digitorum muscle.

from the TrP and needle towards the TrP using a shallow to deeper needling approach.

- *Precautions:* The radial nerve crosses over the extensor digitorum muscle and the extensor carpi radialis brevis and should be avoided.

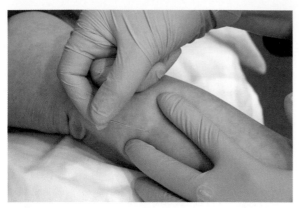

FIG. 9.11 Dry needling of the extensor carpi ulnaris muscle.

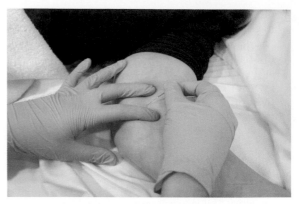

FIG. 9.12 Dry needling of the pronator teres muscle (proximal).

Pronator Teres Muscle

- *Anatomy:* The humeral head of the pronator teres muscle originates from the medial epicondyle, whereas the ulnar head originates from the medial side of the coronoid process of the ulnar bone. Both heads insert over the radius distally from the insertion of the supinator muscle.
- *Function:* The pronator teres muscle pronates the forearm and assists the pronator quadratus, the primary pronator, in fast movements and to overcome resistance.
- *Innervation:* Median nerve, via the lateral cord and upper and middle trunks of the brachial plexus from spinal roots C6 and C7. In fact, the median nerve runs in between the two heads of the pronator teres muscle (Lee & LaStayo, 2004).
- *Referred pain:* TrPs in the pronator teres muscle refer deep in the volar radial region of the wrist and of the forearm over the carpal tunnel.
- *Needling technique:* The patient lies in supine position with the forearm supinated. The muscle can be needled at the proximal, medial portion approximately 1 to 2 cm below the medial epicondyle to avoid the median and ulnar nerves. The muscle is palpated with flat palpation. The needle is inserted perpendicular to the skin and directed towards the ulna (Fig. 9.12). The muscle can also be needled in its distal portion with needling towards the radius (Fig. 9.13).
- *Precautions:* The median nerve runs between the two heads of the muscle and should be avoided.

Wrist and Finger Flexor Muscles

- *Anatomy:* The wrist–finger flexor muscles, including the flexor carpi radialis, palmaris longus, flexor digitorum superficialis, flexor digitorum

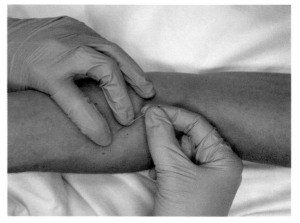

FIG. 9.13 Dry needling of the pronator teres muscle (distal).

profundus, and flexor carpi ulnaris muscles, originate from the lateral supracondylar ridge of the humerus, the medial epicondyle, and the intermuscular septa via a common tendon. The flexor pollicis longus originates from the radius, the interosseous membrane, and the humerus, and attaches to the base of the distal phalanx of the thumb. The muscle is covered by the flexor digitorum superficialis. The attachments of the other flexor muscles are the palmar aspect of the second metacarpal bone for the flexor carpi radialis muscle, the base of the palmar fascia for the palmaris longus muscle, the ulnar aspect of the base of the fifth metacarpal bone for the flexor carpi ulnaris muscle, the second phalanx of the second to fourth fingers for the flexor digitorum superficialis muscle, and the third phalanx of the second to fourth fingers for the flexor digitorum profundus muscle. It should be noted that the palmaris longus muscle is not present in all subjects.

- *Function:* The wrist–finger flexor muscles flex the wrist. The flexor carpi radialis muscle provides radial abduction of the hand at the wrist, and the flexor carpi ulnaris muscle provides ulnar abduction. The flexor digitorum communis muscle flexes the phalanges. The primary function of the flexor pollicis longus is flexion of the terminal phalanx of the thumb.

- *Innervation:* Median nerve, via the lateral cord and upper-middle trunks of the brachial plexus from spinal roots C6 and C7; ulnar nerve, via the medial cord and lower trunk of the brachial plexus from spinal roots C8 and T1. In fact, the median nerve can be entrapped by the flexor digitorum profundus and superficialis muscles and the ulnar nerve can be entrapped by the flexor carpi ulnaris and flexor digitorum profundus muscles (Chaitow & Delany, 2008).

- *Referred pain:* TrPs in the flexor carpi radialis muscle refer pain to the volar aspect of the wrist. TrPs in the palmaris longus muscle project superficial, needle-like pain over the volar area of the palm. TrPs in the flexor carpi ulnaris muscle refer pain to the ulnar side of the volar aspect of the wrist, whereas TrPs in the flexor digitorum superficialis and profundus muscles refer pain to the same digit that the fibres activate (e.g., the fibres of the middle finger flexor muscle refer pain through the length of the middle finger). TrPs in the flexor pollicis longus refer to the thumb.

- *Needling technique:* The patient lies in supine or sidelying position with the forearm supinated. The muscles are needled with a flat palpation. The needle is inserted perpendicular to the skin and directed towards the ulna and the interosseous for the flexor carpi radialis and palmaris muscle (Fig. 9.14). For the flexor pollicis longus muscle, the needle is directed towards the palmar aspect of the middle third of the radius (Fig. 9.15). For the flexor digitorum muscles, the needle is directed more towards the interosseous membrane (Fig. 9.16). For the flexor carpi ulnaris, the needle is directed towards the ulna (Fig. 9.17).

- *Precautions:* The median nerve, which runs between the flexor digitorum profundus and superficialis muscles, and the ulnar nerve, which runs between the flexor carpi ulnaris and flexor digitorum profundus muscles, should be avoided.

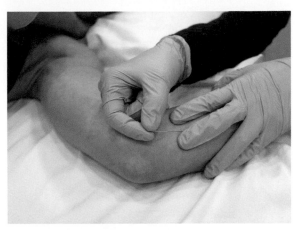

FIG. 9.14 Dry needling of the flexor carpi radialis, palmaris, and flexor digitorum superficialis muscle.

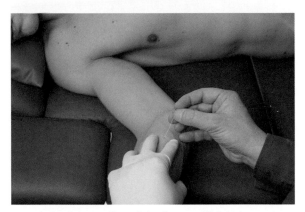

FIG. 9.15 Dry needling of the flexor pollicis longus muscle.

Extensor Pollicis Longus and Brevis and Abductor Pollicis Longus Muscles

- *Anatomy:* The extensor pollicis longus muscle extends from the dorsal surface of the ulna bone and the interosseous membrane to the base of the distal phalanx of the thumb. The abductor pollicis longus muscle originates from the ulnar side of the middle third of the radius and the lateral side of the dorsal surface of the ulna; it inserts into the radial side of the base of the first metacarpal bone.

- *Function:* The extensor pollicis longus and brevis muscles extend the terminal phalanx of the thumb and help to extend and abduct the wrist, whereas the abductor pollicis longus muscle abducts the first metacarpal bone and also helps to abduct the wrist.

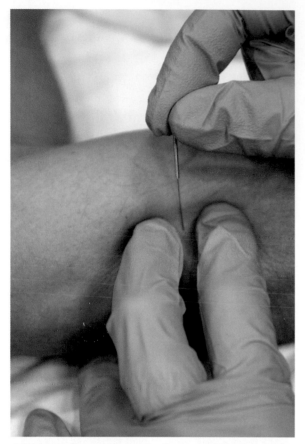

FIG. 9.16 Dry needling of the flexor carpi ulnaris muscle.

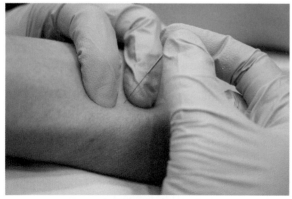

FIG. 9.17 Dry needing of the flexor digitorum profundus muscle.

- *Innervation:* The extensor pollicis longus and brevis and abductor pollicis longus muscles are innervated by the posterior interosseous nerve, the deep branch of the radial nerve, via the posterior cord of the brachial plexus from spinal roots C7 and C8.

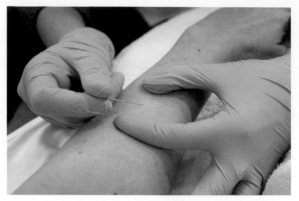

FIG. 9.18 Dry needling of the extensor pollicis longus and abductor pollicis longus muscles.

- *Referred pain:* TrPs in the extensor pollicis longus muscle refer pain to the dorsal aspect of the thumb; TrPs in the abductor pollicis longus muscle refer pain to the radial aspect of the wrist and the dorsal aspect of the third and fourth fingers (Hwang et al., 2005).
- *Needling technique:* The patient lies in supine position. All muscles are needled with a flat palpation. For the extensor pollicis longus and brevis and abductor pollicis longus muscles, the needle is inserted perpendicular to the skin and directed towards the dorsal aspect of the radius (Fig. 9.18). Hwang and colleagues (2005) used a midpoint between the lateral epicondyle and radial styloid for needling the abductor pollicis longus muscle.
- *Precautions:* The median nerve runs between the flexor digitorum profundus and superficialis muscles and should be avoided. Branches of the radial nerve run over the extensor pollicis longus and abductor pollicis longus muscles but rarely interfere with DN procedures.

Extensor Indicis Muscle

- *Anatomy:* The extensor indicis muscle extends from the dorsal–lateral surface of the ulna and interosseous membrane to the dorsal aspect of the second metacarpal bone.
- *Function:* The extensor indicis muscle extends the second finger.
- *Innervation:* The extensor indicis muscle is innervated by the posterior interosseous nerve via the posterior cord of the brachial plexus from spinal roots C7 and C8.
- *Referred pain:* TrPs in the extensor indicis muscle refers pain to the dorsal aspect of the second finger.
- *Needling technique:* The needle is inserted perpendicular to the skin towards the dorsal aspect of the

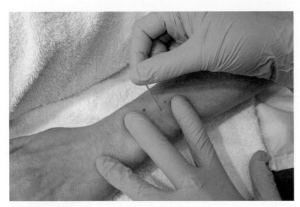

FIG. 9.19 Dry needling of the extensor indices muscle.

middle third of the radius, similar to the needling procedures for the extensor pollicis longus and abductor pollicis longus muscles (Fig. 9.19). The referred pain and the muscle contraction will assist the clinician to focus the needling in one or other muscle.

- *Precautions:* Branches of the radial nerve rarely interfere with DN procedures.

The Thenar Muscles

- *Anatomy:* The adductor pollicis muscle has two sections. The transverse head originates from the palmar surface of the third metacarpal. The oblique head originates from the palmar aspect of the bases of the second and third metacarpals and their adjacent trapezoid and capitate bones. Both heads attach to the base of the ulnar side of the proximal phalanx of the thumb. The opponens pollicis muscle extends from the trapezium bone of the wrist and the flexor retinaculum in the heel of the hand to wrap partially around and attaches to the first metacarpal bone. The flexor pollicis brevis muscle extends from the trapezium, trapezoid, and capitate bones, and the flexor retinaculum to the palmar aspect of the first metacarpal and sesamoid bone. The abductor pollicis brevis muscle originates in the scaphoid bone and the flexor retinaculum and inserts to the lateral aspect of the first metacarpal and sesamoid bones.
- *Function:* The adductor pollicis muscle adducts the thumb towards the index finger. The opponens pollicis muscle opposes the thumb towards the ring and little fingers. The flexor pollicis brevis muscle flexes the thumb towards the palm and the abductor pollicis brevis muscle abducts the thumb away from the palm.

- *Innervation:* The adductor pollicis muscle is supplied by the deep palmar branch of the ulnar nerve via the medial cord and lower trunk of the brachial plexus from spinal roots C8 and T1, whereas the opponens pollicis, flexor pollicis brevis, and abductor pollicis brevis muscles are supplied by a branch of the median nerve via the lateral cord and upper-middle trunks of the brachial plexus from spinal roots C6 and C7.
- *Referred pain:* TrPs in the adductor pollicis muscle refer pain to the ulnar aspect of the thumb. TrPs in the opponens pollicis muscle and flexor pollicis brevis muscle project pain to the palmar aspect of the thumb. TrPs in the abductor pollicis brevis muscle projects pain to the radial aspect of the thumb. It is debatable whether the adductor pollicis brevis and opponens pollicis muscles can be distinguished with manual palpation, which questions the notion of distinct and different referred pain patterns.
- *Needling technique:* Generally, a short but thin needle is used for the thenar muscles, such as a 0.16 × 15 mm needle. In the hand, needles are used only once. The patient lies in supine position with the forearm pronated for the adductor pollicis muscle or supinated for the remaining muscles. The adductor pollicis muscle is needled with a pincer palpation. The needle is inserted perpendicular to the skin and directed to the muscle. For the adductor pollicis muscle the needle is usually inserted between the first and second metacarpal bones (Fig. 9.20), but TrPs in this muscle can also be needled on the volar side of the hand with the forearm in supination. The abductor pollicis brevis, opponens pollicis (Fig. 9.21), and flexor pollicis brevis (Fig. 9.22) muscles are needled from the volar side of the thenar eminence using flat palpation. Taut bands in these muscles are very thin and resemble the thickness of a small paperclip. Alternatively, the needle is inserted via the radial aspect of the first metacarpal if the palmar fascia would be too sensitive (Fig. 9.23).
- *Precautions:* None

Interosseous and Lumbrical Muscles

- *Anatomy:* The dorsal and palmar interosseous muscles lie between the adjacent metacarpal bones. The lumbrical muscles attach proximally to the four tendons of the flexor digitorum profundus in the mid-palm, distally to the radial side of the aponeurosis on each of the four fingers.
- *Function:* The dorsal interosseous muscles move a finger away from the midline of the middle finger (abduction); the palmar interosseous muscles adduct each of the other fingers towards the middle

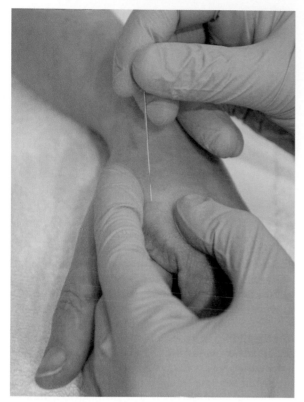

FIG. 9.20 Dry needling of the adductor pollicis muscle.

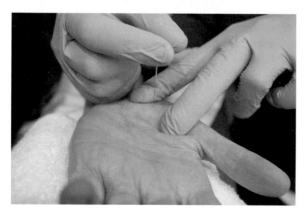

FIG. 9.21 Dry needling of the abductor pollicis brevis and opponens pollicis muscles.

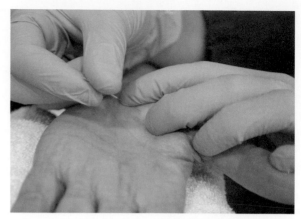

FIG. 9.22 Dry needling of the flexor pollicis muscles.

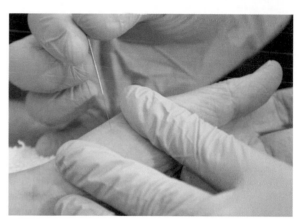

FIG. 9.23 Alternate dry needling approach for the thenar muscles.

finger (adduction); the lumbricals inhibit flexion of a distal phalanx via the extensor mechanism.

- *Innervation:* The interosseous and the third and fourth lumbricals muscles are supplied by branches of the ulnar nerve via the medial cord and lower trunk of the brachial plexus from spinal roots C8 and T1. The first and second lumbricals are supplied by the median nerve via the lateral cord and upper-middle trunks of the brachial plexus from spinal roots C6 and C7.

- *Referred pain:* TrPs in the dorsal and palmar interosseous muscles project their pain along the side of the finger to which that interosseous muscle attaches. TrPs in the first dorsal interosseous also refer to the dorsum of the hand and ulnar side of the little finger. The referred pain patterns from the lumbricals are thought to be similar to the referred pain patterns of the interossei.

- *Needling technique:* The patient lies in supine position with the forearm pronated. All muscles are needled with flat palpation. The needle is inserted perpendicular to the skin from the dorsal aspect of the hand, directed towards the practitioner's finger. For the lumbrical, palmar, and dorsal interosseous muscles, the

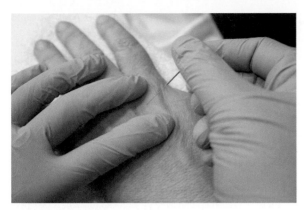

FIG. 9.24 Dry needling of lumbrical, palmar, and dorsal interosseous muscles.

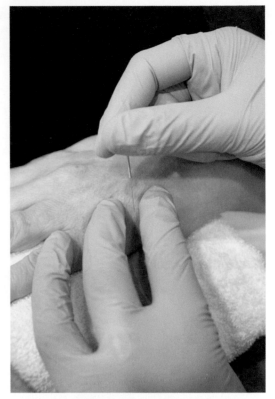

FIG. 9.25 Dry needling of the abductor digiti minimus muscle.

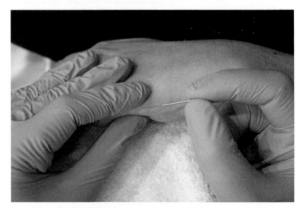

FIG. 9.26 Dry needling of the abductor digiti minimus muscle.

needle is directed towards the muscle belly between the metacarpal bones (Fig. 9.24), although the palmar and lumbrical muscles can also be approached from the volar side of the hand using a thinner needle.

- *Precautions:* None

The Hypothenar Muscles

- *Anatomy:* The hypothenar group of intrinsic hand muscles consists of the abductor digiti minimus, the opponens digiti minimus, and flexor digiti minimus muscles. The abductor digiti minimus muscle arises proximally from the pisiform bone and attaches distally to the ulnar side of the base of the first phalanx of the little finger. The opponens digiti minimus and flexor digiti minimus muscles originate from the hamate bone and flexor retinaculum and inserts at the medial border of the fifth metacarpal bone. The opponens digiti minimus muscle lies mostly underneath the flexor digiti minimus.
- *Function:* The abductor digiti minimus muscle abducts the little finger. The opponens digiti minimus and flexor digiti minimus muscles flex and rotate the fifth metacarpal and assist with opposition of the little finger.
- *Innervation:* The hypothenar muscles are supplied by branches of the ulnar nerve via the medial cord and lower trunk of the brachial plexus from spinal roots C8 and T1.
- *Referred pain:* TrPs in the abductor digiti minimus muscle refer pain along the lateral side of the little finger. The referred pain patterns of TrPs in the opponens digiti minimus and flexor digiti minimus muscles have not yet been described.
- *Needling technique:* The abductor digiti minimus muscle is needled either with a pincer palpation

towards the thumb (Fig. 9.25), or shallow towards the fifth metacarpal in between the palpating fingers (Fig. 9.26). The opponens digiti minimus and flexor digiti minimus muscles are needled with a flat palpation (Fig. 9.27).

- *Precautions:* None

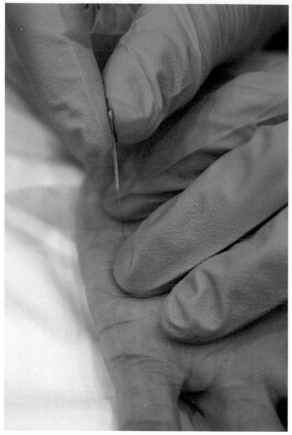

FIG. 9.27 Dry needling of the flexor and opponens digiti minimus muscles.

REFERENCES

Alonso-Blanco, C., Fernández-de-las Peñas, C., Morales-Cabezas, M., et al. (2011). Multiple active myofascial trigger points reproduce the overall spontaneous pain pattern in women with fibromyalgia and are related to widespread mechanical hypersensitivity. *The Clinical Journal of Pain, 27,* 405–413.

Chaitow, L., & Delany, J. (2008). Clinical application of neuromuscular techniques: the upper body. In *Shoulder, arm and hand* (2nd ed., p. 445). London: Elsevier.

Clavert, P., Lutz, J. C., Adam, P., et al. (2009). Frohse's arcade is not the exclusive compression site of the radial nerve in its tunnel. *Orthopaedics & Traumatology, Surgery & Research, 95,* 114–118.

Ferguson, L., & Gerwin, R. (2005). Shoulder dysfunction and frozen shoulder. In L. Ferguson & R. Gerwin (Eds.), *Clinical mastery in the treatment of myofascial pain* (pp. 91–121). Baltimore: Lippincott Williams & Wilkins.

Fernández-Carnero, J., Fernández-de-las Peñas, C., De-la-Llave-Rincón, A. I., et al. (2007). Prevalence of and referred pain from myofascial trigger points in the forearm muscles in patients with lateral epicondylalgia. *Clinical Journal of Pain, 23,* 353–360.

Fernández-Carnero, J., Fernández-de-las Peñas, C., De-la-Llave-Rincón, A. I., et al. (2008). Bilateral myofascial trigger points in the forearm muscles in chronic unilateral lateral epicondylalgia: a blinded controlled study. *Clinical Journal of Pain, 24,* 802–807.

Fernández-de-las Peñas, C., Gröbli, C., Ortega Santiago, R., et al. (2012). Referred pain from myofascial trigger points in head, neck, shoulder and arm muscles reproduces pain symptoms in blue-collar (manual) and white-collar (office) workers. *The Clinical Journal of Pain, 28,* 511–518.

González-Iglesias, J., Cleland, J. A., Gutiérrez-Vega, M. R., & Fernández-de-las Peñas, C. (2011). Multimodal management of lateral epicondylalgia in rock climbers: a prospective case series. *Journal of Manipulative and Physiological Therapeutics, 34,* 635–642.

Hwang, M., Kang, Y. K., Shin, J. Y., & Kim, D. H. (2005). Referred pain pattern of the abductor pollicis longus muscle. *American Journal of Physical Medicine & Rehabilitation, 84,* 593–597.

Kheradmandi, A., Ebrahimian, M., Ghaffarinejad, F., Ehyaii, V., & Farazdaghi, Reza. (2015). The effect of dry needling of the trigger points of shoulder muscles on pain and grip strength in patients with lateral epicondylitis: a pilot study. *J.R.S.R., 3,* 58–62.

Lee, M. J., & LaStayo, D. (2004). Pronator syndrome and other nerve compressions that mimic carpal tunnel syndrome. *Journal of Orthopaedic & Sports Physical Therapy, 34,* 601–609.

McManus, R., & Cleary, M. (2018). *BMJ Case Rep.* 14 January 2018. https://doi.org/10.1136/bcr-2017-221302.

Maeda, S., Kawai, K., Koizumi, M., et al. (2009). Morphological study of the communication between the musculo-cutaneous and median nerves. *Anatomical Science International, 84,* 34–40.

Mekhail, A. O., Checroun, A. J., Ebraheim, N. A., Jackson, W. T., & Yeasting, R. A., (1999). Extensile approach to the anterolateral surface of the humerus and the radial nerve. *Journal of Shoulder and Elbow Surgery, 8,* 112–118.

Mora-Relucio, R., Núñez-Nagy, S., Gallego-Izquierdo, T., Rus, A., Plaza-Manzano, G., Romero-Franco, N., et al. (2016). Experienced versus inexperienced inter-examiner reliability on location and classification of myofascial trigger point palpation to diagnose lateral epicondylalgia: an observational cross-sectional study. *Evidence-Based Complementary and Alternative Medicine, 2016.* 6059719.

Qerama, E., Kasch, H., & Fuglsang-Frederiksen, A. (2009). Occurrence of myofascial pain in patients with possible carpal tunnel syndrome: a single-blinded study. *European Journal of Pain, 13,* 588–591.

Rezzouk, J., Durandeau, A., Vital, J. M., & Fabre, T. (2002). Long head of the triceps brachii in axillary nerve injury: anatomy and clinical aspects. *Revue de Chirurgie Orthopédique et Réparatrice de l'Appareil Moteur, 88,* 561–564.

Schneider, M. (2005). Tennis elbow. In L. Ferguson & R. Gerwin (Eds.), *Clinical mastery in the treatment of myofascial pain* (pp. 122–144). Baltimore: Lippincott Williams & Wilkins.

Shmushkevich, Y., & Kalichman, L. (2013). Myofascial pain in lateral epicondylalgia: a review. *Journal of Bodywork and Movement Therapies, 17,* 434–439.

Simons, D. G., Travell, J. G., & Simons, L. S. (1999). *Travell & Simons' Myofascial pain and dysfunction: the trigger point manual. Vol. 1* (2nd ed., pp. 278–307). Baltimore: Lippincott William & Wilkins.

Slater, H., Arendt-Nielsen, L., Wright, A., & Graven-Nielsen, T. (2003). Experimental deep tissue pain in wrist extensors: a model of lateral epicondylalgia. *European Journal of Pain, 7,* 277–288.

Tatar, I., Kocabiyik, N., Gayretli, O., & Ozan, H. (2009). The course and branching pattern of the deep branch of the radial nerve in relation to the supinator muscle in fetus elbow. *Surgical and Radiologic Anatomy, 31,* 591–596.

Uygur, E., Aktaş, B., Özkut, A., Erinç, S., & Yilmazoglu, E. G. (2017). Dry needling in lateral epicondylitis: a prospective controlled study. *International Orthopaedics, 41,* 2321–2325.

Villafañe, J. H., & Herrero, P. (2016). Conservative treatment of myofascial trigger points and joint joint mobilization for management in patients with thumb carpometacarpal osteoarthritis. *Journal of Hand Therapy, 29,* 89–92.

CHAPTER 10

Deep Dry Needling of the Trunk Muscles

MICHELLE FINNEGAN • JAN DOMMERHOLT •
CÉSAR FERNÁNDEZ-DE-LAS-PEÑAS

INTRODUCTION

Muscles of the trunk, linked intimately to vital human functions, aid in breathing, digestion, and locomotion and provide upright postural support. Myofascial trigger points (TrPs) located in the trunk region can influence movement patterns, reflect breathing and visceral dysfunction, and contribute to a wide array of commonly diagnosed musculoskeletal pain syndromes. Pain from trunk muscle TrPs may be local or diffuse, referring anteriorly, posteriorly, or into the upper or lower extremities. For example, referred pain from TrPs in the quadratus lumborum muscle may be confused with trochanteric bursitis, sacroiliac joint dysfunction, or coccydynia. In addition, the referred pain pattern of TrPs in the serratus anterior muscle to the medial aspect of the arm can easily be mistaken for the pain pattern associated with cervical radiculopathy.

Several researchers have examined the efficacy of deep dry needling (DN) on TrPs of the muscles of the lumbar spine. Deep DN may be more effective in reducing pain compared with standard acupuncture therapy or superficial needling in elderly patients presenting with chronic low back pain (Itoh et al., 2004). More recently, Itoh and colleagues (2006) found similar findings with DN being superior to sham needling in the short term for elderly patients with low back pain. It should be noted that both studies had small sample sizes, and therefore definitive conclusions cannot be drawn. When evaluating the effects of DN compared with the effects of anaesthetic injections and percutaneous electrical nerve stimulation, DN was equally successful in inactivating TrPs in low back muscles and reducing pain (Perez-Palomares et al., 2010). Comparing DN with DN combined with neuroscience education showed that, although both groups exhibited similar decreases in pain and in scores on the Roland-Morris Disability Questionnaire and Oswestry Low Back Pain Disability Index, the group that received DN and neuroscience education demonstrated greater improvement of pressure sensitivity at the L3 transverse

process and a greater reduction of kinesiophobia. The researchers found similar increases in pressure sensitivity at all assessed areas (Téllez-García et al., 2015). A Cochrane review by Furlan and colleagues (2005) of 35 randomised controlled trials of acupuncture and DN for chronic low back pain concluded that DN may be a useful adjunct to conventional therapies. Most studies were of lower methodological quality than recommended by the Cochrane Back Review Group (Furlan et al., 2005). In a recent systematic review, Boyles and colleagues (2015) reported limited benefit of DN to the lumbar paraspinal muscles; however, only one study met the inclusion and exclusion criteria of the paper. For other areas of the body DN has been shown to be effective (Liu et al., 2015; Morihisa et al., 2016; Gattie et al., 2017), especially for short-term pain relief, increased range of motion, and improved quality of life compared with no intervention, sham, and placebo (Espejo-Antúnez et al., 2017). A recent study confirmed that the benefits of three sessions of DN TrPs in cervical muscles persisted for at least 6 weeks (Gerber et al., 2015, 2017) with objective tissue improvements assessed by ultrasound vibration elastography lasting as long as 8 weeks (Turo et al., 2015). Overall, there is a promising trend toward better myofascial pain and DN studies with improved methodological quality (Gattie et al., 2017; Stoop et al., 2017).

Two recent studies examined the physiological changes in lumbar muscle function after DN. Both studies demonstrated improvements in muscle activation after DN with changes in the thickness of the lumbar multifidus muscle (Koppenhaver et al., 2015a; Dar & Hicks, 2016). However, Koppenhaver and colleagues (2015a) also reported a decrease in nociceptive sensitivity. A limitation of both studies is that subjects received only one DN treatment, which is not common in clinical practice. Further work has been done to examine whether there are particular clinical predictors that would determine which patients would most likely benefit from DN of the lumbar multifidus muscle.

Among multiple variables, pain with the multifidus lift test was the strongest predictor of improved disability after DN. The multifidus lift test is used to examine the activation of the lumbar multifidus muscle at the L4-L5 and L5-S1 levels based on palpation by the therapist. In this study, the multifidus lift test was performed by asking prone patients to lift their abducted arm of the table as the clinician palpated the contralateral lumbar multifidi muscles. Subjects who had pain that worsened with standing had a 23% smaller improvement in disability than those who had pain that was not aggravated by standing (Koppenhaver et al., 2015b).

Although thoracic spine pain has a lifetime prevalence of almost 20% in the general population (Briggs et al., 2009), there is limited evidence of the efficacy of DN for thoracic spine pain (Fernández-de-las-Peñas et al., 2015). Currently, there is only one report of two patients with thoracic spine pain, motor control dysfunction, and tightness and pain in the thoracic paraspinal muscles who showed improvements in pain and range of motion after two sessions of DN (Rock & Rainey, 2014). Another paper, although not exclusively pertaining to the thoracic spine region, compared the effectiveness of DN in the thoracic, lumbar spine, and sacral regions versus cross tape in patients with fibromyalgia (Castro-Sanchez et al., 2017). DN was directed to TrPs in the thoracic, lumbar, and sacral multifidus and iliocostalis muscles, the quadratus lumborum muscle, and the latissimus dorsi muscle both in the axilla and on the rib cage. The DN group showed a significant decrease in the number of TrPs compared with the cross tape group along with a major improvement in pain intensity. Both groups demonstrated changes in spinal mobility, but the effect sizes were negligible to small. Mahmoudzadeh and colleagues established that DN was a valuable addition to a more traditional treatment approach for patients with discogenic low back pain (Mahmoudzadeh et al., 2016). Anandkumar and Manivasagam presented a case of a 42-year-old female with complaints of diffuse pain in her thoracic paraspinal region from T2 to T7. The patient was treated with DN targeting the fascia twice weekly for 2 weeks with reported improvements in pain, range of motion, and functional activities (Anandkumar & Manivasagam, 2017).

Currently there is no direct evidence to support DN of thoracic muscles for pain in the lumbar region other than the established referred pain patterns of the lower thoracic multifidus and longissimus thoracis muscles into the lumbar region (Simons et al., 1999). There is, however, one DN study of the lower trapezius muscle to treat mechanical neck pain (Pecos-Martin et al., 2015).

DN of a TrP was compared with DN of a non-TrP region of the same muscle with improvements of pain, pressure pain threshold testing, and disability in the needling group compared with the control group and baseline measurements. Although no other studies have looked at needling of thoracic spine muscles for neck pain, empirically, needling of the upper thoracic multifidi can improve cervical, thoracic and lumbar pain and dysfunction.

A recent study showed that DN might be useful in patients with cancer-related trunk pain. Hasuo and colleagues (2016) described five patients with terminal cancer and intractable pain, who initially responded to opioid pain medications. When pain control became less effective, the opioid dosages were increased, but patients became delirious. Based on diagnostic imaging, the increase in pain was thought to be due to either the primary cancer lesion or metastases; however, when specific muscles were examined, the patients' familiar pain was reproduced. DN of TrPs reduced the patients' pain, delirium, and pain medication intake (Hasuo et al., 2016). Vas and colleagues (2016) reported a significant decrease of pain in subjects with intractable pain due to pancreatic cancer after DN of the abdominal and paravertebral muscles. Subjects received DN if they still experienced pain greater than a 5 of 10 on a Visual Analog Scale after having either a neurolytic coeliac plexus block or a splanchnic nerve radiofrequency ablation.

Although the literature to date supports the inclusion of deep DN for mitigation of pain related to TrPs of the trunk, studies are limited in scope, quality, and quantity. Ongoing research, including high quality randomised controlled trials, is warranted for improved clinical decision making.

CLINICAL RELEVANCE OF TRIGGER POINTS IN SYNDROMES RELATED TO THE TRUNK

The most prevalent syndrome associated with the trunk is low back pain. Throughout the world low back pain continues to be a major concern with the highest prevalence among women and those aged 40 to 80 years (Manchikanti et al., 2014). The prevalence of low back pain is also on the rise. The overall prevalence has increased by 162%, with increases in non-Hispanic blacks as high as 226%. Furthermore, the number of individuals who sought healthcare for back pain increased from 73.1% to 84% (Manchikanti et al., 2014). Although pain with a myofascial origin was the primary cause of pain in 85% of patients going to a tertiary pain clinic (Chu et al., 2016), the role of muscles, specifically TrPs, in the aetiology of low back pain appears to be overlooked in favour of structural disorders that can be seen on imaging (Hendler & Kozikowski, 1993). Attempting to identify a single source of pain may cause practitioners to ignore the potential contribution of other tissues to the overall pain presentation. Low back pain should be considered a summation of dysfunctions with ligamentous instability and facet joint degeneration occurring in conjunction with development of motor control dysfunction and muscle TrPs formation (Kirkaldy-Willis, 1990; Chaitow, 1997; Paris, 1997; Waddell, 1998; Bajaj et al., 2001a, 2001b; Fernández-de-las-Peñas, 2009). Fernández-de-las-Peñas (2009) examined the relationship between TrPs and facet joint hypomobility. He postulated that increased tension from taut bands may maintain abnormal facet joint compression and displacement and, conversely, abnormal sensory input from dysfunctional facet joints may reflexively activate TrPs. Persistent nociceptive input from any number of tissues of the spine leads to an increase in responsiveness of the corresponding dorsal horn neurons (Mense, 2008; Taguchi et al., 2008) and, through antidromic mechanisms, sensitisation of the tissues at the same segmental levels. Hoheisel and colleagues (2011) established that, in anaesthetised rats, the nociceptive input from the thoracolumbar fascia increased significantly from 4% to 15% in animals with an experimentally induced inflammation of the lumbar multifidus muscle.

Several studies have examined the role of TrPs in the aetiology and maintenance of low back pain. Teixera and colleagues (2011) identified the presence of TrPs in 85.7% of patients diagnosed with failed back surgery pain syndrome primarily in the quadratus lumborum and gluteus medius muscles. Similarly, Njoo and van der Does (1994) reported a greater number of TrPs in the quadratus lumborum and gluteus medius muscles in patients with nonspecific low back pain versus control patients. Iglesias-González and colleagues (2013) examined the quadratus lumborum, iliocostalis lumborum, psoas major, piriformis, gluteus minimus, and gluteus medius muscles in patients with nonspecific low back pain. They confirmed the prevalence of active TrPs in the quadratus lumborum, gluteus medius, and iliocostalis lumborum muscles. There is a strong correlation between the prevalence of TrPs and persistent back pain (Chen & Nizar, 2011). The trapezius, piriformis, and quadratus lumborum muscles were most commonly involved with a favourable outcome after DN interventions. These findings suggest that the persistence of pain may in fact be due to unresolved

TrPs. Cornwall and colleagues (2006) injected the lumbar multifidus muscles with hypertonic saline at the L4 level to examine their referral patterns. All subjects reported local pain with 87% reporting referred pain into the anterior or posterior thigh. Samuel and colleagues (2007) established the connection between muscle-induced pain and lumbar disc disease in a study of 60 subjects with lumbar disc prolapse. There was a significant association between disc disease and the presence of TrPs in muscles innervated by the corresponding segmental level, i.e., L4-L5 lesions with anterior tibialis TrPs. In a similar type of study, Hsueh and colleagues (1998) found an association between the level of disc lesion and cervical and trunk muscles with TrPs. The latissimus dorsi muscle was involved with lesions at the C3-C4, C5-C6, and C6-C7 levels, and the rhomboid minor muscle was involved with lesions of C4-C5, C5-C6, and C6-C7 levels.

A less recognised contributing factor to low back pain and, indeed, to pain throughout the body is dysfunctional breathing. Dysfunctional breathing includes breathing pattern disorders such as hyperventilation, periodic deep sighing, thoracic-dominant breathing, forced abdominal breathing, and thoracoabdominal asynchrony, which is better known as paradoxical breathing (Boulding et al., 2016). Breathing pattern disorders can adversely affect posture and can induce muscle pain (Chaitow, 1997, 2004; Hodges & Richardson, 1999; Hodges et al., 2001; Courtney, 2009; Neiva et al., 2017), which can subsequently lead to the development of TrPs due to overuse of certain muscles. Beeckmans and colleagues (2016) reported a significant correlation between low back pain and the presence of respiratory disorders such as asthma, dyspnea, respiratory infections, and different forms of allergy. To date, no articles have been published on the correlation between hyperventilation syndrome and low back pain (Beeckmans et al., 2016); however, hyperventilation is the most commonly researched and described type of dysfunctional breathing (Boulding et al., 2016).

Hyperventilation is associated with a variety of conditions, including asthma (Ogata et al., 2006; D'alba et al., 2015), anxiety (Howell, 1997), panic disorder (Hasler et al., 2005; Meuret & Ritz, 2010), endocrine diseases (Lencu et al., 2016), and mouth breathing (Han et al., 1997). A primary symptom of hyperventilation is dyspnea or difficulty in breathing (Boulding et al., 2016), which can cause an increase in the respiratory rate leading to hyperventilation. Several medical conditions are associated with dyspnea, including mental disorders and asthma (Berliner et al., 2016), and these conditions have an established relationship with hyperventilation. Others conditions such as liver disease (Kaltsakas et al., 2013), lung disease, and cardiovascular system disorders (Berliner et al., 2016) are also associated with dyspnea but have not been specifically considered with hyperventilation, although the physiological changes that occur support a correlation.

Hyperventilation leads to respiratory alkalosis (primary hypocapnia), an increase in the body's pH, decreases in partial pressure of carbon dioxide ($PaCO_2$), and compensatory decreases in blood bicarbonate (HCO_3) levels (Porth, 2011; Greger & Windhorst, 2013; Johnson, 2017). This, in turn, results in a host of neurophysiological changes, including an increased affinity of haemoglobin for oxygen, sympathetic nervous system dominance, anxiety and panic, vasoconstriction, and smooth and skeletal muscle spasm and constriction (Porth, 2011; Greger & Windhorst, 2013). With reduced blood flow and diminished availability of oxygen, muscles become prone to fatigue and the formation of TrPs. The hypoxic environment stimulates the release of nociceptive substances, for example, bradykinin, calcitonin gene-related peptide, and prostaglandins, among others; these substances in turn perpetuate TrP sensitisation and pain (Dommerholt & Shah, 2010). Deleterious effects on spinal stability and skeletal alignment may occur. Studies in which strenuous exercise was simulated revealed reduced postural functions of both the transverse abdominus and diaphragm as respiratory demands increased. Spinal stabilisers become overloaded, making them more vulnerable to injury. Hyperactivity of accessory muscles of respiration such as the pectoralis major and minor, upper trapezius, levator scapula, and sternocleidomastoid may occur with resulting rib cage stiffness, forward head posture, suboccipital compression, headaches, and temporomandibular joint disease (Hruska, 1997, 2002; Courtney, 2009; Bartley, 2010). Inactivation of TrPs of the neck, thorax, abdominal wall, and low back may assist in restoring normal breathing mechanics. Conversely, breathing retraining may help prevent the development of TrPs in the first place. All 29 subjects with neck or back pain, who had plateaued with manual therapy and exercise, had a low end tidal CO_2, which is an indication of arterial CO_2 in people with normal cardiopulmonary function (Mclaughlin et al., 2011). All patients experienced improved pain, function, and end tidal CO_2 with breathing retraining.

Muscle pain related to visceral disease occurs in more predictable, specific patterns than that of breathing dysfunction. Muscle hyperalgesia is triggered by a reflex arc known as the visceral-somatic reflex. Noxious signals from a distended organ are thought to trigger neuroplastic changes in the dorsal horn of both sensory neurons and of neighbouring efferent neurons. The resultant efferent signals create neurogenic inflammation, hyperalgesia, and TrPs in somatic structures sharing the same segmental level (Gerwin, 2002; Giamberadino et al., 2002; Montenegro et al., 2009). Examples of visceral disease and their associated pain referral include myocardial infarction with the left pectoralis major, ureteral colic with the iliocostalis, dysmenorrhea and interstitial cystitis with the lower abdominals, cholecystectomy with the latissimus dorsi, and pleurisy with thoracic multifidi (Boissonault & Bass, 1990). A single session of DN to the thoracolumbar multifidi and iliocostalis lumborum in a patient with constipation resulted in a complete resolution of his symptoms. DN of the abdominal muscles in patients with endometriosis can quickly relieve the symptoms (Jarrell et al., 2005). Furthermore, wet needling of the abdominal muscles can improve the severity of chronic pelvic pain (Montenegro et al., 2015) and dysmenorrhea (Huang & Liu, 2014). Because myofascial pain syndromes may predict, outlast, or mimic visceral disease, a detailed knowledge and awareness of visceral-induced pain patterns is essential for accurate differential diagnosis.

DRY NEEDLING OF THE TRUNK MUSCLES

Some of the muscles on the trunk are covered in other chapters. The pectoralis major and minor muscles are discussed in Chapter 8. The iliacus muscle, gluteal muscles, and pelvic muscles are reviewed in Chapter 11.

Rhomboid Major and Minor Muscles

- Anatomy:
  1. The rhomboid major muscle arises from the spinous processes and supraspinous ligaments of the second to fifth thoracic vertebrae and descends laterally to the medial border of the scapula between the root of the spine and the inferior angle with direct attachments to the serratus anterior muscle (Porterfield & DeRosa, 1995). Anatomical variations of the origin of this muscle have been reported (Lee & Jung, 2015) with the upper end of the origin of the ligamentum nuchae between C5 and C6 on the left and the ligamentum nuchae of C6 on the right. The lower end of the origin of this muscle was the spinous process of T4 on the left and the spinous process of T2 on the right.
  2. The rhomboid minor muscle runs from the distal ligamentum nuchae and the spines of the 7th cervical and first thoracic vertebrae to the base of

the triangular surface of the medial end of the scapula spine. An anatomical variation of the origin of this muscle has also been described, with it coming from the ligamentum nuchae between C5 and C6 on the left and the ligamentum nuchae at C6 on the right (Lee & Jung, 2015).

- *Function:* Both muscles retract the medial border of the scapula superiorly and medially.
- *Innervation:* Dorsal scapular nerve C4-C5, via the upper trunk of the brachial plexus.
- *Referred pain:* Pain is projected to the medial border of the scapula and superiorly over the supraspinatus muscle. However, in clinical practice, the referred pain pattern of the rhomboid muscles appears to include the referred pain patterns originally attributed to the serratus superior posterior muscle with pain projecting as a deep ache to the anterior surface of the scapula, posterior aspect of the scapula and shoulder, triceps region, olecranon, ulnar side of the forearm and hand, and the entire fifth digit.
- *Needling techniques:*
  1. The patient lies prone with the arm at the side hanging off the table or in the hammerlock position. Secure the TrP over a rib between the proximal phalangeal joints of the index and middle fingers, which are placed in the intercostal spaces above and below. Insert the needle perpendicular to the skin in between the distal phalangeal joints, and angle it tangentially toward the TrP, while staying over the rib (Fig. 10.1). If the TrP cannot be positioned directly over a rib, needle the muscle over the closest rib without aiming for the TrP.

  2. Using a 5-cm needle, insert the needle perpendicular to the skin close to the TrP. Direct the needle perpendicular to the direction of the individual ribs in a shallow to gradually deeper fashion toward the TrP (Fig. 10.2). This technique is always performed in a 'downhill' fashion, which, depending on the curvature of the spine at the TrP location, is either in a caudal or cranial direction.

- *Precautions:* The lungs can easily be penetrated if the intercostal spaces are not blocked with the fingers with the first technique. The needle should always be directed toward the rib, with the fingers remaining in the intercostal spaces. With the second technique, the lungs can be reached when a needle shorter than 5 cm is being used or when the needling is performed in an 'uphill' direction.

Serratus Posterior Superior Muscle

- *Anatomy:* The serratus posterior superior muscle arises from the distal portion of the nuchal ligament, the spinous processes and supraspinous ligaments of the 7th cervical, and first two or three thoracic vertebrae. It descends laterally and ends in four digitations attached to the upper borders and external surfaces of the second, third, fourth, and fifth ribs, just lateral to their angles. This muscle can be absent in some individuals.
- *Function:* The muscle attachments suggest that the muscle could elevate the ribs; however, its function has not been established. Several studies have confirmed that the muscle has no respiratory function (Vilensky et al., 2001; Loukas et al., 2008), and it may be primarily a proprioceptive muscle (Vilensky et al., 2001).

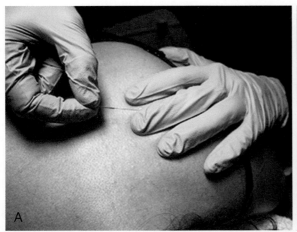
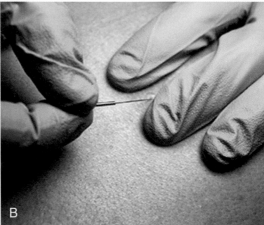

FIG. 10.1 Dry needling of trigger points in the rhomboid muscles.

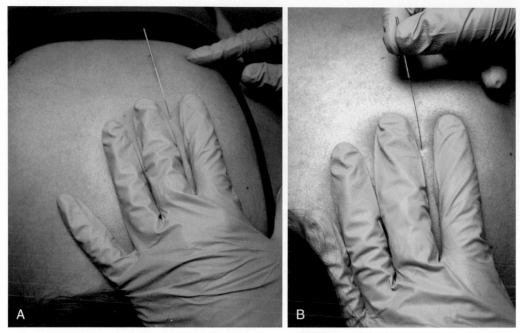

FIG. 10.2 Dry needling of trigger points in the rhomboid muscles—second technique.

- *Innervation:* Second, third, fourth, and fifth intercostal nerves.
- *Referred pain:* Pain is projected as a deep ache to the anterior surface of the scapula, posterior aspect of the scapula and shoulder, triceps region, olecranon, ulnar side of the forearm and hand, and the entire fifth digit. It can also refer pain to the pectoralis region.
- *Needling techniques:* The needling techniques are identical to the techniques for the rhomboid muscles.
- *Precautions:* The lungs can easily be penetrated if the intercostal spaces are not blocked with the fingers with the first technique. The needle should always be directed toward the rib with the fingers remaining in the intercostal spaces. With the second technique, the lungs can be reached when a needle shorter than 5 cm is being used or when the needling is performed in an uphill direction.

Middle Trapezius Muscle

- *Anatomy:* The middle trapezius muscle attaches medially to the spinous processes and the supraspinous ligaments of C7-T3. Its fibres run transversally to attach laterally to the superior lip of the scapular spine and to the acromion. Johnson and colleagues (1994) described that the muscle originates from C7 and T1

with the C7 fascicle attaching to the acromion and the T1 fascicle attaching to the scapular spine.
- *Function:* The superior fibres assist with scapular adduction and serve as part of the force couple for upward rotation of the scapula. The inferior fibres adduct the scapula. The entire muscle assists with scapular stabilisation during flexion and abduction of the arm.
- *Innervation:* The spinal portion of the spinal accessory nerve (cranial nerve XI) supplies motor fibres (Standring, 2016). The spinal accessory nerve forms an anastomosis with fibres from C2-C4 (Caliot et al., 1989; Kim et al., 2014; Lanisnik et al., 2014; Brennan et al., 2015). Although it is thought that these fibres carry sensory information, there is electromyographic (Pu et al., 2008; Kim et al., 2014) and histochemical (Pu et al., 2008) data that shows that the nerves have both sensory and motor functions, thereby contributing to some degree to contraction of the three portions of the trapezius muscle. The motor input from the C2-C4 nerves is not consistently present or is irregularly innervated to the three parts of the muscle when it is present (Kim et al., 2014).
- *Referred pain:* TrPs may refer to the acromion. A superficial burning pain may be felt in the interscapular region.

- *Needling techniques:*
  1. The patient lies prone with the arm at the side hanging off the table or in the hammerlock position. Secure the TrP over a rib between the proximal phalangeal joints of the index and middle fingers, which are placed in the intercostal spaces above and below. Insert the needle perpendicular to the skin in between the distal phalangeal joints, and angle it tangentially toward the TrP, while staying over the rib (Fig. 10.3). If the TrP cannot be positioned directly over a rib, needle the muscle over the closest rib without aiming for the TrP.
  2. Another technique involves securing the taut band via a pincer grip with the TrP between the index finger and the thumb. The needle is inserted perpendicular to the skin in between the index and middle finger and directed toward the TrP and the underlying thumb (Fig. 10.4).

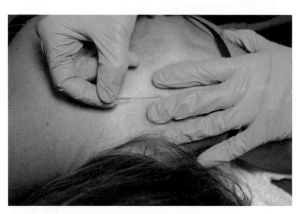

FIG. 10.3 Dry needling of trigger points in the middle trapezius muscle.

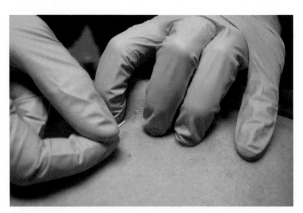

FIG. 10.4 Dry needling of trigger points in the middle trapezius muscle using pincer palpation.

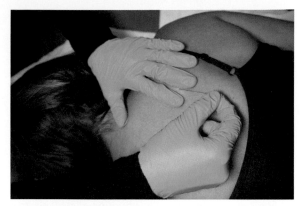

FIG. 10.5 Dry needling of trigger points in the middle trapezius muscle.

  3. Using a 5-cm needle, insert the needle perpendicular to the skin close to the TrP. Direct the needle perpendicular to the direction of the individual ribs in a shallow to gradually deeper fashion toward the TrP. This technique is always performed in a downhill fashion, which, depending on the curvature of the spine at the TrP location, is either in a caudal or cranial direction, similar to needling the rhomboid muscles (Fig. 10.5).
- *Precautions:* With the first approach, the lungs can easily be penetrated if the intercostal spaces are not blocked with the fingers or the muscle held in a pincer palpation. The needle should always be directed toward the rib with the fingers remaining in the intercostal spaces or towards the thumb. The second technique has no specific lung field precautions; however, with the third technique, the lungs can be reached when a needle shorter than 5 cm is being used or when the needling is performed in an uphill direction.

Lower Trapezius Muscle

- *Anatomy:* The lower trapezius muscle attaches medially to the spinous processes and the supraspinous ligaments of T4-T12. Its fibres run supero-laterally and attach to an aponeurosis on the medial end of the spine of the scapula. Johnson and colleagues (1994) concluded that the lower part of the trapezius muscle starts at T2 with fascicles arising from the spinous processes. The fascicles from T2 to T5 converge to a common aponeurotic tendon that attach on the scapula at the deltoid tubercle. According to the authors, fascicles from T6 to about T10 insert into the medial border of the deltoid tubercle. Lower fascicles insert into the lower edge of the deltoid tubercle.

- *Function:* The muscle acts synergistically with the lower portion of the serratus anterior and the upper trapezius muscles in upward rotation of the glenoid fossa. Electromyographic studies support that the muscle is active during upward rotation activities along with the upper and middle trapezius (Ebaugh et al., 2005; Pizzari et al., 2014).
- *Innervation:* The spinal portion of the spinal accessory nerve (cranial nerve XI) supplies motor fibres (Standring, 2016). The spinal accessory nerve forms an anastomosis with fibres from C2-C4 (Caliot et al., 1989; Kim et al., 2014; Lanisnik et al., 2014; Brennan et al., 2015). Although it is often thought that these fibres carry only sensory information, there is electromyographic (Pu et al., 2008; Kim et al., 2014) and histochemical (Pu et al., 2008) evidence that the nerves have both sensory and motor functions, thereby contributing to some degree to contractions of the three portions of the trapezius muscle. The motor input from the C2-C4 nerves is, however, not consistently present or is irregularly innervated to the three parts of the muscle when it is present (Kim et al., 2014).
- *Referred pain:* TrPs may refer to the posterior neck and adjacent mastoid region, to the acromion, and to the suprascapular and interscapular regions.
- *Needling technique:*
  1. The patient is positioned in prone with the arm at the side hanging off the table or in the hammerlock position. Secure the TrP over a rib between the proximal phalangeal joints of the index and middle fingers, which are placed in the intercostal spaces above and below. Insert the needle perpendicular to the skin in between the distal phalangeal joints, and angle it tangentially toward the TrP, while staying over the rib (Fig. 10.6). If the TrP cannot be positioned

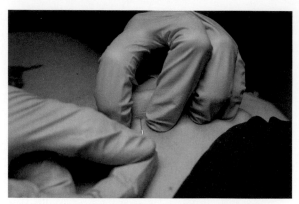

FIG. 10.7 Dry needling of trigger points in the lower trapezius muscle using a pincer palpation.

directly over a rib, needle the muscle over the closest rib without aiming for the TrP.
  2. Another technique involves securing the taut band via a pincer grip with the TrP between the index finger and the thumb. The needle is inserted perpendicular to the skin in between the index and middle finger and directed toward the TrP and the underlying thumb (Fig. 10.7).
- *Precautions:* The lungs and pleura can easily be penetrated if the intercostal spaces are not blocked with the fingers or the muscle held in a pincer palpation. The needle should always be directed toward the rib with the fingers remaining in the intercostal spaces or towards the thumb depending on the approach.

Latissimus Dorsi Muscle

- *Anatomy:* The latissimus dorsi muscle arises from the spinous processes of the lower six thoracic vertebrae, from the posterior layer of the thoracolumbar fascia (which is attached to the spinous processes and supraspinous ligaments of the lumbar and sacral vertebrae), and from the posterior iliac crest. It also has fibres from the iliac crest, lateral to the erector spine, and slips from the three or four lower ribs, interdigitating with the external oblique muscle. From this extensive attachment, fibres pass laterally with different degrees of obliquity to overlap the inferior scapular angle. In a study of 100 cadavers, Pouliart and Gagey (2005) found muscular attachments to the scapula 43% of the time. On others they noted a small fibrous attachment or an intervening bursa with no connecting tissue. It attaches to the intertubercular sulcus of the humerus anterior to the teres major. Rarely, a variant axillary arch muscle has been identified as a slip of muscle extending from

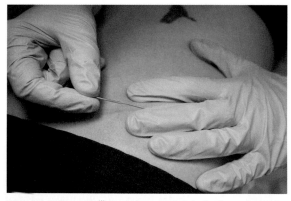

FIG. 10.6 Dry needling of trigger points in the lower trapezius muscle.

the latissimus dorsi's upper border to the humerus where it inserts deep to the pectoralis major tendon (Bakirci et al. 2010).

- *Function:* The muscle adducts, extends, and medially rotates the humerus (Standring, 2016). Alizadehkhaiyat and colleagues (2015) found the greatest activity of the latissimus dorsi with internal rotation at 155 degrees of shoulder elevation in the scapular plane. It can also influence shoulder depression (Park & Yoo, 2014).
- *Innervation:* Thoracodorsal nerve, from the posterior cord of the brachial plexus, C6, C7, C8.
- *Referred pain:* TrPs may project pain to the inferior angle of the scapula and surrounding midthoracic area, to the posterior aspect of the shoulder, to the medial aspect of the arm and forearm, and to the fourth and fifth fingers. They can also refer pain to the anterior shoulder and over the lower lateral aspect of the trunk above the iliac crest.
- *Needling techniques—trunk:*
  1. The patient lies prone with the arm resting at the side or off the table or in the sidelying position. Secure the TrP over a rib, between the proximal phalangeal joints of the index and middle fingers, which are placed in the intercostal spaces above and below. Insert the needle perpendicular to the skin in between the distal phalangeal joints, and angle it tangentially toward the TrP, while staying over the rib (Fig. 10.8). If the TrP cannot be positioned directly over a rib, needle the muscle over the closest rib without aiming for the TrP.
  2. Position the patient in the sidelying position with the side to be treated facing up and the arm placed in front of the patient or in the prone position.

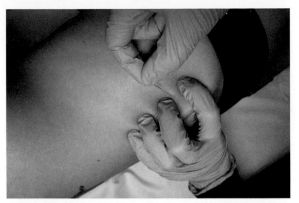

FIG. 10.9 Dry needling of trigger points in the latissimus dorsi muscle in sidelying position.

Secure the taut band via a pincer grip with the TrP between the index finger and the thumb. The needle is inserted perpendicular to the skin in between the index and middle finger and directed toward the TrP and the underlying thumb. The muscle may be followed caudally as long as it can be lifted away from the chest wall (Fig. 10.9).

- *Needling techniques—axilla:* The axillar part of the latissimus dorsi muscle can be treated with the patient in the prone, supine, or sidelying position. In the prone position, the arm is either off the table or on the table with the hand under the pillow (Fig. 10.10). In supine position the arm is abducted to give better access to the axilla (Fig. 10.11); in sidelying position the arm is supported by the patient or placed on a pillow (Fig. 10.12). In any of these positions, secure the

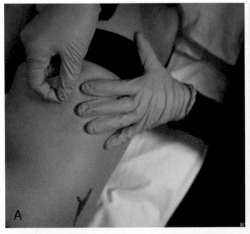
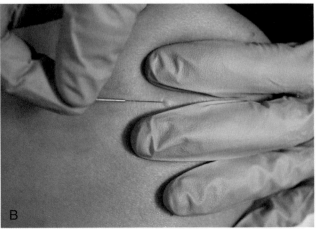

FIG. 10.8 Dry needling of trigger points in the latissimus dorsi muscle.

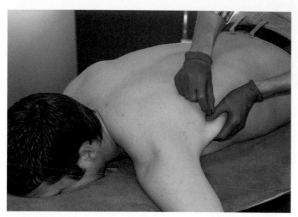

FIG. 10.10 Dry needling of trigger points in the latissimus dorsi muscle in the axilla in prone position.

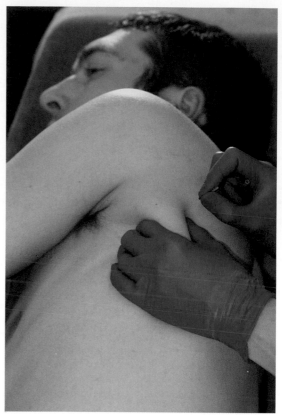

FIG. 10.12 Dry needling of trigger points in the latissimus dorsi muscle in the axilla in sidelying position.

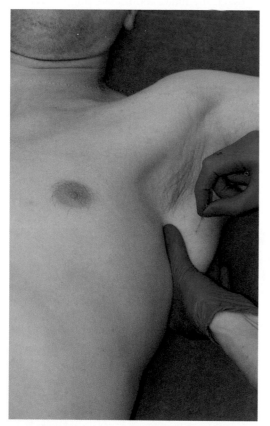

FIG. 10.11 Dry needling of trigger points in the latissimus dorsi muscle in the axilla in supine position.

taut band via a pincer grip with the TrP between the index finger and the thumb or between the middle finger and the thumb with the so-called 'OK sign' pincer palpation. The needle is inserted perpendicular to the skin in between the index and middle finger (pincer) or between the thumb and index finger (OK sign) and directed toward the TrP and the underlying thumb or middle finger. The muscle can be followed caudally as long as it can be lifted away from the chest wall.
- *Precautions:* All trunk needling is performed over a rib with the first approach or away from the chest wall with the second approach to avoid penetrating the lung and the pleura. There are no specific precautions for the axillar approach.

Serratus Anterior Muscle
- *Anatomy:* The serratus anterior muscle arises from an extensive costal attachment and inserts on the

scapula. Fleshy digitations spring anteriorly from the outer surfaces and superior borders of the upper eighth, ninth, or tenth ribs and from the fascia with direct attachments to the pectoralis major and external abdominal oblique muscles, covering the intervening intercostal muscles. The first digitations spring from the first and second ribs and intercostal fascia. Various combinations of the first digitations have been reported, going to the first, second, and third ribs (Smith et al., 2003; Webb et al., 2016). It attaches to the medial angle, vertebral border, and inferior angle of the scapula with direct attachments to the rhomboid major muscle (Porterfield & DeRosa, 1995).

- *Function:* With the pectoralis minor muscle, the muscle protracts the scapula, serving as a prime mover in all pushing and reaching movements. The muscle also draws the ribs posteriorly, assisting with pushing movements. The superior portion, with the levator scapulae and upper fibres of the trapezius, suspends the scapula. The inferior portion pulls the inferior scapular angle antero-laterally around the thorax, assisting the trapezius in upward rotation, an action that is essential to raising the arm above the head. In the initial stages of abduction, the muscle aids in securing and stabilising the scapula to allow the deltoid muscle to act effectively on the humerus.
- *Innervation:* Long thoracic nerve, C5 to C7, which descends on the external surface of the muscle.
- *Referred pain:* TrPs can refer antero-laterally at mid-chest level, posteriorly to the inferior angle of the scapula, and down the medial aspect of the arm, extending to the palm and ring finger. It can also contribute to abnormal breast sensitivity.
- *Needling technique:* Position the patient in sidelying position with the side to be treated facing upwards and the arm resting in front of the patient. Secure the TrP over a rib (by passively moving the arm) between the proximal phalangeal joints of the index and middle fingers, which are placed in the intercostal spaces above and below. Insert the needle perpendicular to the skin in between the distal phalangeal joints, and angle it tangentially toward the TrP, while staying over the rib (Fig. 10.13). As an alternative, the muscle can also be needled from the medial aspect of the scapula as described for the subscapularis muscles (Fig. 8.7 and 8.8).
- *Precautions:* The lungs and pleura can easily be penetrated if the intercostal spaces are not blocked with the fingers. The needle should always be directed toward the rib with the fingers remaining in the intercostal spaces.

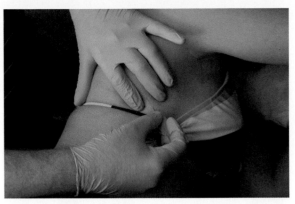

FIG. 10.13 Dry needling of trigger points in the serratus anterior muscle.

Longissimus Thoracis Muscle

- *Anatomy:* The longissimus thoracis muscle attaches to the tips of the transverse processes of all of the thoracic vertebrae and ribs 3 or 4 through 12 between their tubercles and angles. In the lumbar region, the muscle blends with the iliocostalis lumborum. Some of its fibres are attached to the entire posterior surface of the transverse processes, to the accessory processes of the lumbar vertebrae, and to the middle layer of the thoracolumbar fascia. Fascicles range in length from approximately 5 to 12 cm (Delp et al., 2001).
- *Function:* The muscle works in conjunction with the iliocostalis thoracis and lumborum to extend and laterally flex the spine against gravity. Together, they contract eccentrically to control the movement as the spine is flexed forward or laterally with the aid of gravity.
- *Innervation:* Lateral and intermediate branches of the dorsal rami of the thoracic spinal nerves.
- *Referred pain:* The inferior portions of this muscle refer pain several segments caudally into the lumbar spine and into the buttock region. The muscle can also refer to the anterior trunk and abdomen.
- *Needling technique:* The patient lies prone with the arm at the side. The TrP is identified via flat palpation. In some cases, the muscle can be squeezed together to bring a TrP farther away from the underlying surface. Insert the needle slightly superior to the TrP, perpendicular to the skin, and direct the needle longitudinally in a shallow to gradual deeper fashion toward the TrP (Fig. 10.14). This technique is usually performed in a caudal and slightly medial direction; however, in the upper thoracic spine

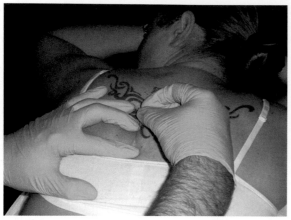

FIG. 10.14 Dry needling of trigger points in the longissimus thoracis muscle.

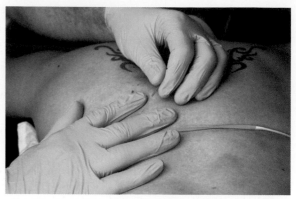

FIG. 10.15 Dry needling of trigger points in the iliocostalis thoracis muscle.

it may have to be performed in a cranial direction, depending on the curvature of the spine, at the TrP location to maintain the principle of needling downhill.

- *Precautions:* Maintain a shallow angle to avoid penetration of the lungs and the pleura.

Iliocostalis Thoracis and Lumborum Muscles

- *Anatomy:* The iliocostalis thoracis muscle attaches proximally to the upper borders of the angles of the lower six ribs, medial to the tendons of the insertion of iliocostalis lumborum, and to the superior borders of the angles of the upper six ribs and transverse process of the seventh cervical vertebrae. The iliocostalis lumborum muscle attaches to the inferior borders of the angles of the lower six or seven ribs. Both muscles attach inferiorly to the anterior surface of a broad aponeurosis. The aponeurosis attaches to the spinous processes of the lumbar and 11th and 12th thoracic vertebrae and their supraspinous ligaments and laterally to the medial aspect of the posterior iliac crest and to the lateral sacral crest, where it blends with the sacrotuberous and dorsal sacroiliac ligaments. In some cases, the longissimus thoracis muscle and the iliocostalis thoracis muscle appear as one muscle.
- *Function:* Together, these muscles extend and laterally flex the spine against gravity. They contract eccentrically as the spine flexes forward or laterally.
- *Innervation:* Lateral and intermediate branches of the dorsal rami of the thoracic and lumbar spinal nerves.
- *Referred pain:* The iliocostalis thoracis muscle refers pain superiorly, inferiorly, and anteriorly from its

TrP. It can mimic the pain of angina, pleurisy, or visceral pathology. The iliocostalis lumborum muscle refers into the lumbar spine, buttock region, and posterior hip.

- *Needling technique:*
    1. Thoracis—The patient lies prone. Secure the TrP over a rib (by passively moving the arm) between the proximal phalangeal joints of the index and middle fingers, which are placed in the intercostal spaces above and below. Insert the needle perpendicular to the skin in between the distal phalangeal joints, and angle it tangentially toward the TrP, while staying over the rib (Fig. 10.15).
    2. Lumborum—The patient lies prone. Identify the TrP via flat palpation. Insert the needle slightly superior and lateral to the TrP, perpendicular to the skin; then angle it in a caudal medial direction (Fig. 10.16). TrPs in the iliocostalis

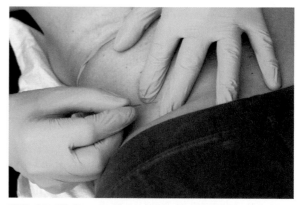

FIG. 10.16 Dry needling of trigger points in the iliocostalis lumborum muscle.

lumborum muscle can also be needled with the patient in the sidelying position with a lateral to medial needle direction.

- *Precautions:*
  1. Thoracis—The lungs and pleura can easily be penetrated if the intercostal spaces are not blocked properly with the fingers. The needle should always be directed toward the rib, with the fingers remaining in the intercostal spaces.
  2. Lumborum: none.

Thoracic and Lumbar Multifidus Muscles

- *Anatomy:* The multifidus muscle group consists of fasciculi that attach most caudally to the back of the sacrum at the level of the fourth sacral foramen and to the posterior superior iliac spine and dorsal sacroiliac ligaments. In the lumbar spine they attach to the mammillary processes; in the thoracic spine they attach to the transverse processes. Each fasciculus runs superiorly and medially, attaching to the base or to the tip of the spinous process of the vertebrae above. The most superficial fasciculi attach three to four levels above. Deeper fasciculi connect two to three levels up, and the deepest layers attach to the adjacent vertebrae. DN of the lumbar multifidi muscles caused a decreased resting thickness and an increased contraction thickness of the transverse abdominis muscle in asymptomatic participants (Puentedura et al., 2017).
- *Function:* The primary action of the multifidi muscles is stabilisation of the spine. Acting bilaterally, the muscles extend the spine. Acting unilaterally, they rotate the vertebrae to the contralateral side.
- *Innervation:* Dorsal rami of spinal nerves, usually by medial branches.
- *Referred pain:* The thoracic and lumbar multifidus muscles refer pain to the spinous process, the adjacent area of that segment, and anteriorly to the chest and abdomen. The lumbar multifidi muscles also refer inferiorly to the anterior and posterior thigh.
- *Needling technique:*
  1. Thoracic—The patient lies prone. The muscle is palpated via flat palpation in the valley next to the spinous processes, which is referred to as the 'safe needling zone' (Fig. 10.17). Staying within the safe needling zone, which is approximately 1 finger-breadth or 1 cm wide, the needle is inserted perpendicular to the skin, then angled in a caudal medial direction towards the lamina of the vertebral body (Fig. 10.18).
  2. Lumbar—The patient lies prone. The muscle is palpated via flat palpation in the valley next to the spinous processes. There is no safe needle zone in

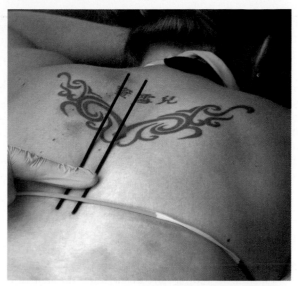

FIG. 10.17 The 1 cm of one finger-breath safety zone in the thoracic spine region. Note that the right line is over the spinous processes and the left line is 1 cm lateral. Of course, there is a safety zone on both sides of the spine.

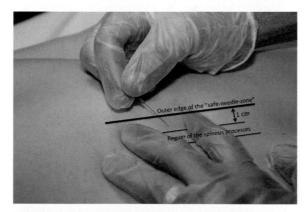

FIG. 10.18 Dry needling of trigger points in the thoracic multifidi muscles within the 1 cm safety zone.

this region; therefore the needle can be inserted perpendicular to the skin, just lateral to the finger. The needle is angled in a caudal medial direction towards the lamina of the vertebral body in a similar fashion as in the thoracic area without concerns for staying within the safety zone.

- *Precautions:* Inserting the needle outside of the 1 finger-breadth (1 cm) safe needle zone may cause the needle to penetrate the lung. Needling in a cranial medial direction may cause an epidural hematoma with paralysis and loss of bladder control (Chen et al., 2006; Lee et al., 2011).

Serratus Posterior Inferior Muscle

- *Anatomy:* The serratus posterior inferior muscle lies deep to the latissimus dorsi muscle. Medially, it attaches to the spinous processes of T11 through L2 or L3 and its supraspinous ligaments by a thin aponeurosis. It passes obliquely in a superior and lateral direction and divides into four flat digitations. These digitations attach to the inferior borders and outer surfaces of the last four ribs, just lateral to their angles. In some people, there are fewer digitations (usually the two attaching to the 9th and 12th ribs) or the entire muscle is missing.
- *Function:* The muscle draws the lower ribs posteriorly and inferiorly. It does not have an established role in respiration (Loukas et al., 2008). Vilensky and colleagues (2001) showed that the muscle has primarily a proprioceptive function.
- *Innervation:* Ventral rami of the ninth through 12th thoracic spinal nerves.
- *Referred pain:* Active TrPs may produce a nagging ache in the lower thoracic region, which may extend across the back over the lower ribs.
- *Needling technique:* The patient lies prone or on the contralateral side to be treated. Secure the TrP over the 9th, 10th, 11th, or 12th rib, depending on the involved digitation, between the proximal phalangeal joints of the index and middle fingers, which are placed in the intercostal spaces above and below. Insert the needle perpendicular to the skin in between the distal phalangeal joints, and angle it tangentially toward the TrP, while staying over the rib (Fig. 10.19).
- *Precautions:* The lungs and pleura can easily be penetrated if the intercostal spaces are not blocked with the fingers. The needle should always be directed toward the rib with the fingers remaining in the intercostal spaces.

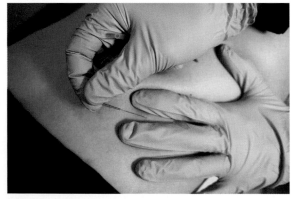

FIG. 10.19 Dry needling of trigger points in the serratus posterior inferior muscle.

Quadratus Lumborum Muscle

- *Anatomy:* The quadratus lumborum muscle attaches inferiorly by aponeurotic fibres to the iliolumbar ligament and the adjacent portion of the iliac crest. It attaches superiorly to the medial half of the lower border of the 12th rib, to the transverse processes of L1 through L4, and, occasionally, to the transverse process or body of T12. A second layer of this muscle occasionally is present. It attaches inferiorly to the transverse processes of the lower three or four lumbar vertebrae and superiorly to the lower border of the 12th rib.
- *Function:* The quadratus lumborum muscle is commonly considered to be a hip hiker; however, research does not necessarily support this function. Instead, it is shown to have several other functions. By stabiising the 12th rib and the lower attachments of the diaphragm, the quadratus lumborum muscle acts as a muscle of inspiration (Park et al., 2013; Standring, 2016) and forced exhalation (Standring, 2016). Acting bilaterally, it extends the spine (Standring, 2016). With the pelvis fixed, the muscle performs ipsilateral side bending of the spine (Park et al., 2013, 2014; Standring, 2016). During ipsilateral side bending of the spine the contralateral quadratus lumborum muscle is also active, serving a stabilising role (Park et al., 2013, 2014). When carrying a load in one upper extremity, the contralateral quadratus lumborum muscle will contract for stabilisation (Park et al., 2014).
- *Innervation:* The ventral rami of the 12th thoracic and upper three or four lumbar spinal nerves.
- *Referred pain:* Referred pain from the quadratus lumborum muscle tends to be deep and aching or sharp and severe. The most lateral TrPs refer along the iliac crest, to the lower portion of the abdomen, and into the groin, labia, and testicles. They may refer to the greater trochanter and outer, lateral thigh. The most medial TrPs refer to the sacroiliac joint and to the lower buttock. Pain that extends across the upper sacral region may be referred from bilateral quadratus lumborum TrPs.
- *Needling technique:* The patient is in the sidelying position with the side to be treated facing up. If needed, the patient can bring the ipsilateral arm overhead with a pillow placed under the torso to improve access to the muscle. The 'true trunk' is identified by finding the anterior pelvis and ribs along with the posterior pelvis and ribs. This region is then bisected, staying in

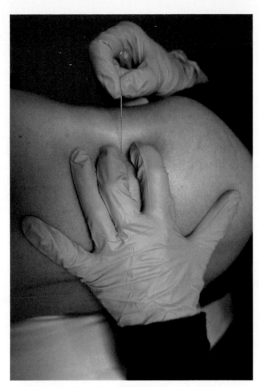

FIG. 10.20 Dry needling of trigger points in the quadratus lumborum muscle.

between the 12th rib and iliac crest. Next, the fingers move slightly posterior and press deeply with a flat palpation to identify the lateral border of the quadratus lumborum muscle, which is just lateral and ventral to the iliocostalis lumborum muscle. Note that the muscle is only directly palpable at the L4 level. Higher than this level, the latissimus dorsi muscle lies between the quadratus lumborum muscle and the skin. The needle must be long enough to reach the depth of the muscle toward its attachments at the transverse processes. Initially, the needle is aimed straight downward in the direction of the transverse process, followed by slight anterior, posterior, and caudal needling to explore the entire muscle. Depression of the subcutaneous tissue is required to reduce the distance from the skin to the muscle (Fig. 10.20).

- *Precautions:* To avoid penetration of the kidney, as well as the more cephalic diaphragm and pleura, do not direct the needle in a cephalic direction.

Psoas Major Muscle

- *Anatomy:* The psoas major muscle attaches at the 12th thoracic and all lumbar vertebral bodies, intervertebral discs, and anterior and inferior portions of the lumbar transverse processes. It is divided into an anterior and posterior mass (Gibbons et al., 2002; Standring, 2016). The posterior mass of the psoas major muscle attaches to the anterior surface of all lumbar vertebrae as well as the lower borders of the transverse processes (Gibbons et al., 2002; Standring, 2016). The anterior mass of the psoas major muscle has two different sets of attachments (Standring, 2016). The first part consists of five digitations of the muscle attached to the bodies of two adjoining vertebrae and the associated intervertebral disc. The highest level comes from the T12-L1 segment and the lowest is from the L4-L5 segment. The second part is a series of tendinous arches that extend across the narrow portions of the bodies of all five lumbar vertebrae between the digitations of the first part. The muscle passes anterior to the sacroiliac joint. The muscle shares a common tendinous insertion with the iliacus muscle at the lesser trochanter on the posteromedial surface of the femur. The muscle is palpated via the abdomen.
- *Function:* The primary function of the psoas major muscle is generally thought to be flexion of the hip (Hu et al., 2011; Standring, 2016); however, Yoshio and colleagues (2002) found that the psoas major is only an effective hip flexor between 45 degrees and 60 degrees of flexion. Several researchers have confirmed that the primary function of the psoas major is axial compression on the lumbar spine and stabilisation of the trunk (Rab et al., 1977; Bogduk et al., 1992; Santaguida & McGill, 1995). This is partially due to its anatomical connections at the diaphragm and pelvic floor (Gibbons et al., 2002; Sajko & Stuber, 2009). Park and colleagues (2013) reported that differences in function exist between the two portions of the muscle—the fascicles that arise from the transverse processes and those from the vertebral bodies, not from higher versus lower levels. The activities of the fascicles of the psoas major muscle that attach to the transverse processes were greater in extension of the trunk versus trunk flexion or hip flexion to 90 degrees. The fascicles from the portion of the psoas major muscle attaching to the vertebral bodies had greater activity in hip flexion than flexion of the trunk. The muscle also has a stabilising function at the hip. Yoshio and colleagues (2002) found that when the hip was flexed 0 to 15 degrees, the psoas muscle stabilises the femoral head onto the acetabulum in hip flexion and maintains erection of the lumbar column. In sitting, the psoas major is active in balancing the trunk (Standring, 2016).
- *Innervation:* The ventral rami of mainly L1 and L2, with some contribution from L3 (Standring, 2016).

Other variations, however, have been reported. Posterior fibres of the psoas major can be innervated by the ventral rami of spinal nerves T12-L4; the anterior fibres can be supplied by branches of the femoral nerve from L2-L4 (Gibbons et al., 2002).

- *Referred pain:* Pain is projected in a vertical pattern along the lumbar spine and may include the sacroiliac region and buttock and the anterior thigh up into the groin. When bilateral, it causes pain across the low back. Frequently, the patient will report having pain deep in the lower back. Muscolino (2013) described this muscle as also contributing to abdominal pain and nausea. Cummings (2003) described a referred pain pattern to the knee.

- *Needling technique:* It is not possible to direct the needle toward a TrP in the psoas major muscle even when TrPs were identified with abdominal palpation of the muscle. Therefore needling the psoas major muscle is a nonspecific technique whereby only the belly of the psoas major muscle can be treated. The patient is the sidelying position, possibly with a bolster or pillow underneath the patient's flank to increase the available space between the ilium and 12th rib. There are two approaches.

  1. In the lateral approach, the quadratus lumborum muscle serves as the anatomical landmark; therefore, the quadratus lumborum muscle is identified first. The needle technique is similar to needling the quadratus lumborum muscle; however, the needle is directed approximately 10 degrees to 30 degrees anteriorly into the psoas muscle (Fig. 10.21). An increase in resistance can

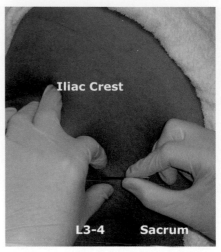

FIG. 10.22 Dry needling of the psoas major muscle— posterior approach.

be felt when the needle reaches the epimysium of the psoas major muscle.

  2. In the posterior approach, the muscle is also accessed in the sidelying position, at the level of L3 to L4, which is well below the level of the kidney (usually above L2). The psoas major muscle lies alongside the vertebrae anterior to the transverse processes. Palpate the spinal processes of L3-L4 and the adjacent longissimus and iliocostalis muscles. The needle is placed just lateral to the lumbar longissimus muscle and transverse processes. The needle is directed anteriorly, staying parallel to the table. If the needle would touch the transverse process, the needle placement is too medial and should be redirected. The optimal length of the needle depends entirely on the individual dimensions of the patient (Fig. 10.22).

- *Precautions:* Even though needling the kidney does not cause harm, every effort should be made to avoid penetrating the kidney, as well as the more cephalic diaphragm and pleura.

Rectus Abdominus Muscle

- *Anatomy:* The rectus abdominus muscle attaches inferiorly along the crest of the pubic bone via a medial and lateral tendon. The medial tendon interlaces with the contralateral muscle and attaches to the symphysis pubis. Superiorly, the muscle attaches to the fifth, sixth, and seventh costal cartilages. Occasionally there may be attachments to the third or fourth ribs. The paired recti are separated in the midline by the linea alba. Three transverse fibrous bands, or tendinous inscriptions, interrupt

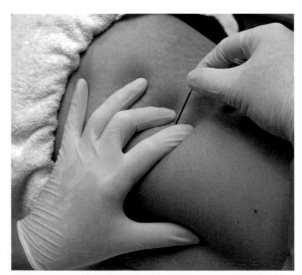

FIG. 10.21 Dry needling of the psoas major muscle— lateral approach.

the rectus abdominus muscle. Anita and colleagues (2015) reported variations with four or five intersections typically situated at the level of the umbilicus, near the tip of the xyphoid process, and midway between the umbilicus and the xyphoid process. The intersections are rarely full-thickness inscriptions.

- *Function:* The rectus abdominus muscle flexes the trunk and increases the intraabdominal pressure during activities such as exhalation, defecation, micturition, parturition, coughing, and vomiting.
- *Innervation:* Branches of the ventral rami of the lower six or seven spinal via the lower intercostal and subcostal nerves.
- *Referred pain:* The rectus abdominus muscle refers pain to the entire low back region; the upper rectus abdominus muscle refers pain horizontally across the back in the thoracolumbar region and the xiphoid process. Somatovisceral symptoms caused by upper rectus abdominus TrPs may include abdominal fullness, heartburn, indigestion, nausea, and vomiting. Muscolino (2013) described a patient with TrPs in the rectus abdominus muscle that caused nausea and abdominal pain. Peri-umbilical TrPs may cause abdominal cramping or colic. The lower rectus abdominus muscle refers pain across the low back and sacral regions and to the groin, penis, perineum, rectum, and suprapubic area. Somatovisceral symptoms include spasm of the detrusor and urinary sphincter muscles, diarrhoea, and dysmenorrhea. A TrP located in the lower right quadrant, known as McBurney's point, may mimic symptoms of appendicitis.
- *Needling technique:* For the midportion of the muscle, the patient lies supine with the clinician positioned contralateral to the side to be needled. Depress the abdominal wall just lateral to the taut band in the muscle and create a shelf or 'wall' by pulling the muscle toward you. The needle is inserted perpendicular to the skin and directed medially toward the linea alba, staying tangential to the abdominal wall (Fig. 10.23). For lower rectus abdominus TrPs, place the needle slightly cranially from the TrP and direct the needle in a shallow to gradual deeper fashion toward the pubic bone (Fig. 10.24).
- *Precautions:* Avoid entering the abdominal cavity.

Pyramidalis Muscle

- *Anatomy:* The pyramidalis muscles are small triangular muscles just above the pubic bone on both sides of the midline within the aponeurosis of the transverse abdominal muscle underneath the rectus abdominus muscle. The muscle attaches at the anterior surface of the superior ramus and symphysis of the pubic bone with tendinous connections to the suspensory

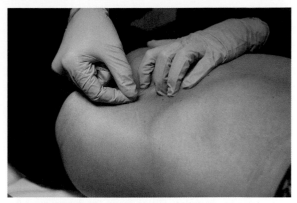

FIG. 10.23 Dry needling of trigger points in the rectus abdominus muscle.

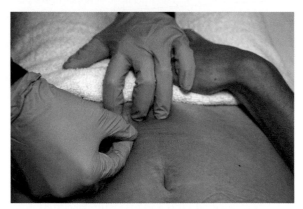

FIG. 10.24 Dry needling of trigger points in the lower portion of the rectus abdominus muscle.

ligament of the penis. The muscle blends into the linea alba approximately halfway between the pubis and the umbilicus. The muscle may be entirely absent on one or both sides, especially in females. According to Ashley-Montagu (1939), the muscle is present on one or both sides of the body in 82.6% of cases, ranging from 79% in Caucasians to 96% in Asians. Of interest is that the muscle is being used as a small muscle free flap in the treatment of small chronic wounds on the foot or ankle (Van Landuyt et al., 2003). The pyramidalis muscle cannot be distinguished from the rectus abdominus muscle by palpation, even though Simons and associates (1999) described a unique referred pain pattern to the muscle.

- *Function:* The pyramidalis muscle tenses the linea alba.
- *Innervation:* The 7th to 12th intercostal nerves.
- *Referred pain:* According to Simons and associates (1999), the pyramidalis muscle refers pain to the region between the symphysis pubis and the umbilicus.

- *Needling technique:* The needling technique is identical to the technique for TrP in the lower rectus abdominus muscle.
- *Precautions:* Avoid entering the abdominal cavity.

External and Internal Oblique Abdominal Muscles

- Anatomy:
  1. The external oblique abdominal muscle is the largest and most superficial of the lateral abdominal muscles. It attaches superiorly to the external, inferior border of the lower eight ribs, interdigitating with the latissimus dorsi and the lower serratus anterior muscles. Fibres from the lower two ribs pass nearly vertically to attach to the anterior half of the iliac crest. The middle and upper fibres pass obliquely medially and caudally to join the abdominal aponeurosis, which attaches to the linea alba.
  2. The internal oblique abdominal muscle lies deep to the external oblique. Its fibres arise from the lateral two-thirds of the inguinal ligament, the anterior two-thirds of the iliac crest, and the lower portion of the thoracolumbar fascia. The posterior fibres pass vertically to attach to the cartilages of the last three or four ribs. The fibres attached to the anterior iliac crest pass superiorly and medially to attach to the lines alba via the anterior and posterior rectus sheath. The medial fibres pass horizontally and arch downwards. These fibres become tendinous and fuse with the corresponding aponeurosis of the transverse abdominus muscle, forming the conjoint tendon. This tendon attaches to the pubic crest and pectineal line. Posteriorly, the common tendon of the transverse abdominis and internal oblique muscles are linked through the aponeurosis of the thoracolumbar fascia and contribute to complex matrix stabilising the lumbosacral spine (Willard et al., 2012; Vleeming et al., 2014).
- *Function:* Both the internal and external oblique abdominal muscles contribute lateral flexion of the trunk against resistance. With the transverse abdominus muscle, they maintain abdominal tone and increase intraabdominal pressure for defecation, micturition, parturition, forced exhalation, coughing, and vomiting. Together with the paraspinal muscles, the abdominal muscles contribute to lumbosacral stability.
- *Innervation:* The external and internal obliques are innervated by the intercostal nerves of T8-T12 and the subcostal nerves of T7-T12. The internal oblique is also supplied by branches of the iliohypogastric and iliolingual nerves from L1.

- *Referred pain:* TrPs located in either oblique muscle refer pain to the groin and genitals. Somatovisceral responses to TrPs located in the external oblique include deep epigastric pain, chronic diarrhoea and, in the posterior region just below the 12th rib, belching. The lower internal oblique muscle along with the lower rectus abdominus may contribute to spasm of the detrusor and urinary sphincter muscles.
- *Needling technique:* The patient is either in the side-lying position or in supine. Staying in between the 12th rib and iliac crest, grasp the oblique muscles between your fingers to ensure that the abdominal contents remain medial. The hand position should reflect the fibre direction of the two muscles. The needle is inserted anteriorly and directed posteriorly toward the thumb. Only the muscle tissue between your fingers is needled (Figs. 10.25 and 10.26).
- *Precautions:* Avoid entering the abdominal cavity.

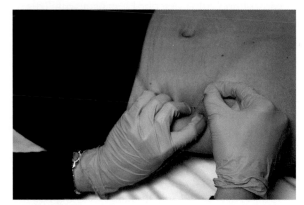

FIG. 10.25 Dry needling of trigger points in the external oblique abdominal muscle.

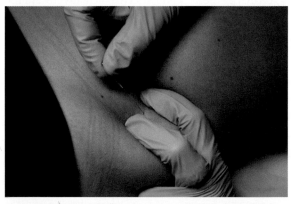

FIG. 10.26 Dry needling of trigger points in the internal oblique abdominal muscle.

REFERENCES

Alizadehkhaiyat, O., Hawkes, D. H., Kemp, G. J., & Frostick, S. P. (2015). Electromyographic analysis of shoulder girdle muscles during common internal rotation exercises. *International Journal of Sports Physical Therapy, 10*(5), 645–654.

Anandkumar, S., & Manivasagam, M. (2017). Effect of fascia dry needling on non-specific thoracic pain—a proposed dry needling grading system. *Physiotherapy Theory and Practice, 33*(5), 420–428.

Anita, M., Haque, Gupta, A., & Nasar, A. (2015). Variation in tendinous intersections of rectus abdominus muscle in northern Indian population with clinical implications. *Journal of Clinical and Diagnostic Research, 9*(6), 10–12.

Ashley-Montagu, M. F. (1939). Anthropological significance of the musculus pyramidalis and its variability in man. *American Journal of Physical Anthropology, 25*, 435–490.

Bajaj, P., Bajaj, P., Graven-Nielsen, T., & Arendt-Nielsen, L. (2001a). Trigger points in patients with lower limb osteoarthritis. *Journal of Musculoskeletal Pain, 9*, 17–33.

Bajaj, P., Bajaj, P., Graven-Nielsen, T., & Arendt-Nielsen, L. (2001b). Osteoarthritis and its association with muscle hyperalgesia: an experimental controlled study. *Pain, 93*, 107–114.

Bakirci, S., Kafa, I. M., Uysal, M., & Sendemir, E. (2010). Langer's axillary arch (axillopectoral muscle): a variation of latissimus dorsi muscle. *International Journal of Anatomical Variations, 3*, 91–92.

Bartley, J. (2010). Breathing and temporomandibular joint disease. *Journal of Bodywork and Movement Therapies, 15*, 291–297.

Beeckmans, N., Vermeersch, A., Lysens, R., Van Wambeke, P., Goossens, N., Thys, T., et al. (2016). The presence of respiratory disorders in individuals with low back pain: a systematic review. *Manual Therapy, 26*, 77–86.

Berliner, D., Schneider, N., Welte, T., & Bauersachs, J. (2016). The differential diagnosis of dyspnea. *Deutsches Ärzteblatt International, 113*(49), 834–845.

Bogduk, N., Pearcy, M., & Hadfield, G. (1992). Anatomy and biomechanics of psoas major. *Clinical Biomechanics (Bristol, Avon), 7*, 109–119.

Boissonault, W., & Bass, C. (1990). Pathological origins of trunk and neck pain: part 1- pelvic and abdominal visceral disorders. *The Journal of Orthopaedic and Sports Physical Therapy, 12*, 192–221.

Boulding, R., Stacey, R., Niven, R., & Fowler, S. J. (2016). Dysfunctional breathing: a review of the literature and proposal for classification. *European Respiratory Review, 25*(141), 287–294.

Boyles, R., Fowler, R., Ramsey, D., & Burrows, E. (2015). Effectiveness of trigger point dry needling for multiple body regions: a systematic review. *The Journal of Manual & Manipulative Therapy, 23*(5), 276–293.

Brennan, P. A., St, J., Blythe, J., Alam, P., Green, B., & Parry, D. (2015). Division of the spinal accessory nerve in the anterior triangle: a prospective clinical study. *The British Journal of Oral & Maxillofacial Surgery, 53*(7), 633–636.

Briggs, A. M., Smith, A. J., Straker, L. M., & Bragge, P. (2009). Thoracic spine pain in the general population: prevalence, incidence and associated factors in children, adolescents and adults. A systematic review. *BMC Musculoskeletal Disorders, 10*, 77.

Caliot, P., Bousquet, V., Midy, D., & Cabanié, P. (1989). A contribution to the study of the accessory nerve: surgical implications. *Surgical and Radiologic Anatomy, 11*, 11–15.

Castro-Sanchez, A. M., Garcia-Lopez, H., Mataran-Penarrocha, G. A., Fernandez-Sanchez, M., Fernandez-Sola, C., Granero-Molina, J., et al. (2017). Effects of dry needling on spinal mobility and trigger points in patients with fibromyalgia syndrome. *Pain Physician, 20*(2), 37–52.

Chaitow, L. (1997). Breathing pattern disorders and back pain. In A. Vleeming, V. Mooney, & T. Dorman, et al. (Eds.), *Movement, stability and low back pain* (pp. 563–571). Edinburgh: Churchill Livingstone.

Chaitow, L. (2004). Breathing pattern disorders, motor control, and low back pain. *Journal of Osteopathic Medicine, 7*, 34–41.

Chen, J. C., Chen, Y., Lin, S. M., Yang, H. J., Su, C. F., & Tseng, S. H. (2006). Acute spinal epidural hematoma after acupuncture. *The Journal of Trauma, 60*, 414–416.

Chen, C. K., & Nizar, A. J. (2011). Myofascial pain syndrome in chronic back pain patients. *The Korean Journal of Pain, 24*, 100–104.

Chu, J., Bruyninckx, F., & Neuhauser, D. V. (2016). Chronic refractory myofascial pain and denervation supersensitivity as global public health disease. *BML Case Reports*. 13 Jan;2016. pii: bcr2015211816.

Cornwall, J., Harris, A. J., & Mercer, S. R. (2006). The lumbar multifidus muscle and patterns of pain. *Manual Therapy, 11*, 40–45.

Courtney, R. (2009). The functions of breathing and its dysfunctions and their relationship to breathing therapy. *International Journal of Osteopathic Medicine, 12*, 78–85.

Cummings, M. (2003). Referred knee pain treated with electroacupuncture to iliopsoas. *Acupuncture in Medicine, 21.1-2*, 32–35.

D.Alba, I., Carloni, I., Ferrante, A. L., Gesuita, R., Palazzi, M. L., & de Benedictis, F. M. (2015). Hyperventilation syndrome in adolescents with and without asthma. *Pediatric Pulmonology, 50*(12), 1184–1190.

Dar, G., & Hicks, G. E. (2016). The immediate effect of dry needling on multifidus muscles' function in healthy individuals. *Journal of Back and Musculoskeletal Rehabilitation, 29*(2), 273–278.

Delp, S., Suryanarayanan, S., Murray, W. M., Uhlir, J., & Triolo, R. J. (2001). Architecture of the rectus abdominis, quadratus lumborum, and erector spinae. *Journal of Biomechanics, 34*, 371–375.

Dommerholt, J., & Shah, J. (2010). Myofascial pain syndrome. In J. C. Ballantyne, J. P. Rathmell, & S. M. Fishman (Eds.), *Bonica's management of pain* (pp. 450–471). Baltimore: Lippincott, Williams, & Wilkins.

Ebaugh, D. D., McClure, P. W., & Karduna, A. R. (2005). Three-dimensional scapulo-thoracic motion during active and passie arm elevation. *Clinical Biomechanics, 20*, 700–709.

Espejo-Antúnez, L., Fernández-Huertas Tejeda, J., Albornoz-Cabello, M., Rodríguez-Mansilla, J., De La Cruz-Torres, B., Ribeiro, F., et al. (2017). Dry needling in the management of myofascial trigger points: a systematic review of randomized controlled trials. *Complementary Therapies in Medicine, 33*, 46–57.

Fernández-de-las-Peñas, C. (2009). Interaction between trigger points and joint hypomobility: a clinical perspective. *The Journal of Manual & Manipulative Therapy, 17,* 74–77.

Fernández-de-las-Peñas, C., Layton, M., & Dommerholt, J. (2015). Dry needling for the management of thoracic spine pain. *The Journal of Manual & Manipulative Therapy, 23*(3), 147–153.

Furlan, A. D., van Tulder, M. W., Cherkin, D. C., Tsukayama, H., Lao, L., Koes, B., et al. (2005). Acupuncture and dry-needling for low back pain. *The Cochrane Database of Systematic Review, 1,* 386.

Gattie, E., Cleland, J. A., & Snodgrass, S. (2017). The effectiveness of trigger point dry needling for musculoskeletal conditions by physical therapists: a systematic review and meta-analysis. *The Journal of Orthopaedic and Sports Physical Therapy, 47*(3), 133–149.

Gerber, L. H., Shah, J., Rosenberger, W., Armstrong, K., Turo, D., Otto, P., et al. (2015). Dry needling alters trigger points in the upper trapezius muscle and reduces pain in subjects with chronic myofascial pain. *PM&R, 7*(7), 711–718.

Gerber, L. H., Sikdar, S., Aredo, J. V., Armstrong, K., Rosenberger, W. F., Shao, H., et al. (2017). Beneficial effects of dry needling for treatment of chronic myofascial pain persist for 6 weeks after treatment completion. *PM&R, 9,* 105–112.

Gerwin, R. (2002). Myofascial and visceral pain syndromes: visceral-somatic pain representations. *Journal of Musculoskeletal Pain, 10,* 165–175.

Giamberardino, M. A., Affaitati, G., Lerza, R., & De Laurentis, S. (2002). Neurophysiological basis of visceral pain. *Journal of Musculoskeletal Pain, 10,* 151–163.

Gibbons, S., Comerford, M. J., & Emerson, P. (2002). Rehabilitation of the stability function of psoas major. *Orthopaedic Division Review Jan/Feb.*

Greger, R., & Windhorst, U. (2013). *Comprehensive human physiology: from cellular mechanisms to integration. Ebook.* Springer Science & Business Media.

Han, J. N., Stegen, K., Simkens, K., Cauberghs, M., Schepers, R., Van den Bergh, O., et al. (1997). Unsteadiness of breathing in patients with hyperventilation syndrome and anxiety disorders. *The European Respiratory Journal, 10*(1), 167–176.

Hasler, G., Gergen, P. J., Kleinbaum, D. G., et al. (2005). Asthma and panic in young adults: a 20-year prospective community study. *American Journal of Respiratory and Critical Care Medicine, 171,* 1224–1230.

Hasuo, H., Ishihara, T., Kanbara, K., & Fukunaga, M. (2016). Myofascial trigger points in advanced cancer patients. *Indian Journal of Palliative Care, 22*(1), 80–84.

Hendler, N. H., & Kozikowski, J. G. (1993). Overlooked physical diagnoses in chronic pain patients involved in litigation. *Psychosomatics, 34,* 494–501.

Hodges, P., & Richardson, C. (1999). Altered trunk muscle recruitment in people with LBP with upper limb movement at different speeds. *Archives of Physical Medicine and Rehabilitation, 80,* 1005–1012.

Hodges, P., Heinjnen, I., & Gandevia, S. (2001). Postural activity of the diaphragm is reduced in humans when respiratory demand increases. *The Journal of Physiology, 537,* 999.

Hoheisel, U., Taguchi, T., Treede, R. D., & Mense, S. (2011). Nociceptive input from the rat thoracolumbar fascia to lumbar dorsal horn neurones. *European Journal of Pain, 15,* 810–815.

Howell, J. B. (1997). The hyperventilation syndrome: a syndrome under threat? *Thorax, 52*(Suppl 3), S30–S34.

Hruska, R. J. (1997). Influences of dysfunctional respiratory mechanics on orofacial pain. *Dental Clinics of North America, 41,* 211–227.

Hruska, R. J. (2002). Management of pelvic-thoracic influences on temporomandibular dysfunction. *Orthop Phys Ther Clin N Am, 11,* 263–284.

Hsueh, T. C., Yu, S., Kuan, T. S., & Hong, C. Z. (1998). Association of active myofascial trigger points and cervical disc lesions. *Journal of the Formosan Medical Association, 97*(3), 174–180.

Hu, H., Meijer, O. G., Dieen, J. H., Hodges, P. W., Bruijn, S. M., Strijers, R. L., Nanayakkara, Prabath W.B., Royen, Barend J., Wu, Wen Hua, & Xia, Chun. (2011). Is the psoas a hip flexor in the active straight leg raise? *European Spine Journal, 20*(5), 759–765.

Huang, Q. M., & Liu, L. (2014). Wet needling of myofascial trigger points in abdominal muscles for treatment of primary dysmenorrhea. *Acupuncture in Medicine, 32*(4), 346–349.

Iglesias-González, J. J., Muñoz-García, M. T., Rodrigues-de-Souza, D. P., Alburquerque-Sendín, F., & Fernández-de-las-Peñas, C. (2013). Myofascial trigger points, pain, disability, and sleep quality in patients with chronic nonspecific low back pain. *Pain Medicine, 14*(12), 1964–1970.

Itoh, K., Katsumi, Y., & Kitakoji, H. (2004). Trigger point acupuncture treatment of chronic low back pain in elderly patients—a blinded RCT. *Acupuncture in Medicine, 22*(4), 170–177.

Itoh, K., Katsumi, Y., Hirota, S., & Kitakoji, H. (2006). Effects of trigger point acupuncture on chronic low back pain in elderly patients-a sham-controlled randomised trial. *Acupuncture in Medicine, 24*(1), 5–12.

Jarrell, J. F., Vilos, G. A., Allaire, C., Burgess, S., Fortin, C., Gerwin, R., et al. (2005). Consensus guidelines for the management of chronic pelvic pain. *Journal of Obstetrics and Gynaecology Canada, 27,* 781–826.

Johnson, G., Bogduk, N., Nowitzke, A., & House, D. (1994). Anatomy and actions of the trapezius muscle. *Clinical Biomechanics (Bristol, Avon), 9,* 44–50.

Johnson, R. A. (2017). A quick reference on respiratory alkalosis. *The Veterinary Clinics of North America Small Animal Practice, 47*(2), 181–184.

Kaltsakas, G., Antoniou, E., Palamidas, A. F., Gennimata, S. A., Paraskeva, P., Smyrnis, A., et al. (2013). Dyspnea and respiratory muscle strength in end-stage liver disease. *World Journal of Hepatology, 5*(2), 56–63. 27.

Kim, J. H., Choi, K. Y., Lee, K. H., Lee, D. J., Park, B. J., & Rho, Y. S. (2014). Motor innervation of the trapezius muscle: intraoperative motor conduction study during neck dissection. *ORL: Journal for Otorhinolaryngology and Its Related Specialties, 76,* 8–12.

Kirkaldy-Willis, W. H. (1990). *Segmental instability: the lumbar spine.* Philadelphia, PA: WB Saunders.

Koppenhaver, S. L., Walker, M. J., Smith, R. W., Booker, J. M., Walkup, I. D., Su, J., et al. (2015a). Baseline examination factors associated with clinical improvement after dry needling in individuals with low back pain. *The Journal of Orthopaedic and Sports Physical Therapy, 45*(8), 604–612.

Koppenhaver, S. L., Walker, M. J., Su, J., McGowen, J. M., Umlauf, L., Harris, K. D., et al. (2015b). Changes in lumbar multifidus muscle function and nociceptive sensitivity in low back pain patient responders versus non-responders after dry needling treatment. *Manual Therapy, 20*(6), 769–776.

Lanisnik, B., Zargi, M., & Rodi, Z. (2014). Identification of three anatomical patterns of the spinal accessory nerve in the neck by neurophysiological mapping. *Radiology and Oncology, 48,* 387–392.

Lee, J., & Jung, W. (2015). A pair of atypical rhomboid muscles. *The Korean Journal of Physical Anthropology, 28*(4), 247–251.

Lee, J. H., Lee, H., & Jo, D. J. (2011). An acute cervical epidural hematoma as a complication of dry needling. *Spine (Phila Pa 1976), 36,* E891–893.

Lencu, C., Alexescu, T., Petrulea, M., & Lencu, M. (2016). Respiratory manifestations in endocrine diseases. *Clujul Med, 89*(4), 459–463.

Liu, L., Huang, Q. M., Liu, Q. G., Ye, G., Bo, C. Z., Chen, M. J., et al. (2015). Effectiveness of dry needling for myofascial trigger points associated with neck and shoulder pain: a systematic review and meta-analysis. *Archives of Physical Medicine and Rehabilitation, 96*(5), 944–955.

Loukas, M., Louis, R. G., Jr., Wartmann, C. T., Tubbs, R. S., Gupta, A. A., Apaydin, N., et al. (2008). An anatomic investigation of the serratus posterior superior and serratus posterior inferior muscles. *Surgical and Radiologic Anatomy, 30*(2), 119–123.

Mahmoudzadeh, A., Rezaeian, Z. S., Karimi, A., & Dommerholt, J. (2016). The effect of dry needling on the radiating pain in subjects with discogenic low back pain: a randomized control trial. *Journal of Research in Medical Sciences, 21,* 94.

Manchikanti, L., Singh, V., Falco, F. J., Benyamin, R. M., & Hirsch, J. A. (2014). Epidemiology of low back pain in adults. *Neuromodulation, 17*(Suppl 2), 3–10.

Mclaughlin, L., Goldsmith, C. H., & Coleman, K. (2011). Breathing evaluation and retraining as an adjunct to manual therapy. *Manual Therapy, 16,* 51–52.

Mense, S. (2008). Muscle pain: mechanisms and clinical significance. *Deutsches Ärzteblatt International, 105,* 214–219.

Meuret, A. E., & Ritz, T. (2010). Hyperventilation in panic disorder and asthma: empirical evidence and clinical strategies. *International Journal of Psychophysiology, 78*(1), 68–79.

Montenegro, M. L., Gomide, L. B., Mateus-Vasconcelos, E. L., Rosa-e-Silva, J. C., Candido-dos-Reis, F. J., Nogueira, A. A., et al. (2009). Abdominal myofascial pain syndrome must be considered in the differential diagnosis of chronic pelvic pain. *European Journal of Obstetrics, Gynecology, and Reproductive Biology, 147,* 21–24.

Montenegro, M. L., Braz, C. A., Rosa-e-Silva, J. C., Candido-dos-Reis, F. J., Nogueira, A. A., & Poli-Neto, O. B. (2015). Anaesthetic injection versus ischemic compression for the pain relief of abdominal wall trigger points in women with chronic pelvic pain. *BMC Anesthesiology, 15,* 175.

Morihisa, R., Eskew, J., McNamara, A., & Young, J. (2016). Dry needling in subjects with muscular trigger points in the lower quarter: a systematic review. *International Journal of Sports Physical Therapy, 11*(1), 1–14.

Muscolino, J. E. (2013). Abdominal wall trigger point case study. *Journal of Bodywork and Movement Therapies, 17*(2), 151–156.

Neiva, P. D., Kirkwood, R. N., Mendes, P. L., Zabjek, K., Becker, H. G., & Mathur, S. (2017). Postural disorders in mouth breathing children: a systematic review. *Brazilian Journal of Physical Therapy.* [Epub ahead of print]

Njoo, K. H., & van der Does, E. (1994). The occurrence and inter-rater reliability of myofascial trigger points in the quadratus lumborum and gluteus medius: a prospective study in non-specific low back pain patients and controls in general practice. *Pain, 58*(3), 317–323.

Ogata, N., Bapat, U., Darby, Y., & Scadding, G. (2006). Prevalence of hyperventilation syndrome in an allergy clinic, compared with routine ENT clinc. *The Journal of Laryngology and Otology, 120*(11), 924–926.

Park, R. J., Tsao, H., Claus, A., Cresswell, A. G., & Hodges, P. W. (2013). Changes in regional activity of the psoas major and quadratus lumborum with voluntary trunk and hip tasks and different spinal curvatures in sitting. *The Journal of Orthopaedic and Sports Physical Therapy, 43*(2), 74–82.

Park, S., & Yoo, W. (2014). Differential activation of parts of the latissimus dorsi with various isometric shoulder exercises. *Journal of Electromyography and Kinesiology, 24*(2), 253–257.

Paris, S. (1997). Differential diagnosis of lumbar, back, and pelvic pain. In A. Vleeming, V. Mooney, & T. Dorman, et al. (Eds.), *Movement, stability and low back pain.* Edinburgh: Churchill Livingstone.

Pecos-Martín, D., Montañez-Aguilera, F. J., Gallego-Izquierdo, T., Urraca-Gesto, A., Gómez-Conesa, A., Romero-Franco, N., et al. (2015). Effectiveness of dry needling on the lower trapezius in patients with mechanical neck pain: a randomized controlled trial. *Archives of Physical Medicine and Rehabilitation, 96*(5), 775–781.

Perez-Palomares, S., Olivan-Blazquez, B., Magallon-Botaya, R., et al. (2010). Percutaneous electrical nerve stimulation versus dry needling: effectiveness in the treatment of chronic low back pain. *Journal of Musculoskeletal Pain, 18*(1), 23–30.

Pizzari, T., Wickham, J., Balster, S., Ganderton, C., & Watson, L. (2014). Modifying a shrug exercise can facilitate the upward rotator muscles of the scapula. *Clinical Biomechanics, 29,* 201–205.

Porterfield, J. A., & DeRosa, C. (1995). *Mechanical neck pain; perspectives in functional anatomy.* Philadelphia: W.B. Saunders.

Porth, C. (2011). *Essentials of pathophysiology: concepts of altered health states* (4th ed.). Baltimore: Lippincott, Williams & Wilkins.

Pouliart, N., & Gagey, O. (2005). Significance of the latissimus dorsi for shoulder instability. I. Variations in its anatomy around the humerus and scapula. *Clinical Anatomy, 18*(7), 493–499.

Pu, Y. M., Tang, E. Y., & Yang, X. D. (2008). Trapezius muscle innervation from the spinal accessory nerve and branches of the cervical plexus. *International Journal of Oral and Maxillofacial Surgery, 37,* 567–572.

Puentedura, E. J., Buckingham, S. J., Morton, D., Montoya, C., & Fernandez de las Penas, C. (2017). Immediate changes in resting and contracted thickness of transversus abdominis after dry needling of lumbar multifidus in healthy participants: a randomized controlled crossover trial. *Journal of Manipulative and Physiological Therapeutics, 40,* 615–623.

Rab, G. T., Chao, E. Y. S., & Stauffer, R. N. (1977). Muscle force analysis of the lumbar spine. *The Orthopedic Clinics of North America, 8*(1), 193–199.

Rock, J. M., & Rainey, C. E. (2014). Treatment of nonspecific thoracic spine pain with trigger point dry needling and intramuscular electrical stimulation: a case series. *International Journal of Sports Physical Therapy, 9*(5), 699–711.

Sajko, S., & Stuber, K. (2009). Psoas major: a case report and review of its anatomy, biomechanics, and clinical implications. *The Journal of the Canadian Chiropractic Association, 53*(4), 311–318.

Samuel, S., Peter, A., & Ramanathan, K. (2007). The association of active trigger points with lumbar disc lesions. *Journal of Musculoskeletal Pain, 15*(2), 11–18.

Santaguida, P. L., & McGill, S. M. (1995). The psoas major muscle: a three-dimensional geometric study. *Journal of Biomechanics, 28,* 339–345.

Simons, D. G., Travell, J. G., & Simons, L. S. (1999). *Travell & Simons' myofascial pain and dysfunction: the trigger point manual, the upper half of the body. Vol.1.* Baltimore: Lippincott, Williams & Wilkins.

Smith, R., Jr., Nyquist-Battie, C., Clark, M., & Rains, J. (2003). Anatomical characteristics of the upper serratus anterior: cadaver dissection. *The Journal of Orthopaedic and Sports Physical Therapy, 33*(8), 449–454.

Standring, S. (Ed.), (2008). *Gray's anatomy: the anatomical basis of clinical practice* (40th ed.). London: Churchill Livingstone Elsevier.

Standring, S. (Ed.), (2016). *Gray's anatomy: the anatomical basis of clinical practice* (41st ed.). London: Churchill Livingstone Elsevier.

Stoop, R., Clijsen, R., Leoni, D., Soldini, E., Castellini, G., Redaelli, V., et al. (2017). Evolution of the methodological quality of controlled clinical trials for myofascial trigger point treatments for the period 1978–2015: a systematic review. *Musculoskelet Sci Pract, 30,* 1–9.

Taguchi, T., Hoheisel, U., & Mense, S. (2008). Dorsal horn neurons having input from low back structures in rats. *Pain, 138,* 119–129.

Téllez-García, M., de-la-Llave-Rincón, A. I., Salom-Moreno, J., Palacios-Ceña, M., Ortega-Santiago, R., & Fernández-de-las-Peñas, C. (2015). Neuroscience education in addition to trigger point dry needling for the management of patients with mechanical chronic low back pain: a preliminary clinical trial. *Journal of Bodywork and Movement Therapies, 19*(3), 464–472.

Teixeira, M. J., Yeng, L. T., Garcia, O. G., Fonoff, E. T., Paiva, W. S., & Araujo, J. O. (2011). Failed back surgery pain syndrome: therapeutic approach descriptive study in 56 patients. *Revista da Associação Médica Brasileira, 57,* 282–287.

Turo, D., Otto, P., Hossain, M., Gebreab, T., Armstrong, K., Rosenberger, W. F., et al. (2015). Novel use of ultrasound elastography to quantify muscle tissue changes after dry needling of myofascial trigger points in patients with chronic myofascial pain. *Journal of Ultrasound in Medicine, 34,* 2149–2161.

Van Landuyt, K., Hamdi, M., Blondeel, P., & Monstrey, S. (2003). The pyramidalis muscle free flap. *British Journal of Plastic Surgery, 56,* 585–592.

Vas, L., Phanse, S., & Pai, R. (2016). A new perspective of neuromyopathy to explain intractable pancreatic cancer pains; dry needling as an effective adjunct to neurolytic blocks. *Indian Journal of Palliative Care, 22*(1), 85–93.

Vilensky, J. A., Baltes, M., Weikel, L., Fortin, J. D., & Fourie, L. J. (2001). Serratus posterior muscles: anatomy, clinical relevance, and function. *Clinical Anatomy, 14,* 237–241.

Vleeming, A., Schuenke, M. D., Danneels, L., & Willard, F. H. (2014). The functional coupling of the deep abdominal and paraspinal muscles: the effects of simulated paraspinal muscle contraction on force transfer to the middle and posterior layer of the thoracolumbar fascia. *Journal of Anatomy, 225,* 447–462.

Waddell, G. (1998). *The back pain revolution.* Edinburgh: Churchill Livingstone.

Webb, A. L., O'Sullivan, E., Stokes, M., & Mottram, S. (2016). A novel cadaveric study of the morphometry of the serratus anterior muscle: one part, two parts, three parts, four? *Anatomical Science International.* 18 Oct [Epub ahead of print].

Willard, F. H., Vleeming, A., Schuenke, M. D., Danneels, L., & Schleip, R. (2012). The thoracolumbar fascia: anatomy, function and clinical considerations. *Journal of Anatomy, 221,* 507–536.

Yoshio, M., Murakami, G., Sato, T., Sato, S., & Noriyasu, S. (2002). The function of the psoas major muscle: passive kinetics and morphological studies using donated cadavers. *Journal of Orthopaedic Science, 7*(2), 199–207.

CHAPTER 11

Deep Dry Needling of the Hip and Pelvic Muscles

BLAIR H. GREEN • JAN DOMMERHOLT

INTRODUCTION

The pelvis is the region of the body bound by the innominate bones, sacrum, and coccyx. Within this bony framework lie the contents of the pelvic floor. The pelvic floor is comprised not only of muscular structures, but also all of the structures in the pelvic cavity (Hartman & Sarton, 2014). The muscles of the abdominal–pelvic region serve many roles, including control of the urinary and anal sphincters, sexual arousal and orgasm, support for the pelvic viscera, local spinal stability, and motor control. Muscles contributing to pelvic girdle pain may not be limited to the intrinsic muscles of the pelvic floor.

The American College of Obstetricians and Gynaecologists describes chronic pelvic pain (CPP) as pain located in the pelvis, abdominal wall at or below the umbilicus, lumbar, sacral, and buttock regions (Vercellini et al., 2009). Several pain syndromes are included within the CPP terminology, including bladder pain syndrome, endometriosis pain syndrome, interstitial cystitis, prostatic pain syndrome, dysmenorrhoea, and vulvodynia (Fall et al., 2010). CPP remains a somewhat enigmatic diagnosis. Pastore and Katzman (2012) commented that 40% of all laparoscopies are performed to determine a cause of CPP. Vleeming and colleagues (2008) suggested that, from a biomechanical point of view, there is a connection between chronic sacroiliac dysfunction and CPP, which is evidenced by many patients with SI pain, who also suffer from CPP. In addition, Vleeming and colleagues (2008) reported that the prevalence of pelvic girdle pain in pregnancy is 20%. According to Zondervain and colleagues (2001), the lifetime occurrence of CPP is 33%. In a recent study researchers found a significant relationship between the presence of spine and hip movement diagnoses and pelvic floor muscle diagnoses (Wente & Spitznagle 2017). Cohen and colleagues (2016) described the relationship between pelvic floor muscle dysfunction in males with sexual dysfunction, chronic prostatitis,

and CPP. These authors found a significant overlap of signs and symptoms of these disorders with a common thread of muscular dysfunction in the muscles of the pelvic floor, which implies that treating these muscles may result in improved function in men with chronic pelvic pain, chronic prostatitis, and sexual dysfunction (Cohen et al., 2016).

Moreover, pelvic floor muscle dysfunction is associated with impairments of the lumbar spine and hip regions. A functional relationship exists between the pelvic floor, diaphragm and transverse abdominus (Sapsford et al., 2001; Hodges et al., 2014). Smith and colleagues (2006) reported that the association between incontinence and low back pain is greater than the association between low back pain and body mass index. Several studies reported an association between hip pathology, including end-stage hip osteoarthritis and femoroacetabular impingement, and pelvic floor disorders such as vulvodynia and urinary incontinence (Podschun et al., 2013; Baba et al., 2014; Tamaki et al., 2014; Prather & Camacho-Soto 2014; Coady & Futterman, 2015).

Pain from visceral organs is often similar to myofascial pain and described as a poorly localised, dull, aching pain. Both myofascial and visceral pain are known causes of secondary hyperalgesia or referred pain. Of interest is that visceral-induced referred pain can persist even after the dysfunctions or the disease has been resolved. For example, referred pain from kidney stones to the quadratus lumborum muscle may continue to cause low back pain even after the kidney stones are no longer present. Little is known about the referred pain from muscles to the viscera, although there is an established somatovisceral pathway. A study of injections of an acidic saline solution in the gastrocnemius of a rat caused more distention of the colon and increased muscle activity in the ipsilateral external abdominal oblique muscle (Miranda et al., 2004; Peles et al., 2004); however, it is not known whether such patterns are common. Luz and colleagues (2015) found that lamina I of the spinal cord is the first site in the central nervous system in an animal model at which somatic and visceral pathways converge onto individual projection and local circuit neurons, explaining potential somatovisceral interactions. Abdominal and pelvic TrPs may be secondary to visceral disease or dysfunction through a visceral–somatic convergence pathway; however, myofascial impairments, including myofascial trigger points (TrPs), are also common pain contributors to CPP (Pastore & Katzman 2012) and other types of pelvic floor dysfunction (Doggweiler-Wiygul, 2004).

CLINICAL RELEVANCE OF TRIGGER POINTS IN SYNDROMES RELATED TO THE PELVIS

Myofascial dysfunction is one of the most common contributing factors to pelvic pain (Itza et al., 2010). Patients with visceral pain and cutaneous hyperalgesia in the abdominal wall are likely to present with abdominal TrPs (Giamberardino et al., 1999; Jarrell, 2011). Close to 90% of patients with interstitial cystitis, pelvic pain, and incontinence present with myofascial pain and TrPs (Wesselman, 2001; Fitzgerald & Kotarinos, 2003; Pastore & Katzman, 2012). Jarrell (2011) described abdominal TrPs in patients with endometriosis. TrPs are also a common finding in patients with provoked vestibulodynia, which is another type of a CPP disorder (Hartman & Sarton, 2014). Moldwin and Fariello (2013) found that TrPs are associated with high tone pelvic floor dysfunction. Men with chronic prostatitis and CPP presented with pain in the scrotal, perineal, inguinal, and bladder areas in 54% of cases, and 88% of the cases had myofascial pain (Zermann et al., 2001). TrPs in the puborectalis, pubococcygeus, and rectus abdominus muscles reproduced penile pain 75% of the time, whereas TrPs in the external oblique elicited suprapubic, groin, and testicular pain in 80% of the cases (Anderson et al., 2009). Another study showed that 78.5% of patients with interstitial cystitis had myofascial pain, and 67.9% of those patients had six or more identifiable TrPs (Bassaly et al., 2010). TrPs were most commonly found in the obturator internus, puborectalis, iliococcygeus muscles, and the arcus tendineus. Farrell and colleagues (2016) studied the effects of physical therapy for chronic scrotal content pain and found that manual physical therapy reduced pain levels in 50% of patients with a complete resolution of pain in 13% of the patients. The number of patients taking pain medication reduced from 73.3%

to 44%. Pelvic floor tension and myofascial pain and tenderness are commonly seen with scrotal pain.

Clinical practice guidelines and recent literature support the treatment of TrPs as part of a multidisciplinary approach to treating patients with pelvic floor dysfunction. The European Association of Urology and the Society of Obstetricians and Gynaecologists of Canada recommend that TrPs be considered in the diagnosis of pelvic pain (Jarrell et al., 2005; Fall et al., 2010), which is supported in studies by Jarrell, who demonstrated that abdominal TrPs have a 93% positive predictive value for visceral disease, particularly CPP (Jarrell, 2011; Jarrell et al., 2011). The presence of abdominal TrPs along with abdominal and perineal cutaneous allodynia discriminated visceral from somatic sources of pain (Jarrell et al., 2011). However, of interest is that in spite of the recommendations, obstetrics and gynaecology residency training programs rarely include the examination of the pelvic floor muscles (Bonder et al., 2017). The American Urological Association (2014) lists release of TrPs as a second-line treatment for interstitial cystitis/bladder pain syndrome (IC/BPS), after self-care and patient education (Qaseem et al., 2014), whereas the Canadian Urological Association considers that 'looking for tenderness, spasm/tight bands, and/or trigger points, is important for both diagnosis and treatment recommendations' as part of the mandatory physical examination of patients with IC/BPS (Cox et al., 2016). IC/BPS is defined as 'an unpleasant sensation (pain, pressure, discomfort) perceived to be related to the urinary bladder, associated with lower urinary tract symptoms for more than 6 weeks duration, in the absence of infection or other identifiable causes'.

Fitzgerald and colleagues (2013) utilised TrP treatment in addition to other specific manual therapy techniques to treat women with IC/BPS and compared this approach with generalised massage. Their findings demonstrated greater reduction in pain and urinary urgency in the myofascial group. Other studies demonstrated similar results incorporating TrP release into a comprehensive plan to address pelvic floor dysfunction (Weiss, 2001; Anderson et al., 2009). Goldstein and colleagues (2016) recommend physical therapy treatment to the pelvic floor, including internal muscle treatment, for the treatment of vulvodynia. Several studies have confirmed that physical therapy interventions are useful in the treatment of patients with sexual dysfunction such as erectile dysfunction (Lavoisier et al., 2014; Pelayo-Nieto et al., 2015; Yüksela et al., 2015; Bechara et al., 2016; Rudolph et al., 2017).

Pain in the pelvic girdle may be referred from other muscles in the spine and hip regions. Examination of the patient with pain or other symptoms in the pelvis should include an assessment of the lower thoracic and lumbar segments, the sacroiliac and hip joints, and the pubic region. Careful consideration should be given to muscle, fascia, and nerves in addition to the joints of these regions. Muscle or fascia innervated by the 10th thoracic to the sacral segments can refer pain to the lower abdomen, pubic region, groin, buttocks, and ischial tuberosities (Baker, 1993; Brookhoff & Bennett, 2006; Longbottom, 2009). Treatment of TrPs in the pelvic floor muscles as well as the spine, hips, and lower extremities is an integral part of any physical therapy plan of care to address pelvic pain and dysfunction.

CLINICAL RELEVANCE OF TRIGGER POINTS IN SYNDROMES RELATED TO THE HIP AND THIGH

Several studies have reported that TrPs in hip muscles such as the gluteus medius or piriformis can be involved in patients with low back pain. Teixera and colleagues (2011) identified the presence of active TrPs in the gluteus medius and the quadratus lumborum muscles in 85.7% of patients suffering from postlaminectomy pain syndrome. Iglesias-Gonzalez and colleagues (2013) found that active TrPs in the gluteus medius and piriformis were present in almost 35% of patients with nonspecific low back pain. TrPs in the gluteus muscles have been identified in 76% of patients with lumbar radiculopathy (Adelmanesh et al., 2015), and their presence has been considered a highly specific indicator of radiculopathy with a specificity of 0.91 and a sensitivity of 0.74 (Adelmanesh et al., 2016).

There is a lack of studies investigating the effects of dry needling (DN) in the hip muscles. Rainey (2013) reported a case report study of a patient with low back pain who received DN into the lumbar multifidus and gluteus maximus and gluteus medius muscles with a positive outcome on pain and related disability. Huguenin and colleagues (2005) observed that DN of the gluteal muscles was effective for decreasing symptoms and tightness in athletes with posterior thigh pain; however, no changes in the straight leg raise test were found. Anandkumar (2017) recently described the positive effects of DN of the quadratus femoris muscle in a case report of a patient with posterior thigh pain managed unsuccessfully with other conventional treatments.

Due to the interregional dependence principle, the hip and the knee are clearly interconnected. In fact, several hip muscles can refer pain to the knee. Roach and colleagues (2013) found an increase in the prevalence of TrPs in the gluteus medius and quadratus lumborum muscles in patients with patellofemoral pain. Additionally, the role of TrPs in knee pain syndromes has been recently confirmed. Torres-Chica and colleagues (2015) observed that the referred pain elicited by active TrPs of the knee muscles reproduced symptoms in individuals with postmeniscectomy knee pain. The review of Dor and Kalichman (2017) concluded that there is preliminary evidence suggesting a potential role of TrPs in knee osteoarthritis, but more research is clearly needed. In fact, one study included in this review found that the higher number of active TrPs was associated with higher intensity of ongoing knee pain in a sample of elder people with knee osteoarthritis (Alburquerque-García et al., 2015). This hypothesis is also supported by a case series showing that the combination of TrP DN and therapeutic exercises was effective for improving pain, range of motion, and related disability in patients who had chronic pain after total knee arthroplasty (Núñez-Cortés et al., 2017). Similarly, Mayoral and colleagues (2013), in a double-blind study, reported that a single DN treatment under anaesthesia reduced pain in the first month in patients receiving a total knee arthroplasty for knee osteoarthritis. The randomised clinical trial conducted by Espí-López and colleagues (2017) showed that the inclusion of three sessions of DN into the vastus medialis and lateralis muscles in a manual therapy and exercise program did not result in improved outcomes for pain and disability in individuals with patellofemoral pain at the 3-month follow-up. It is important to consider that only two muscles received the needling intervention, explaining the lack of effects. In fact, a recent randomised, controlled trial observed that application of DN into TrPs on the vastus medialis combined with a rehabilitation protocol was effective for increasing range of motion and function in subacute patients with surgical reconstruction of complete anterior cruciate ligament rupture (Velázquez-Saornil et al., 2017).

Hamstrings injuries also represent a significant problem for the population. Some case reports have observed that the combination of DN with eccentric exercises of the lower extremity was effective for pain and function outcomes for the treatment of hamstring tendinopathy (Jayaseelan et al., 2014) or hamstring strain (Dembowski et al., 2013). However, these results were not replicated in posterior clinical trials. Geist and colleagues (2016) analysed the effects of DN into a sample of asymptomatic individuals with hamstring extensibility deficits and observed that DN did not result in increased extensibility beyond that of stretching alone. It should be noted that the authors did not mention TrPs in the hamstring muscles. (Geist et al., 2016). Similarly, Mason and colleagues (2016) also did not observe any significant effect on hamstring range of motion after application of two session of DN compared with sham needling in a young active population with nontraumatic knee pain.

DRY NEEDLING OF THE ABDOMINAL, HIP, PELVIS, AND THIGH MUSCLES

Some of the muscles on the hip and pelvis are covered in other chapters. The abdominal muscles are discussed in Chapter 10. The referred pain patterns are mostly based on the descriptions by Simons and colleagues (1999), with substitutions and additions by Dalmau-Carola (2005) and Longbottom (2009).

Hip Muscles

Gluteus maximus muscle

- *Anatomy:* The gluteus maximus muscle originates at the posterior aspect of the ilium, the lower part of the sacrum and coccyx inferior and lateral across the greater trochanter to the iliotibial band of the tensor fascia lata and the gluteal tuberosity. Of importance is that there are extensive connections between the gluteus maximus muscle, the latissimus dorsi muscle, and the thoracolumbar fascia (Carvalhais et al., 2013). Lieberman and colleagues (2006) found that more cranial fibres of the muscle terminate in a thick laminar tendon, which inserts into the iliotibial band. Recent research confirms that the iliotibial band is, in fact, a reinforcement of the fascia lata (Fairclough et al., 2006; Stecco et al., 2008) and, as such, can be viewed as a tendon of insertion of the gluteus maximus muscle, which may explain the

functional force relationship between the thoracolumbar fascia and the knee (Stecco et al., 2013).
- *Function:* The gluteus maximus muscle is a hip extensor, lateral rotator and contributes to stabilisation of the iliotibial tract.
- *Innervation:* Inferior gluteal nerve from L5, S1, and S2.
- *Referred pain:* Pain referral is along the inferior or inferior-lateral aspect of the sacrum, the gluteal fold, or insertion along the iliotibial tract. TrPs in the gluteus maximus muscle can imitate sacroiliac pain.
- *Needling technique:* Position the patient in the side-lying with the affected side up and a pillow placed between the knees. The muscle is needled with flat palpation towards the TrP (Fig. 11.1). Strong depression of the subcutaneous tissue is required to reduce the distance from the skin to the muscle.
- *Precautions:* Avoid needling the sciatic nerve. The depth of penetration is dependent on the amount of adipose tissue.

Gluteus medius muscle

- *Anatomy:* The gluteus medius muscle is found between the gluteus maximus and the tensor fascia latae. It originates between the posterior and anterior gluteal lines of the ilium and inserts with two distinct and consistent insertions onto the lateral border of the greater trochanter (Robertson et al., 2008). A bursa lies under the tendinous portion over the surface of the trochanter. In the region of overlap between the gluteus medius and gluteus minimus muscles, the individual muscles cannot be identified with palpation.
- *Function:* The gluteus medius muscle is the main hip abductor and medial rotator. Insufficiency of the gluteus medius muscle results in a positive

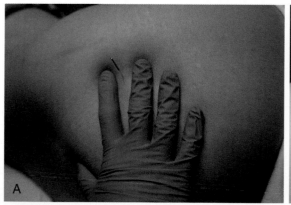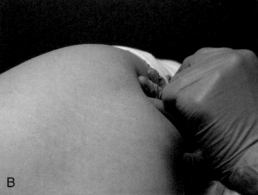

FIG. 11.1 Dry needling of trigger points in the gluteus maximus muscle: A. upper fibres; B. lower fibres.

Trendelenburg test. Commonly, the gluteus medius muscle becomes insufficient when active TrPs are present in the quadratus lumborum muscle. The gluteus medius muscle activation patterns may be useful in identifying patients at risk for developing low back pain (Nelson-Wong et al., 2008).

- *Innervation:* Superior gluteal nerve from L4, L5, and S1.
- *Referred pain:* TrPs may be found throughout the entire muscle with referral to the sacroiliac joint, gluteal and lumbosacral regions, and along the iliotibial band, gluteal region, posterior thigh, and posterior lower leg. It is not possible to separate the referred pain patterns from the gluteus minimus muscle in the area where the two muscles overlap.
- *Needling technique:* The patient is in the sidelying position with a pillow between the knees. The muscle is needled with flat palpation along the contour of the iliac crest towards the TrP. Strong depression of the subcutaneous tissue is required to reduce the distance from the skin to the muscle. Needle contact at the periosteum of the ilium is common (Fig. 11.2).
- *Precautions:* There are deep branches of the superior gluteal vessels and nerve between the gluteus medius and minimus muscles, but these cannot be always be avoided. The depth of penetration is dependent on the amount of adipose tissue.

Gluteus minimus muscle

- *Anatomy:* The gluteus minimus muscle is found deep to the gluteus medius muscle. It originates between the anterior and inferior gluteal lines of the anterior aspect of the ilium and inserts on the anterior aspect of the greater trochanter. It also has a bursa between the tendon and the insertion at the greater trochanter.
- *Function:* The gluteus minimus muscle is a hip abductor and medial rotator. Insufficiency of this muscle along with the gluteus medius results in a positive Trendelenburg test. The muscle supports the body in single leg stance with the tensor fascia latae.
- *Innervation:* Superior gluteal nerve from L4, L5, and S1.
- *Referred pain:* Referred pain from the gluteus minimus muscle is into the iliotibial band, gluteal region, posterior thigh, and posterior one-third of the lower leg. It is not possible to separate referred pain patterns from the gluteus medius muscle in the area where the two muscles overlap.
- *Needling technique:* The patient is in the sidelying position with a pillow between the knees. The muscle is needled with flat palpation along the contour of the iliac crest towards the TrP. Strong depression of the subcutaneous tissue is required to reduce the distance from the skin to the muscle. Needle contact at the periosteum is common (Fig. 11.3).
- *Precautions:* There are deep branches of the superior gluteal vessels and nerve between the gluteus medius and minimus muscles, but these cannot be always be avoided. The depth of penetration is dependent on the amount of adipose tissue.

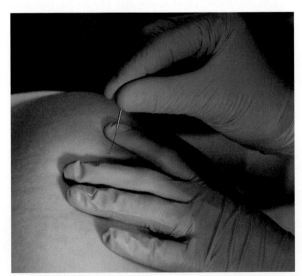

FIG. 11.2 Dry needling of trigger points in the gluteus medius muscle.

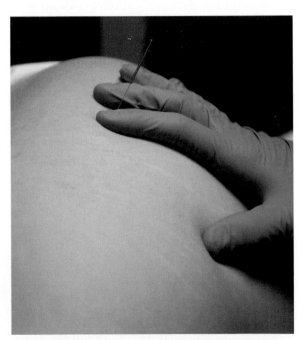

FIG. 11.3 Dry needling of trigger points in the gluteus minimus muscle.

Tensor fascia latae muscle

- *Anatomy:* The tensor fascia latae muscle originates from the anterior outer aspect of the iliac crest and the anterior superior iliac spine (ASIS), between the gluteus medius and sartorius, and from the deep surface of the fascia latae. It inserts between the two layers of the iliotibial band of the fascia latae of the middle and upper thirds of the thigh.
- *Function:* Via the iliotibial band, the tensor fascia latae muscle contributes to knee extension, lateral rotation of the leg, knee flexion, hip abduction, and medial hip rotation. Its main functions are pelvic stabilisation and posture control.
- *Innervation:* Superior gluteal nerve from L4, L5, and S1.
- *Referred pain:* The referred pain from the tensor fascia latae muscle travels along the iliotibial band, gluteal region, and posterior lateral thigh.
- *Needling technique:* The patient is supine or in the sidelying position with a pillow between the knees. The muscle is needled with flat palpation towards the TrP (Fig. 11.4).
- *Precautions:* None

Iliacus muscle

- *Anatomy:* The iliacus muscle originates from the upper two-thirds of the inner surface of the iliac fossa, inner lip of the iliac crest, the iliolumbar and ventral sacroiliac ligaments, and the upper surface of the lateral portion of the sacrum. It comes forward as far as the anterior superior and anterior inferior iliac spines. Many of the fibres of the iliacus muscle join the psoas major tendon, and together they insert into the lesser trochanter of the femur. Some fibres also attach to the femur and in front of the trochanter.

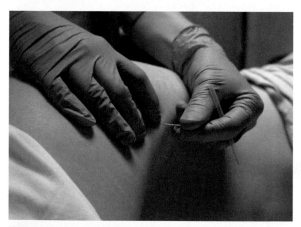

FIG. 11.4 Dry needling of trigger points in the tensor fascia latae muscle.

The muscle also receives some fibres from the upper portion of the hip joint capsule (Standring, 2015). Anatomical variations have been reported for the iliacus muscle. Jelev and colleagues (2005) as well as D'Costa and associates (2008) reported the presence of an accessory iliacus muscle, covered by a separate fascia, which attached at the middle third of the iliac crest and inserted on the lesser trochanter with the iliopsoas tendon. Rao and colleagues (2008) reported another variation of the iliacus muscle: two defined variant muscles, an iliacus minimus and an accessory slip of the iliacus muscle, were identified on one side; on the contralateral side, an additional single slip of the iliacus muscle fused with the iliopsoas tendon distally. Fabrizio (2011) reported a variation that originated from the superior–lateral aspect of the iliac fascia and travelled nearly horizontally to insert into the psoas major muscle, forming a blended iliacus–psoas muscle. Another variation, reported by Aleksandrova and colleagues (2013), described slips missing from the middle and anterior parts of the muscle (due to not developing). The posterior portion of the muscle started unusually high from the iliolumbar ligament. There are also reported variations of the iliopsoas tendon at the level of the hip joint. Philippon and colleagues (2014) examined 52 cadavers and found that in only 28% of the specimens were the tendons single banded. Sixty-four percent of the specimens featured double banded tendons, and 7.5% were triple banded.

- *Function:* One of the primary functions of the muscle is flexion of the hip. When acting from below and contracting bilaterally, the iliacus muscles and the psoas major muscle are able to bend the trunk and pelvis forward against resistance, as when performing a sit-up (Standring, 2015).
- *Innervation:* Branches from the femoral nerve in the pelvic region (L2-L3). The accessory iliacus muscle is innervated by the L4 root of the femoral nerve when present (D'Costa et al., 2008).
- *Referred pain:* The iliacus muscle refers pain to the sacroiliac region and may continue to include the sacrum and proximal medial buttock. It frequently includes the pelvic floor, groin, and upper anteromedial aspect of the thigh on the same side and should be considered with all pelvic floor pain and dysfunction. The attachment of the iliopsoas muscle (mostly iliacus fibres) on the lesser trochanter of the femur may refer pain both to the back and anteriorly to the thigh. Pain referral to the medial knee has been reported in the literature (Cummings, 2003) and frequently observed in clinical practice.

- *Needling technique:* The iliacus muscle should be approached from below the iliac crest with the patient in the sidelying position. Wrap the fingers of the nonneedling hand around the iliac crest and 'hook on' to the bone. Insert the needle approximately 5 mm from the bone into the abdominal external oblique muscle. Direct the needle towards the ilium and stay close to the inner surface of the ilium to avoid penetrating the abdominal contents. This approach may not be possible in obese individuals (Fig. 11.5).
- *Precautions:* To avoid penetration of the peritoneum, direct the needle towards the inside surface of the ilium.

Obturator internus muscle

- *Anatomy:* The obturator internus muscle has a broad attachment to the anterior lateral wall of the inner pelvic brim, the rim of the obturator foramen, and the obturator membrane, covering most of the obturator foramen. The pelvic surface of the obturator internus and its fascia form the anterior lateral wall of the true pelvis. The muscle exits the pelvis through the lesser sciatic foramen, then makes a right angle turn, posterior to the hip joint capsule, attaching to the anterior medial surface of the greater trochanter in close proximity to the gemelli muscles.
- *Function:* The primary function of the obturator internus muscle is commonly described as lateral or external rotation of the hip joint when the thigh is extended and hip abduction when the hip is flexed to 90 degrees (Travell & Simons, 1992). However, a recent study showed that the muscle consistently showed increased electromyographic activity with hip extension first, followed by external rotation and abduction (Hodges et al., 2014).
- *Innervation:* The muscle is supplied by the nerve to the obturator internus from L5 and S1.
- *Referred pain:* The obturator internus muscle refers pain to the vagina, anococcygeal region, and the posterior thigh. The patient may also have a perception of fullness in the rectum.
- *Needling technique:* The patient is positioned in sidelying on the involved side with hip and knee flexion and a pillow between the knees. Palpate the muscle along the ischial tuberosity. Place the fingers medially around the bony prominence and then angle the needle perpendicular to the muscle surface with a slight anterior superior angle directly into the TrP (Fig. 11.6). An alternate approach is to palpate the TrP along the internal portion of the obturator internus muscle through intrarectal palpation and angle the needle towards the palpating finger (Fig. 11.7). The external portion of the muscle may be needled medial to the greater trochanter with the other hip lateral rotators.
- *Precautions:* Avoid needling towards the pudendal or Alcock canal containing the pudendal and obturator nerve and vessels.

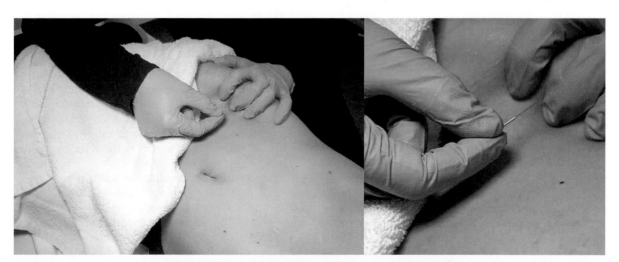

FIG. 11.5 Dry needling of trigger points in the iliacus muscle.

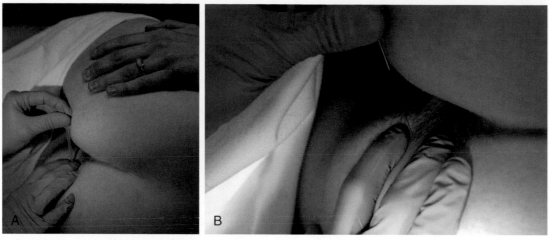

FIG. 11.6 Dry needling of trigger points in the obturator internus muscle.

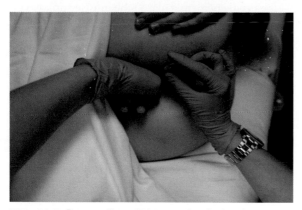

FIG. 11.7 Dry needling of trigger points in the obturator internus muscle with intrarectal palpation.

Obturator externus/gemellus inferior and superior muscles

- *Anatomy:* The obturator externus muscle is a flat triangular muscle that covers the external surface of the obturator membrane and adjacent bone of the ischial and pubic rami laterally and upward to the trochanteric fossa of the femur. The superior gemellus muscle originates at the spine of the ischium and inferior from the ischial tuberosity. Collectively they insert into the medial surface of the greater trochanter of the femur. Functionally, the gemelli muscles can be considered to be part of the obturator internus muscle, and these muscles may actually be fused together (Honma et al., 1998) (Fig. 11.8).
- *Function:* The obturator externus muscle is often described as an external rotator of the hip along

with the gemelli muscles, obturator internus, and quadratus femoris muscles; however, a recent biomechanical study showed that the obturator externus muscle is a primary flexor and adductor of the extended hip (Vaarbakken et al., 2015). It is actually not clear to what degree the obturator externus muscles contribute to external rotation and stability of the hip.

- *Innervation:* The obturator externus muscle is innervated by the posterior branch of the obturator nerve from L3-L4, the gemellus superior muscle by branches of the obturator internus nerve form L5-S2, and the gemellus inferior muscle by branches of the quadratus femoris nerve from L4-S1.
- *Referred pain:* Referred pain patterns from this muscle are not described in detail but are generally thought to include the proximal posterior thigh, hip, and groin and a sciatic-type referral pattern.
- *Needling technique:* The patient is positioned in the sidelying position with the involved side up and a pillow between the knees. Palpate the muscle just medial to the greater trochanter. Insert the needle perpendicular to the muscle surface directly towards the TrP. The obturator externus muscle is found deeper and more posterior to the trochanter (Fig. 11.9).
- *Precautions:* Avoid needling the sciatic nerve.

Quadratus femoris muscle

- *Anatomy:* The quadratus femoris muscle is a flat quadrilateral muscle that originates at the upper part of the external aspect of the ischial tuberosity

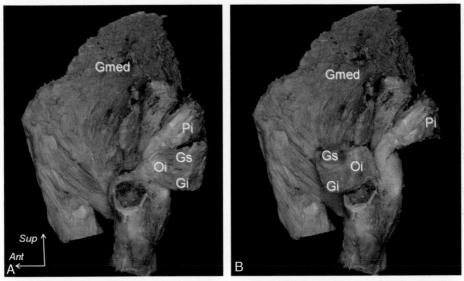

FIG. 11.8 Anatomy of the hip external rotators. (Used with permission from: Tamaki et al. (2004). An Anatomic Study of the Impressions on the greater trochanter: bony geometry indicates the alignment of the short external rotator muscles. *The Journal of Arthroplasty* 29, 2473–2477.)

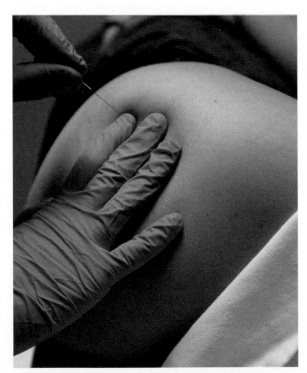

FIG. 11.9 Dry needling of trigger points in the obturator externus/gemelli muscles.

and inserts above the middle of the trochanteric crest of the femur.

- *Function:* As is the case with the obturator externus and gemelli muscles, the quadratus femoris muscle is generally considered to be an external rotator of the hip. However, a recent biomechanical study showed that the quadratus femoris muscle is primarily an extensor of the flexed hip (Vaarbakken et al., 2015). During the late swing phase in running, the quadratus femoris muscle plays a synergistic role with other posterior thigh muscles to control deceleration of the lower extremity (Semciw et al., 2015).
- *Innervation:* Branches from the quadratus femoris nerve from L5 and S1.
- *Referred pain:* Referred pain patterns from this muscle are not described in detail but are generally thought to include the proximal posterior thigh, hip, and groin, along with a sciatic-type referral pattern.
- *Needling technique:* The patient is positioned comfortably in the prone or sidelying position. Palpate the greater trochanter and the ischial tuberosity. The needle can be inserted perpendicular to the muscle surface at the trochanter Dry needling of trigger points or just medial to the ischial tuberosity running parallel to the sciatic nerve directly towards the TrP (Fig. 11.10).
- *Precautions:* Avoid needling the sciatic nerve.

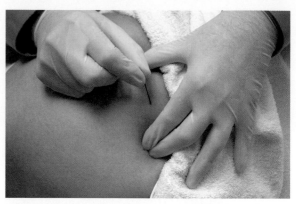

FIG. 11.11 Dry needling of trigger points in the piriformis muscle.

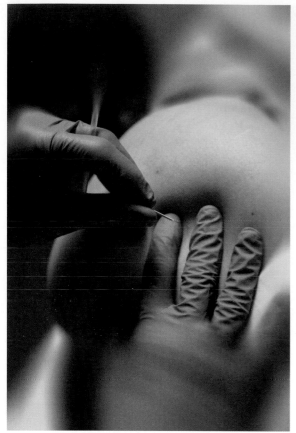

FIG. 11.10 Dry needling of trigger points in the quadratus femoris muscle.

Piriformis muscle

- *Anatomy:* This piriformis muscle originates at the anterior surface of the sacrum at S2-S4, where it passes through and fills the greater sciatic foramen. It inserts on the upper border of the greater trochanter of the femur. The piriformis muscle and the gemellus superior form a canal through which the sciatic nerve travels. A recent study showed that, in 90 out of 102 limbs (89%), the fibular portion of the sciatic nerve passed completely under the piriformis muscle, whereas in 8.8%, the nerve went through the muscle. In the remaining 2.9%, the nerve was in between the piriformis muscle and the gluteus maximus muscle (Lewis et al., 2016). Fibres of the piriformis muscle attach directly to the sacrotuberous ligament (Vleeming et al., 1989).
- *Function:* The piriformis muscle is an external or lateral rotator but also contributes to hip extension and abduction. The muscle functions as an internal or medial rotator when the hip is flexed more than 90 degrees (Michel et al., 2013).

- *Innervation:* The piriformis muscle is innervated by branches from L5, S1, and S2.
- *Referred pain:* Referred pain travels along the path of the sciatic nerve and may include the sacroiliac region, the proximal two-thirds of the thigh, and the inguinal and intrapelvic cavity.
- *Needling technique:* The patient is positioned comfortably in prone or in the sidelying position. Identify the bony landmarks of the greater trochanter and the sacrum at S2-S4. The needle can be inserted perpendicular to the muscle surface in between the sacrum and the greater trochanter. In the region of the sciatic nerve, initially the needle should be advanced slowly to avoid hitting the nerve (Fig. 11.11).
- *Precautions:* Avoid needling the sciatic nerve.

Pelvic Diaphragm Muscles
Ischiocavernosus muscle
- *Anatomy:* The ischiocavernosus muscle is an elongated muscle arising from the inferior lateral aponeurosis over the crus of the penis or clitoris to the medial aspect of the pubic ramus and ischium. The muscle is smaller in the female than the male.
- *Function:* Compression of veins to maintain penile or clitoral erection (Lavoisier et al., 2014; Cohen et al., 2016). Together with the bulbospongiosus muscle, the ischiocavernosus muscle contracts during vaginal distension, which enhances both the clitoris and penile erection during the sexual act (Shafik, 1993). Histochemically, the ischiocavernosus and bulbospongiosus muscles share similarities with striated sphincter muscles (Ravnik & Širca, 1993).
- *Innervation:* Perineal branch of the pudendal nerve S2, S3, and S4.

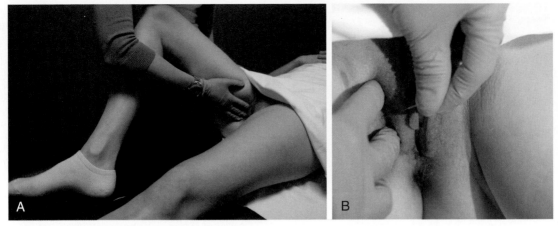

FIG. 11.12 Dry needling of trigger points in the ischiocavernosus muscle (female).

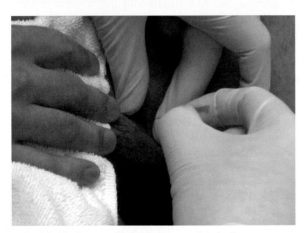

FIG. 11.13 Dry needling of trigger points in the ischiocavernosus muscle (male).

- *Referred pain:* Perineum and the adjacent urogenital region.
- *Needling technique:* In female patients, palpate the TrP via intravaginal palpation in the lithotomy position. Angle the needle perpendicular to the muscle surface, directing it towards the ischiopubic ramus directly into the TrP. In female patients, move the labia to the opposite side you are treating (Fig. 11.12). In male patients, it is helpful to use a towel around the scrotum and have the patient move the scrotum out of the way (Fig. 11.13).
- *Precautions:* Avoid needling the perineal branch of the pudendal nerve, artery, and vein and the perineal branch of the posterior femoral cutaneous nerve.

Bulbospongiosus (bulbocavernosus) muscle

- *Anatomy:* The bulbospongiosus muscle originates at the superficial perineal membrane and dorsal penile or clitoral aponeurosis and attaches at the perineal body in women and at the median raphe over the corpus spongiosum extending one-third of the base of the penis in men. It is a very thin and superficial muscle. Frequently, the bulbospongiosus muscle is connected to the ischiocavernosus muscle anteriorly through a muscle-like or connective tissue-like connection. Dorsally, the muscle is connected to the external anal sphincter (Peikert et al., 2015). The basal electromyographic activity of the bulbospongiosus muscle is elevated in women with vaginismus (Shakif & El-Sibai, 2002).
- *Function:* The bulbospongiosus muscle increases vascular engorgement of the penis or clitoris. In the female, it constricts the vaginal introitus. In the male it assists with emptying urine and ejaculate from the urethra (Cohen et al., 2016).
- *Innervation:* The bulbospongiosus muscle is innervated by the perineal branch of the pudendal nerve from the S2-S4 roots.
- *Referred pain:* The bulbospongiosus muscle refers pain to the perineum and adjacent urogenital structures. Symptoms in the female include dyspareunia; symptoms in the male include pain at the base of the penis, beneath the scrotum, pain with sitting, and difficulty maintaining an erection.
- *Needling technique:* In female patients palpate the TrP via intravaginal palpation in the lithotomy position. Maintain palpation via pincer grasp and angle the needle perpendicular to the muscle surface directly into the TrP (Fig. 11.14). Muscle contraction can

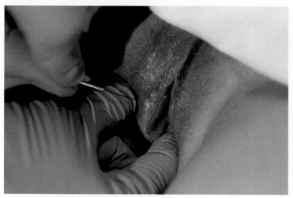

FIG. 11.14 Dry needling of trigger points in the bulbospongiosus muscle.

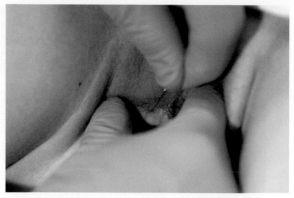

FIG. 11.15 Dry needling of trigger points in the transverse perinei muscles.

confirm placement. For male and female patients the muscle can be treated in a slightly tangential angle, which in women may be preferred in cases of hypersensitivity or when patients do not consent to vaginal insertion. In male patients, it is helpful to use a towel around the scrotum and have the patient move the scrotum out of the way (see Fig. 11.13). In female patients, move the labia to the opposite side you are treating.

- *Precautions:* This muscle is very thin and superficial. It is not recommended to needle the muscle at the base of the penis secondary to the close proximity of the urethra. The perineal artery and vein are located between the superficial and deep transverse perineal muscles and run superiorly.

Superficial and deep transverse perinei muscles

- *Anatomy:* The transverse perinei muscles are part of the external genital muscles and originate from the ischium at the inferior ramus and run medially to the lateral aspect of the vagina or the median line in the male. The superficial transverse perinei is a narrower muscle, which in women blends with the fibres of the external sphincter ani inferiorly and the bulbospongiosus superiorly at the central tendon of the perineal body. In men Stoker (2009) described the presence of a cleavage between the perineal body and the external sphincter. In females the superficial transverse perineal muscle lies directly superior to the external sphincter, whereas in men the muscle lies anterior to the external sphincter. The sphincter urethra in both the male and female lie in the same plane as the transverse perinei near the urethra.
- *Function:* The transverse perinei muscles fix and stabilise the central tendon of the perineal body.

- *Innervation:* Perineal branch of the pudendal nerve via S2-S4 roots.
- *Referred pain:* To the perineum and adjacent urogenital structures. In some cases rectal or coccygeal pain is observed.
- *Needling technique:* In female patients palpate the TrP via intravaginal palpation in the lithotomy position. Angle the needle perpendicular to the muscle surface directly into the TrP in the direction of the palpating finger. As an alternate technique, needle into the muscle with the needle angled towards the ischial tuberosity. In male patients it is helpful to use a towel around the scrotum and have the patient move the scrotum out of the way. In female patients move the labia to the opposite side you are treating (Fig. 11.15).
- *Precautions:* This muscle is very thin and superficial. It is not recommended to needle the muscle at the base of the penis secondary to the close proximity of the urethra. The perineal artery and vein are located between the superficial and deep transverse perineal muscles and run superiorly. Other structures to note are: the deep dorsal vein of the clitoris; a portion of the urethra and the constrictor urethra muscle; the larger vestibular glands and their ducts; the internal pudendal vessels and the dorsal nerves of the clitoris; the arteries and nerves of the bulbi vestibuli; and a plexus of veins.

Pubococcygeus muscle of the pelvic diaphragm

- *Anatomy:* The pubococcygeus muscle originates at the back of the pubis and the anterior part of the obturator fascia. Its direction is posterior in a horizontal fashion to the coccyx and to the most inferior aspect of the sacrum. At the posterior insertion the two pubococcygei muscles come together and form a thick, fibromuscular layer. The puborectalis muscle slings around the rectum to aid in defecation. The pubovaginalis muscle in the female arises for the anterior fibres to the perineal body to aid in vaginal wall support. The levator prostate muscle is the corresponding muscle in the male.

- *Function:* Collectively the pelvic diaphragm muscles constrict and elevate the lower end of the rectum and vagina and support the pelvic viscera. They also aid in forced expiration and spinal stability. The coccygei muscles pull forward and support the coccyx after it has been pressed backward during defecation or parturition.
- *Innervation:* The pubococcygeus muscle is innervated by a branch from the fourth sacral nerve and a branch from the perineal or inferior rectal portion of the pudendal nerve.
- *Referred pain:* Frequently called levator ani syndrome, pain from this region can refer to the any of the areas of the perineum (coccygeal, vaginal, and rectal) or pelvic girdle. Pain with sitting or with bowel movements is common.
- *Needling technique:* The patient should be sidelying on the involved side with the hips flexed to 90 degrees and a pillow between the knees. Ask the patient to lift the gluteal muscles away from the anus. Identify the TrP through intrarectal palpation. Maintain pressure on the TrP with the palpating finger when inserting the needle in the region between the anal sphincter and perineal body, angled towards the palpating finger. The technique is similar to needling the obturator internus with rectal palpation (see Fig. 11.7).
- *Precautions:* Consider the rectum, anus, and anal sphincters.

Iliococcygeus muscle of the pelvic diaphragm

- *Anatomy:* The iliococcygeus muscle originates from the ischial spine and the posterior part of the tendinous arch of the pelvic fascia and inserts into the last two segments of the coccyx and anococcygeal raphe. It is usually thin or may consist largely of fibrous tissue. The iliosacral muscle is an accessory portion at its posterior part.
- *Function:* Collectively the pelvic diaphragm muscles constrict and elevate the lower end of the rectum and vagina and support the pelvic viscera. These muscles also aid in forced expiration and spinal stability.
- *Innervation:* The iliococcygeus muscle is innervated by a branch from the fourth sacral nerve and a branch

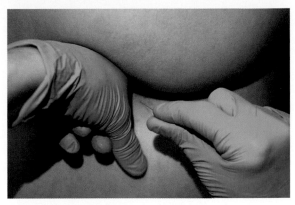

FIG. 11.16 Dry needling of trigger points in the iliococcygeus muscle.

from the perineal or inferior rectal portion of the pudendal nerve.

- *Referred pain and symptoms:* Frequently called levator ani syndrome, pain from this region can refer to the any of the areas of the perineum (coccygeal, vaginal, and rectal) or pelvic girdle. Pain with sitting or with bowel movements is common.
- *Needling technique:* The patient should be sidelying on the involved side with the hips flexed to 90 degrees and a pillow between the knees. Ask the patient to lift the gluteal muscles away from the anus. Identify the TrP through intrarectal palpation. Maintain pressure on the TrP with the palpating finger when inserting the needle in the region between the anal sphincter and perineal body, angled towards the palpating finger (Fig. 11.16). The technique is similar to needling the obturator internus with rectal palpation.
- *Precautions:* Consider the rectum, anus, and anal sphincters.

Coccygeus muscle of the pelvic diaphragm

- *Anatomy:* The coccygeus muscle is a triangular shape muscle that originates from the spine of the ischium and sacrospinous ligament and inserts into the margin of the coccyx and the inferior lateral angle of the sacrum.
- *Function:* Collectively the pelvic diaphragm muscles constrict and elevate the lower end of the rectum and vagina and support the pelvic viscera. These muscles also aid in forced expiration and spinal stability. The coccygei muscles specifically pull the coccyx forward after defecation or parturition and aid in sacroiliac stability.
- *Innervation:* The coccygeus muscle is innervated by a branch from the fourth and fifth sacral nerves.

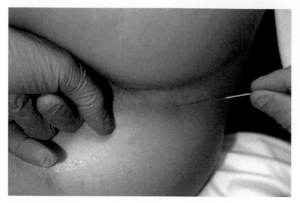

FIG. 11.17 Dry needling of trigger points in the coccygeus muscle.

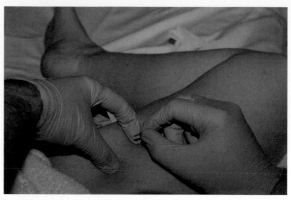

FIG. 11.18 Dry needling of trigger points in the adductor longus muscle.

- *Referred pain:* Coccygeal, hip, sacroiliac, or low back pain.
- *Needling technique:* The patient should be sidely-ing on the involved side with the hips flexed to 90 degrees and a pillow between the knees. Ask the patient to lift the gluteal muscles away from the anus. Identify the TrP through intrarectal pal-pation. Maintain pressure on the TrP with the pal-pating finger when inserting the needle just lateral to the coccyx, angled towards the palpating finger (Fig. 11.17).
- *Precautions:* Consider the rectum, anus, and anal sphincters.

Thigh Muscles
Adductor longus muscle
- *Anatomy:* The adductor longus muscle is a large, fan-shaped muscle that originates from the front of the pubic bone between the crest and symphysis and inserts in the linea aspera in the middle one-third of the femur. Of interest is that the adductor longus muscle and the rectus abdominis muscle are con-nected to each other via a common fascial sheath or aponeurosis with attachments to the capsule of the symphysis pubis and the fibrocartilaginous disk (Pesquera et al., 2015). Superficial fibres of the ad-ductor longus muscle can intersect with fibres of the oblique aponeurosis of the contralateral external oblique muscle (Pesquera et al., 2015).
- *Function:* The adductor longus muscle is active in ad-duction and medial rotation of the thigh and flex-ion with an extended hip. To test the muscle with the adductor squeeze test, a test position with 45 de-grees of hip flexion is optimal for eliciting adductor muscle activity (Delahunt et al., 2011). Hyperalgesia of the adductor longus muscle is commonly seen in

athletes with groin pain (Nevin & Delahunt, 2014; Drew et al., 2016; Hölmich, 2017).
- *Innervation:* The adductor longus muscle is inner-vated by the anterior division of the obturator nerve from L2-L4.
- *Referred pain:* Referred pain not only extends from the femoral triangle to the knee, but also gives rise to intrapelvic pain (Travell & Simons, 1992; Longbottom, 2009).
- *Needling technique:* The patient is supine with slight knee flexion and hip external rotation and the knee supported by a pillow. Secure the taut band via a pincer grip with the TrP between the index finger and the thumb or between the middle finger and the thumb with the so-called 'OK sign' pincer palpation. The needle is inserted perpendicular to the skin in between the index and middle finger (pincer) or be-tween the thumb and index finger (OK sign) and directed towards the TrP and the underlying thumb or middle finger (Fig. 11.18).
- *Precautions:* Avoid the femoral nerve, artery, and vein, and the sciatic nerve.

Adductor brevis muscle
- *Anatomy:* The muscle originates posterior to the pec-tineus and adductor longus with a narrow attach-ment of the external aspect of the body and inferior ramus of the pubis between the gracilis and obturator externus. It inserts posterior laterally into the femur from the lesser trochanter to the linea aspera and di-rectly behind the brevis and upper part of the longus.
- *Function:* Adduction and medial rotation of the thigh as well as hip flexion with an extended hip.
- *Innervation:* Obturator nerve from L2 and L3.
- *Referred pain:* Referred pain may include the area from the femoral triangle to the knee.

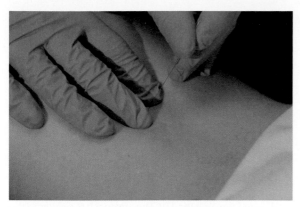

FIG. 11.19 Dry needling of trigger points in the adductor brevis muscle.

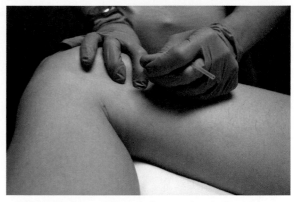

FIG. 11.20 Dry needling of trigger points in the adductor magnus muscle.

- *Needling technique:* The patient is supine with knee flexion and hip external rotation and the knee supported by a pillow. The TrP is identified via flat palpation through or in between the adductor longus and pectineus muscles and medial to the femoral neurovascular bundle. The needle is inserted perpendicular to the skin and directed towards the TrP (Fig. 11.19).
- *Precautions:* Avoid the femoral nerve, artery, and vein, and the sciatic nerve.

Adductor magnus muscle

- *Anatomy:* The adductor magnus muscle is a large, fan-shaped muscle originating from the inferior ramus of the pubis, the conjoined ischial ramus, and the inferior–lateral aspect of the ischial tuberosity. It inserts with horizontal, oblique, and vertical fibres at the gluteal tuberosity and linea aspera deep to the brevis and longus. Goel and colleagues (2015) described the presence of an adductor accessory in between the adductor brevis and the proximal part of adductor magnus.
- *Function:* The functions of the adductor magnus muscle include adduction and internal rotation of the thigh, hip flexion with an extended hip, and possibly even extension of the hip (Benn et al., 2017).
- *Innervation:* The posterior branch of the obturator nerve and the tibial division of the sciatic nerve from L2-L4.
- *Referred pain:* Travell and Simons (1992) described referring pain from the adductor magnus muscle along the anterior medial thigh, but also observed rectal, vaginal, and urethral referred pain. Empirically, the muscle seems to refer pain throughout the medial aspect of the thigh and leg.
- *Needling technique:* The patient is supine with knee flexion and hip external rotation or in the sidelying

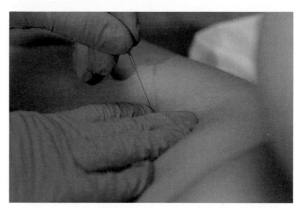

FIG. 11.21 Dry needling of trigger points in the adductor magnus muscle (sidelying).

position. The TrP is identified via flat palpation through or in between the adductor longus and pectineus muscles and medial to the femoral neurovascular bundle. The needle is inserted perpendicular to the skin and directed towards the TrP (Figs. 11.20 and 11.21).
- *Precautions:* Avoid the femoral nerve, artery, and vein along the adductor canal, the sciatic nerve, and, in the most distal portion of the muscle, the saphenous nerve in between the adductor magnus muscle and the vastus medialis muscle and the tendons of the sartorius and gracilis muscles.

Pectineus muscle

- *Anatomy:* The pectineus muscle is a flat quadrangular that originates at the pectin pubis and the pubic bone between the iliopectineal eminence and the tubercle and attaches at the lesser trochanter.
- *Function:* The pectineus muscle contributes to adduction and flexion of the thigh.

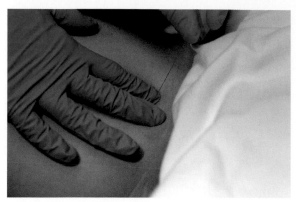

FIG. 11.22 Dry needling of trigger points in the pectineus muscle.

- *Innervation:* The pectineus muscle is innervated by the anterior division of the femoral nerve from L2-L3 and the accessory obturator nerve from L3 when present.
- *Referred pain:* The referred pain pattern involves the anterior medial aspect of the thigh, pubis, lumbopelvic region, and hip and is frequently referred to as athletic pubalgia.
- *Needling technique:* The patient is supine with slight hip external rotation. Locate the femoral artery. The TrP is identified via flat palpation medial to the femoral neurovascular bundle. The needle is inserted perpendicular to the skin and directed towards the TrP (Fig. 11.22).
- *Precautions:* On the lateral aspect of the muscle, avoid needling the femoral nerve, artery, and vein. Medially, there is a slight possibility of reaching the obturator nerve, which lies deep under the muscle just lateral of tendon of the adductor longus muscle.

Gracilis muscle

- *Anatomy:* The gracilis muscle originates from the medial margins of the lower half of the body of the pubis, the inferior pubic ramus, and the ischial ramus and inserts to the upper part of the medial tibia just below the medial condyle. The gracilis muscle is a thin and flat muscle The muscle is often used for gracilis flap reconstruction for a wide variety of indications, ranging from a rectovaginal fistula (Kaoutzanis et al., 2013) to anterior cruciate ligament reconstruction (Häner et al., 2016) and breast reconstruction (Bodin et al., 2015), which may be an indication that the muscle does not have any major functions in the lower extremity.

- *Function:* The functions of the gracilis muscle include flexion and internal rotation of the leg and adduction of the thigh.
- *Innervation:* The gracilis muscle is innervated by the obturator nerve (L2-L3).
- *Referred pain:* TrPs in the gracilis muscle can cause a superficial stinging pain along the inside of the thigh.
- *Needling technique:* The patient is supine with knee flexion and hip external rotation or in the sidelying position. The TrP is identified via flat palpation through or in between the adductor longus and pectineus muscles and medial to the femoral neurovascular bundle. The needle is inserted perpendicular to the skin and directed towards the TrP. The approach is similar to the approach of the adductor magnus muscle.
- *Precautions:* When needling the most distal portion of the muscle, be aware of the saphenous nerve between the tendons of the sartorius and gracilis muscles.

Rectus femoris muscle

- *Anatomy:* The rectus femoris muscle is a fusiform muscle that originates from the anterior inferior iliac spine, from a groove about the acetabulum, and from the capsule of the hip joint. The muscle inserts at the base of the patella via a thick flat tendon. The patellar tendon is a continuation of the main tendon and connects the muscle to the tuberosity of the tibia.
- *Function:* The primary function is knee extension. It also assists with hip flexion. The rectus femoris can perform these two functions simultaneously. The muscle is often described to be active during the swing-to-stance transition (Nene et al., 1999); however, more recent studies showed that the muscle is primarily active during the stance-to-swing transition (Nene et al., 2004).
- *Innervation:* The rectus femoris muscle is innervated by the femoral nerve (L2-L4). The proximal and distal sections of the muscle receive innervation from two different branches of the femoral nerve (Sung et al., 2003).
- *Referred pain:* Anterior thigh and knee pain.
- *Needling technique:* With the patient in the supine position, the TrP is identified via flat palpation. The needle is inserted perpendicular to the skin and directed towards the TrP (Fig. 11.23). It is easy to needle through the rectus femoris muscle into the vastus intermedius muscle.
- *Precautions:* The lateral circumflex femoral artery lies deep underneath the muscle, but in clinical practice, the artery is not a major concern.

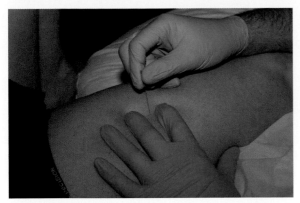

FIG. 11.23 Dry needling of trigger points in the rectus femoris muscle.

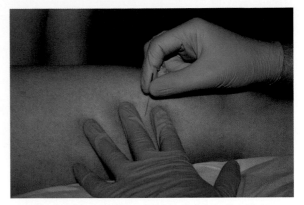

FIG. 11.24 Dry needling of trigger points in the vastus lateralis muscle.

Vastus lateralis muscle

- *Anatomy:* The vastus lateralis muscle is the largest muscle of the quadriceps group. It originates from the upper part of the intertrochanteric line, the anterior and inferior borders of the greater trochanter, the lateral lip of the gluteal tuberosity, and the proximal half of the upper lip of the linea aspera. In addition, fibres may arise from the gluteus maximus tendon and the lateral intermuscular septum. It attaches via a flat tendon to the base and lateral border of the patella, where it joins the compound quadriceps femoris tendon.
- *Function:* The primary function of the vastus lateralis muscle is knee extension. The vastus lateralis and vastus medialis muscles play an important role in maintaining patellar tracking. The activation pattern of the muscle is often delayed with knee pain (Cavazzuti et al., 2010).
- *Innervation:* The vastus lateralis muscle is innervated by the femoral nerve (L2-L4).
- *Referred pain:* The vastus lateralis muscle refers pain throughout the full length of the lateral side of the thigh from the iliac crest to at least midway of the lower leg.
- *Needling technique:* With the patient in the supine position, the TrP in the anterior section of the muscle is identified via flat palpation. The needle is inserted perpendicular to the skin and directed towards the TrP (Fig. 11.24). To needle TrPs in the part of the muscle posterior to the iliotibial tract, the patient is in the sidelying position.
- *Precautions:* None

Vastus medialis muscle

- *Anatomy:* The vastus medialis muscle originates from the lower part of the intertrochanteric line, the linea aspera, the medial intramuscular septum, the medial supracondylar line, and the tendons of the adductor magnus and longus muscles. The muscle inserts at the medial border of the patella.
- *Function:* The primary function is knee extension. The vastus medialis and vastus lateralis muscles play an important role in maintaining patellar tracking. Changes in patellar tracking and patellofemoral joint contact pressures are often due to weakness of the vastus medialis muscle (Sawatsky et al., 2012).
- *Innervation:* Femoral nerve (L2-L4).
- *Referred pain:* TrPs in the vastus medialis muscle refer pain to the anteromedial aspect of the thigh down to the medial aspect of the knee.
- *Needling technique:* With the patient in the supine position, the TrP is identified via flat palpation. The needle is inserted perpendicular to the skin and directed towards the TrP (Fig. 11.25).
- *Precautions:* Avoid the saphenous nerve in between the adductor magnus muscle and the vastus medialis muscle and the tendons of the sartorius and gracilis muscles.

Vastus intermedius muscle

- *Anatomy:* The vastus intermedius muscle lies underneath the rectus femoris, vastus medialis, and vastus lateralis muscles. It originates at the anterior and lateral surface of the upper two-thirds of the femoral shaft and from the lower part of the lateral intermuscular septum. The muscle is commonly fused with the vastus medialis muscle. It inserts via the deeper fibres of the quadriceps tendon to the lateral aspect of the patella and the lateral condyle of the tibia.
- *Function:* The primary function of the vastus intermedius muscle is often described as knee extension;

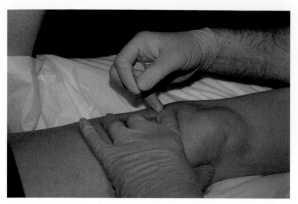

FIG. 11.25 Dry needling of trigger points in the vastus medialis muscle.

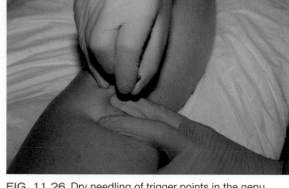

FIG. 11.26 Dry needling of trigger points in the genu articularis muscle.

however, a recent biomechanical study showed that the vastus intermedius muscle may function as a primary antagonistic muscle of the quadriceps femoris muscle during knee flexion and that the muscle may be a main contributor to knee joint stabilisation (Saito et al., 2013).

- *Innervation:* The innervation of the vastus intermedius muscle is the femoral nerve (L2-L4).
- *Referred pain:* The vastus intermedius muscle refers primarily to the anterior aspect of the midthigh.
- *Needling technique:* With the patient in the supine position, the TrP is identified via flat palpation. The needle is inserted perpendicular to the skin and directed towards the TrP. The approach is the same as for the rectus femoris muscle (see Fig. 11.23).
- *Precautions:* None

Genu articularis muscle
- *Anatomy:* The genu articularis muscle is a small muscle underneath the tendon of the rectus femoris muscle. The muscle is rarely described in the myofascial pain literature, but clinically may contribute to anterior knee pain. The muscle may occasionally blend with the vastus intermedius muscle. The muscle originates from the lower part of the femoral shaft and attaches to the synovial membrane of the knee joint.
- *Function:* The only known function of the genu articularis muscle is retraction of the suprapatellar bursa during knee extension likely to prevent compression of synovial folds between the patella and the femur.
- *Innervation:* The genu articularis muscle is innervated by the femoral nerve (L2-L4).
- *Referred pain:* There is no established referred pain pattern for the genu articularis muscle, but empirically, the muscle appears to refer to the anterior knee.

- *Needling technique:* Needling is usually performed from either the medial or lateral side of the rectus femoris tendon towards the underlying femur (Fig. 11.26).
- *Precautions:* None

Biceps femoris muscle
- *Anatomy:* The long head of the biceps femoris muscle originates from the upper part of the ischial tuberosity and may be joining the semitendinosus muscle, but the muscles are still clearly distinguishable from each other. The proximal part of the biceps femoris muscle is comprised of a thick and long tendon, whereas the semitendinosus muscle is mostly muscular with a thin and short tendon. The tendons are covered by a retinaculum, which is continuous with the long head of the biceps femoris, and connected to the semitendinosus muscle via a layer of loose connective tissue (Pérez-Bellmunt et al., 2015). The biceps tendon is directly connected to the sacrotuberous ligament (van Wingerden et al., 1993; Sato et al., 2012). As a side note, the proximal part of the sacrotuberous ligament is directly connected to fibres of the piriformis muscle (Vleeming et al., 1989). The short head of the muscle comes from the lateral lip of the linea aspera but may be totally absent. The two heads merge at the distal end of the muscle and attach to the fibular head, the lateral condyle of the tibia, and the fibular collateral ligament.
- *Function:* The primary function of the biceps femoris muscle is flexion of the knee. With the knee semiflexed, the muscle functions as a lateral rotator of the lower leg on the knee. With the hip extended, the biceps femoris is a lateral rotator of the thigh.

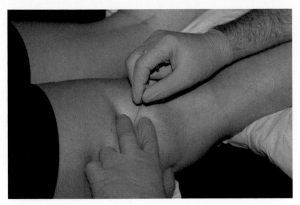

FIG. 11.27 Dry needling of trigger points in the biceps femoris muscle.

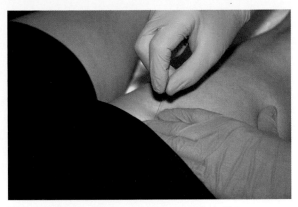

FIG. 11.28 Dry needling of trigger points in the semihamstrings muscles.

- *Innervation:* The biceps femoris muscle is innervated by the sciatic nerve (L5-S2); the long head is innervated by the tibial division and the short head by the common fibular division.
- *Referred pain:* The referred pain pattern of the biceps femoris muscle covers the posterior thigh and knee and the upper one-third of the posterior calf.
- *Needling technique:* With the patient in the prone position with a pillow or bolster under the ankles, the TrP is identified via flat palpation. The needle is inserted perpendicular to the skin and directed towards the TrP (Fig. 11.27).
- *Precautions:* The sciatic nerve lies in the middle of the posterior thigh. Needling the proximal part of the muscle is directed either straight down or slightly medially; needling the distal part of the muscle is directed laterally to avoid the sciatic nerve.

Semimembranosus and semitendinosis muscles
- *Anatomy:*
  1. The semimembranosus muscle originates with a flat tendon from the lateral part of the ischial tuberosity and travels deep to the semitendinosus muscle to divide into five components. The muscle inserts at the tubercle of the medial tibial condyle, the medial margin of the tibia, the fascia over the popliteus muscle, and the lateral femoral condyle where it forms much of the oblique popliteal ligament.
  2. The semitendinosus muscle originates from the inferomedial part of the ischial tuberosity and joins the long head of the biceps femoris muscle via a retinaculum connecting the two muscles (Pérez-Bellmunt et al., 2015). The muscle inserts via a long tendon overlying

the semimembranosus muscle at the upper part of the medial surface of the tibia behind the insertion of the sartorius and distal to the insertion of the gracilis (pes anserine).
- *Function:* The primary function of the semimembranosus and semitendinosus muscles is flexion of the knee. With the knee semiflexed, the muscle functions as medial rotators of the lower leg on the knee. With the hip extended, the semihamstrings are lateral rotators of the thigh.
- *Innervation:* The muscles are innervated by the sciatic nerve (L5-S2) through the tibial division.
- *Referred pain:* The referred pain pattern of the semimembranosus and semitendinosus muscles covers the posterior thigh and knee and the upper one-third of the posterior calf.
- *Needling technique:* With the patient in the prone position with a pillow or bolster under the ankles, the TrP is identified via flat palpation. The needle is inserted perpendicular to the skin and directed towards the TrP (Fig. 11.28).
- *Precautions:* None

Sartorius muscle
- *Anatomy:* The sartorius muscle is the longest muscle in the body. It is a narrow muscle that originates from the anterior superior iliac spine, crosses over the thigh obliquely to the medial side, and inserts at the proximal medial surface of the tibia anteriorly to the insertions of the gracilis and semitendinosus muscles (pes anserine) and to the capsule of the knee joint and the deep fascia.
- *Function:* The sartorius muscle assists in flexion of the leg at the knee, hip flexion, abduction, and lateral rotation of the thigh.
- *Innervation:* Femoral nerve (L2-L3).

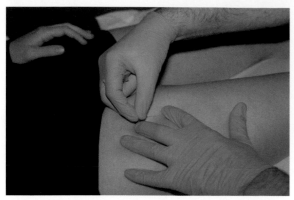

FIG. 11.29 Dry needling of trigger points in the sartorius muscle.

- *Referred pain:* TrPs in the sartorius muscle may give superficial referred pain in the course of the muscle and into the medial knee.
- *Needling technique:* With the patient in supine, direct the needle tangentially to the surface of the muscle (nearly parallel to the skin) (Fig. 11.29).
- *Precautions:* The muscle crosses the femoral nerve, artery and vein.

REFERENCES

Adelmanesh, F., Jalali, A., Jazayeri Shooshtari, S. M., Raissi, G. R., Ketabchi, S. M., & Shir, Y. (2015). Is there an association between lumbosacral radiculopathy and painful gluteal trigger points? *American Journal of Physical Medicine & Rehabilitation, 94,* 784–791.

Adelmanesh, F., Jalali, A., Shirvani, A., Pakmanesh, K., Pourafkari, M., Raissi, G. R., et al. (2016). The diagnostic accuracy of gluteal trigger points to differentiate radicular from nonradicular low back pain. *The Clinical Journal of Pain, 32,* 666–672.

Alburquerque-García, A., Rodrigues-de-Souza, D. P., Fernández-de-las-Peñas, C., & Alburquerque-Sendín, F. (2015). Association between muscle trigger points, ongoing pain, function, and sleep quality in elderly women with bilateral painful knee osteoarthritis. *Journal of Manipulative and Physiological Therapeutics, 38,* 262–268.

Aleksandrova, J. N., Malinova, L., & Jelev, L. (2013). Variations of the iliacus muscle: report of two cases and review of the literature. *International Journal of Anatomical Variations, 6,* 149–152.

American Urological Association (2014). *Diagnosis and treatment interstitial cystitis/bladder pain syndrome.* MD: Linthicum.

Anandkumar, S. (2017). Effect of dry needling on myofascial pain syndrome of the quadratus femoris: A case report. *Physiotherapy Theory and Practice, 18,* 1–8.

Anderson, R. U., Sawyer, T., Wise, D., Morey, A., & Nathanson, B. H. (2009). Painful myofascial trigger points and pain sites in men with chronic prostatitis/chronic pelvic pain syndrome. *The Journal of Urology, 182,* 2753–2758.

Anderson, R. U., Wise, D., Sawyer, T., & Chan, C. (2005). Integration of myofascial trigger point release and paradoxical relaxation training treatment of chronic pelvic pain in men. *The Journal of Urology, 174,* 155–160.

Baba, T., Homma, Y., Takazawa, N., Kobayashi, H., Matsumoto, M., et al. (2014). Is urinary incontinence the hidden secret complications after total hip arthroscopy? *European Journal of Orthopaedic Surgery and Traumatology, 24,* 1455–1460.

Baker, D. (1993). Deficits in innervation of the thoracolumbar fascia have been noted in and can refer pain to the low back, thighs and posterior pelvis. In J. Boyling & G. Jull (Eds.), *Grieve modern manual therapy: the vertebral column.* Churchill Livingstone.

Bassaly, R., Tidwell, N., Bertolino, S., Hoyte, L., Downes, K., & Hart, S. (2010). Myofascial pain and pelvic floor dysfunction in patients with interstitial cystitis. *International Urogynecology Journal, 22,* 413–418.

Bechara, A., Casabe, A., De Bonis, W., & Ciciclia, P. G. (2016). Twelve-month efficacy and safety of low-intensity shockwave therapy for erectile dysfunction in patients who do not respond to phosphodiesterase type 5 inhibitors. *Sexual Medicine, 4*(4), e225–e232.

Benn, M., Tucker, K., Rath, L., Pizzari, T., & Semciw, A. (2017). Adductor magnus and minimus: an EMG investigation into direction specific action. *Journal of Science and Medicine in Sport, 20,* S71.

Bodin, F., Schohn, T., Dissaux, C., Baratte, A., Fiquet, C., & Bruant-Rodier, C. (2015). Bilateral simultaneous breast reconstruction with transverse musculocutaneous gracilis flaps. *Journal of Plastic, Reconstructive & Aesthetic Surgery, 68,* e1–6.

Bonder, J. H., Chi, M., & Rispoli, L. (2017). Myofascial pelvic pain and related disorders. *Physical Medicine and Rehabilitation Clinics of North America, 28,* 501–515.

Brookhoff, D., & Bennett, D. (2006). Neuromodulation in intractable interstitial cystitis and related pelvic pain syndromes. *Pain Medicine, 7,* S166–S184.

Carvalhais, V. O., Ocarino Jde, M., Araújo, V. L., Souza, T. R., Silva, P. L., & Fonseca, S. T. (2013). Myofascial force transmission between the latissimus dorsi and gluteus maximus muscles: an in vivo experiment. *Journal of Biomechanics, 46,* 1003–1007.

Cavazzuti, L., Merlo, A., Orlandi, F., & Campanini, I. (2010). Delayed onset of electro-myographic activity of vastus medialis obliquus relative to vastus lateralis in subjects with patellofemoral pain syndrome. *Gait & Posture, 32,* 290–295.

Claes, H., Bijnens, B., & Baert, L. (1996). The hemodynamic influence of the ischiocavernosus muscles on erectile function. *The Journal of Urology, 156,* 986–990.

Coady, D., Futterman, S., Harris, D., & Coleman, S. H. (2015). Vulvodynia and concomitant femoro-acetabular impingement: long term follow up after hip arthroscopy. *Journal of Lower Genital Tract Disease, 19,* 1–4.

Coady, D., Futterman, S., Harris, D., & Coleman, S. H. (2015). Vulvodynia and concomitant femoro-acetabular impingement: long-term follow-up after hip arthroscopy. *Journal of Lower Genital Tract Disease, 19*(3), 253–256.

Cohen, D., Gonzalez, J., & Goldstein, I. (2016). The role of pelvic floor muscles in male sexual dysfunction and pelvic pain. *Sexual Medicine Reviews, 4*, 53–62.

Cox, A., Golda, N., Nadeau, G., Curtis Nickel, J., Carr, L., Corcos, J., et al. (2016). CUA guideline: diagnosis and treatment of interstitial cystitis/bladder pain syndrome. *Canadian Urological Association Journal, 10*, E136–155.

Cummings, M. (2003). Referred knee pain treated with electroacupuncture to iliopsoas. *Acupuncture in Medicine, 21*(1-2), 32–35.

D'Costa, S., Ramanathan, L. A., Madhyastha, S., et al. (2008). An accessory iliacus muscle: a case report. *Romanian Journal of Morphology and Embryology, 49*, 407–409.

Dalmau-Carola, J. (2005). Myofascial pain syndrome affecting the piriformis and the obturator internus muscle. *Pain Practice, 5*, 361–363.

Delahunt, E., Kennelly, C., McEntee, B. L., Coughlan, G. F., & Green, B. S. (2011). The thigh adductor squeeze test: 45° of hip flexion as the optimal test position for eliciting adductor muscle activity and maximum pressure values. *Manual Therapy, 16*, 476–480.

Dembowski, S. C., Westrick, R. B., Zylstra, E., & Johnson, M. R. (2013). Treatment of hamstring strain in a collegiate polevaulter integrating dry needling with an eccentric training program: a resident's case report. *International Journal of Sports Physical Therapy, 8*, 328–339.

Doggweiler-Wiygul, R. (2004). Urologic myofascial pain syndromes. *Current Pain and Headache Reports, 8*, 445–451.

Dor, A., & Kalichman, L. (2017). A myofascial component of pain in knee osteoarthritis. *Journal of Bodywork and Movement Therapies, 21*, 642–647.

Drew, M. K., Lovell, G., Palsson, T. S., Chiarelli, P. E., & Osmotherly, P. G. (2016). Do Australian Football players have sensitive groins? Players with current groin pain exhibit mechanical hyperalgesia of the adductor tendon. *Journal of Science and Medicine in Sport, 19*, 784–788.

Espí-López, G. V., Serra-Añó, P., Vicent-Ferrando, J., Sánchez-Moreno-Giner, M., Arias-Buría, J. L., Cleland, J., et al. (2017). Effectiveness of inclusion of dry needling in a multimodal therapy program for patellofemoral pain: a randomized parallel-group trial. *The Journal of Orthopaedic and Sports Physical Therapy, 47*, 392–401.

Fabrizio, P. A. (2011). Anatomic variation of the iliacus and psoas muscles. *International Journal of Anatomical Variations, 4*, 28–30.

Fairclough, J., Hayashi, K., Toumi, H., Lyons, K., Bydder, G., Phillips, N., et al. (2006). The functional anatomy of the iliotibial band during flexion and extension of the knee: implications for understanding iliotibial band syndrome. *Journal of Anatomy, 208*, 309–316.

Fall, M., Baranowski, A. P., Elneil, S., Engeler, D., Hughes, J., Messelink, E. J., et al. (2010). EAU guidelines on chronic pelvic pain. *European Urology, 57*, 35–48.

Farrell, M. R., Dugan, S. A., & Levine, L. A. (2016). Physical therapy for chronic scrotal content pain with associated pelvic floor pain on digital rectal exam. *The Canadian Journal of Urology, 23*, 8546–8550.

Fitzgerald, M. P., Anderson, R. U., Potts, J., et al. (2013). Randomized multicenter feasibility trial of myofascial physical therapy for the treatment of urological chronic pelvic pain syndromes. *The Journal of Urology, 182*, 570–580.

Fitzgerald, M. P., & Kotarinos, R. (2003). Rehabilitation of the short pelvic floor. II: Treatment of the patient with the short pelvic floor. *International Urogynecology Journal and Pelvic Floor Dysfunction, 14*, 269–275.

Geist, K., Bradley, C., Hofman, A., et al. (2016). Clinical effects of dry needling among asymptomatic individuals with hamstring tightness: a randomized controlled trial. *Journal of Sport Rehabilitation*, 1–31. [Epub ahead of print].

Giamberardino, M. A., Affaitati, G., Iezzi, S., & Vecchiet, L. (1999). Referred muscle pain and hyperalgesia from viscera. *Journal of Musculoskeletal Pain, 7*, 61–69.

Goel, S., Arora, J., Mehta, V., Sharma, M., Suri, R. K., Rath, G., et al. (2015). Adductor accessorius - an unusual supernumerary adductor muscle of thigh. *La Clinica Terapeutica, 166*, 114–117.

Goldstein, A., Pukall, C., Brown, C., Bergeron, S., Stein, A., & Kellogg-Spadt, S. (2016). Vulvodynia: assessment and treatment. *The Journal of Sexual Medicine, 13*, 572–590.

Häner, M., Bierke, S., & Petersen, W. (2016). Anterior cruciate ligament revision surgery: ipsilateral quadriceps versus contralateral semitendinosus-gracilis autografts. *Arthroscopy, 32*, 2308–2317.

Hartman, D., & Sarton, J. (2014). Chronic pelvic floor dysfunction. *Best Practice & Research Clinical Obstetrics & Gynaecology, 28*, 977–990.

Hodges, P. W., McLean, L., & Hodder, J. (2014). Insight into the function of the obturator internus muscle in humans: observations with development and validation of an electromyography recording technique. *Journal of Electromyography and Kinesiology, 24*, 489–496.

Hölmich, P. (2017). Groin injuries in athletes: new stepping stones. *Sports Orthopaedics and Traumatology, 33*, 106–112.

Honma, S., Jun, Y., & Horiguchi, M. (1998). The human gemelli muscles and their nerve supplies. *Kaibogaku Zasshi, 73*, 329–335.

Huguenin, L., Brukner, P. D., McCrory, P., Smith, P., Wajswelner, H., & Bennell, K. (2005). Effect of dry needling of gluteal muscles on straight leg raise: a randomised, placebo controlled, double blind trial. *British Journal of Sports Medicine, 39*, 84–90.

Iglesias-Gonzalez, J., Munoz-Garcia, M., Rodrigues-de-Souza, D., Alburquerque-Sendin, F., & Fernandez-de-las-Peñas, C. (2013). Myofascial trigger points, pain, disability, and sleep quality in patients with chronic nonspecific low back pain. *Pain Medicine, 14*, 1964–1970.

Itza, F., Zarza, D., Serra, L., Gómez-Sancha, F., Salinas, J., & Allona-Almagro, A. (2010). Myofascial pain syndrome in the pelvic floor: a common urological condition. *Actas Urologicas Españolas, 34*, 318–326.

Jayaseelan, D. J., Moats, N., & Ricardo, C. R. (2014). Rehabilitation of proximal hamstring tendinopathy utilizing eccentric training, lumbopelvic stabilization, and trigger point dry needling: 2 case reports. *The Journal of Orthopaedic and Sports Physical Therapy*, 44, 198–205.

Jarrell, J., Giamberardino, M. A., Robert, M., & Nasr-Esfahani, M. (2011). Bedside testing for chronic pelvic pain: discriminating visceral from somatic pain. *Pain Research and Treatment*, 2011, 692102.

Jarrell, J. (2011). Endometriosis and abdominal myofascial pain in adults and adolescents. *Current Pain and Headache Reports*, 15, 368–376.

Jarrell, J. F., Vilos, G. A., Allaire, C., et al. (2005). Consensus guidelines for the management of chronic pelvic pain. *Journal of Obstetrics and Gynaecology Canada*, 27, 781–826.

Jelev, L., Shivarov, V., & Surchev, L. (2005). Bilateral variations of the psoas major and the iliacus muscles and presence of an undescribed variant muscle—accessory iliopsoas muscle. *Annals of Anatomy*, 187, 281–286.

Kaoutzanis, C., Pannucci, C. J., & Sherick, D. (2013). Use of gracilis muscle as a "walking" flap for repair of a rectovaginal fistula. *Journal of Plastic, Reconstructive & Aesthetic Surgery*, 66, e197–200.

Lavoisier, P., Roy, P., Dantony, E., Watrelot, A., Ruggeri, J., & Dumoulin, S. (2014). Pelvic-floor muscle rehabilitation in erectile dysfunction and premature ejaculation. *Physical Therapy*, 94, 1731–1743.

Lewis, L., Jurak, J., Lee, C., Lewis, R., & Gest, T. (2016). Anatomical variations of the sciatic nerve, in relation to the piriformis muscle. *Translational Research Anatomy*, 5, 1519.

Lieberman, D. E., Raichlen, D. A., Pontzer, H., Bramble, D. M., & Cutright-Smith, E. (2006). The human gluteus maximus and its role in running. *The Journal of Experimental Biology*, 209, 2143–2155.

Longbottom, J. (2009). The treatment of pelvic pain with acupuncture: part 1. *The Journal of Chinese Medicine*, 91, 1–15.

Luz, L. L., Fernandes, E., Sivado, M., Kokai, E., Szucs, P., & Safronov, B. V. (2015). Monosynaptic convergence of somatic and visceral C-fiber afferents on projection and local circuit neurons in lamina I: a substrate for referred pain. *Pain*, 156, 2042–2051.

Mason, J. S., Crowell, M., Dolbeer, J., Morris, J., Terry, A., Koppenhaver, S., et al. (2016). The effectiveness of dry needling and stretching versus stretching alone on hamstring flexibility in patients with knee pain: a randomized controlled trial. *International Journal of Sports Physical Therapy*, 11, 672–683.

Mayoral, O., Salvat, I., Martín, M. T., Martín, S., Santiago, J., Cotarelo, J., et al. (2013). Efficacy of myofascial trigger point dry needling in the prevention of pain after total knee arthroplasty: a randomized, double-blinded, placebo-controlled trial. *Evidence-based Complementary and Alternative Medicine*, 2013, 694941.

Michel, F., Decavel, P., Toussirot, E., Tatu, L., Aleton, E., Monnier, G., Garbuio, P., et al. (2013). The piriformis muscle syndrome: an exploration of anatomical context, pathophysiological hypotheses and diagnostic criteria. *Annals of Physical and Rehabilitation Medicine*, 56, 300–311.

Miranda, A., Peles, S., Rudolph, C., Shaker, R., & Sengupta, J. N. (2004). Altered visceral sensation in response to somatic pain in the rat. *Gastroenterology*, 126, 1082–1089.

Moldwin, R. M., & Fariello, J. Y. (2013). Myofascial trigger points of the pelvic floor: associations with urological pain syndromes and treatment strategies including injection therapy. *Current Urology Reports*, 14, 409–417.

Nelson-Wong, E., Gregory, D. E., Winter, D. A., & Callaghan, J. P. (2008). Gluteus medius muscle activation patterns as a predictor of low back pain during standing. *Clinical Biomechanics*, 23, 545–553.

Nene, A., Byrne, C., & Hermens, H. (2004). Is rectus femoris really a part of quadriceps? Assessment of rectus femoris function during gait in able-bodied adults. *Gait & Posture*, 20, 1–13.

Nene, A., Mayagoitia, R., & Veltink, P. (1999). Assessment of rectus femoris function during initial swing phase. *Gait & Posture*, 9, 1–9.

Nevin, F., & Delahunt, E. (2014). Adductor squeeze test values and hip joint range of motion in Gaelic football athletes with longstanding groin pain. *Journal of Science and Medicine in Sport*, 17, 155–159.

Núñez-Cortés, R., Cruz-Montecinos, C., Vásquez-Rosel, Á., Paredes-Molina, O., & Cuesta-Vargas, A. (2017). Dry needling combined with physical therapy in patients with chronic postsurgical pain following total knee arthroplasty: a case series. *The Journal of Orthopaedic and Sports Physical Therapy*, 47, 209–216.

Pastore, E. A., & Katzman, W. B. (2012). Recognizing myofascial pelvic pain in the female patient with chronic pelvic pain. *Journal of Obstetric, Gynecologic, and Neonatal Nursing*, 41, 680–691.

Peikert, K., Platzek, I., Bessède, T., & May, C. A. (2015). The male bulbospongiosus muscle and its relation to the external anal sphincter. *The Journal of Urology*, 193, 1433–1440.

Pelayo-Nieto, M., Linden-Castro, E., Alias-Melgar, A., Espinosa-Perez Grovas, D., Carreno-de la Rosa, F., Bertrand-Noriega, F., et al. (2015). Linear shock wave therapy in the treatment of erectile dysfunction. *Actas Urologicas Españolas*, 39(7), 456–459.

Peles, S., Miranda, A., Shaker, R., & Sengupta, J. N. (2004). Acute nociceptive somatic stimulus sensitizes neurones in the spinal cord to colonic distension in the rat. *The Journal of Physiology*, 560, 291–302.

Pérez-Bellmunt, A., Miguel-Pérez, M., Brugué, M. B., Cabús, J. B., Casals, M., Martinoli, C., et al. (2015). An anatomical and histological study of the structures surrounding the proximal attachment of the hamstring muscles. *Manual Therapy*, 20, 445–450.

Pesquer, L., Reboul, G., Silvestre, A., Poussange, N., Meyer, P., & Dallaudière, B. (2015). Imaging of adductor-related groin pain. *Diagnostic and Interventional Imaging*, 96, 861–869.

Philippon, M. J., Devitt, B. M., Campbell, K. J., Michalski, M. P., Espinoza, C., Wijdicks, C. A., et al. (2014). Anatomic variance of the iliopsoas tendon. *The American Journal of Sports Medicine*, 42, 807–811.

Podschun, L., Hanney, W. J., Kolber, M. J., Garcia, A., & Rothschild, C. E. (2013). Differential diagnosis of deep gluteal pain in a female runner with pelvic involvement: a case report. *International Journal of Sports Physical Therapy*, 8, 462–471.

Prather, H., & Camacho-Soto, A. (2014). Musculoskeletal etiologies of pelvic pain. *Obstetrics and Gynecology Clinics of North America*, 41, 433–442.

Qaseem, A., Dallas, P., Forciea, M. A., Starkey, M., Denberg, T. D., & Shekelle, P. (2014). Clinical guidelines committee of the American College of Physicians. Nonsurgical management of urinary incontinence in women: a clinical practice guideline from the American College of Physicians. *Annals of Internal Medicine*, 161, 429–440.

Rainey, C. E. (2013). The use of trigger point dry needling and intramuscular electrical stimulation for a subject with chronic low back pain: a case report. *International Journal of Sports Physical Therapy*, 8, 145–161.

Rao, T. R., Vanishree, P. S., Kanyan, & Rao, S. (2008). Bilateral variation of iliacus muscle and splitting of femoral nerve. *Neuroanatomy*, 7, 72–75.

Ravnik, D., & Širca, A. (1993). Histochemical characteristics of bulbospongiosus and ischiocavernosus muscles in man. *Annals of Anatomy*, 175, 135–139.

Roach, S., Sorenson, E., Headley, B., & San Juan, J. G. (2013). Prevalance of myofascial trigger points in the hip in patellofemoral pain. *Archives of Physical Medicine and Rehabilitation*, 94, 522–526.

Robertson, W. J., Gardner, M. J., Barker, J. U., Boraiah, S., Lorich, D. G., & Kelly, B. T. (2008). Anatomy and dimensions of the gluteus medius tendon insertion. *Arthroscopy*, 24, 130–136.

Rudolph, E., Boffard, C., & Raath, C. (2017). Pelvic floor physical therapy for erectile dysfunction fact or fallacy? *The Journal of Sexual Medicine*, 14(6), 765–766.

Saito, A., Watanabe, K., & Akima, H. (2013). The highest antagonistic coactivation of the vastus intermedius muscle among quadriceps femoris muscles during isometric knee flexion. *Journal of Electromyography and Kinesiology*, 23, 831–837.

Sapsford, R. R., Hodges, P. W., Richardson, C. A., Cooper, D. H., Markwell, S. J., & Jull, G. A. (2001). Co-activation of the abdominal muscles and pelvic floor muscles during voluntary exercises. *Neurourology and Urodynamics*, 20, 31–42.

Sato, K., Nimura, A., Yamaguchi, K., & Akita, K. (2012). Anatomical study of the proximal origin of hamstring muscles. *Journal of Orthopaedic Science*, 17, 614–618.

Sawatsky, A., Bourne, D., Horisberger, M., Jinha, A., & Herzog, W. (2012). Changes in patellofemoral joint contact pressures caused by vastus medialis muscle weakness. *Clinical Biomechanics*, 27, 595–601.

Semciw, A. I., Freeman, M., Kunstler, B. E., Mendis, M. D., & Pizzari, T. (2015). Quadratus femoris: an EMG investigation during walking and running. *Journal of Biomechanics*, 48, 3433–3439.

Shafik, A., & El-Sibai, O. (2002). Study of the pelvic floor muscles in vaginismus: a concept of pathogenesis. *European Journal of Obstetrics, Gynecology, and Reproductive Biology*, 105, 67–70.

Shafik, A. (1993). Vaginocavernosus reflex. Clinical significance and role in sexual act. *Gynecologic and Obstetric Investigation*, 35, 114–1147.

Simons, D. G., Travell, J. G., & Simons, L. S. (1999). *Travell and Simons' myofascial pain and dysfunction: the trigger point manual*. Baltimore: Williams and Wilkins.

Smith, M., Russell, A., & Hodges, P. (2006). Disorders of breathing and continence have a stronger association with back pain than obesity and physical activity. *The Australian Journal of Physiotherapy*, 52, 11–16.

Standring, S. (Ed.), (2015). *Gray's anatomy: the anatomical basis of clinical practice* (41st ed.). London: Churchill Livingston Elsevier.

Stecco, C., Porzionato, A., Lancerotto, L., Stecco, A., Macchi, V., Day, J. A., et al. (2008). Histological study of the deep fasciae of the limbs. *Journal of Bodywork and Movement Therapies*, 12, 225–230.

Stecco, A., Gilliar, W., Hill, R., Fullerton, B., & Stecco, C. (2013). The anatomical and functional relation between gluteus maximus and fascia lata. *Journal of Bodywork and Movement Therapies*, 17, 512–517.

Stoker, J. (2009). Anorectal and pelvic floor anatomy. *Best Practice & Research Clinical Gastroenterology*, 23, 463–475.

Sung, D. H., Jung, J. Y., Kim, H. D., Ha, B. J., & Ko, Y. J. (2003). Motor branch of the rectus femoris: anatomic location for selective motor branch block in stiff-legged gait. *Archives of Physical Medicine and Rehabilitation*, 84, 1028–1031.

Tamaki, T., Ouinuma, K., Shiratsuchi, H., et al. (2014). Hip dysfunction-related urinary incontinence: a prospective analysis of 189 female patients undergoing total hip arthroscopy. *International Journal of Urology*, 21, 729–731.

Teixeira, M., Yeng, L. T., Garcia, O., et al. (2011). Failed back surgery pain syndrome: therapeutic approach descriptive study in 56 patients. *Revista da Associação Médica Brasileira*, 57, 282–287.

Torres-Chica, B., Núñez-Samper-Pizarroso, C., Ortega-Santiago, R., et al. (2015). Trigger points and pressure pain hypersensitivity in people with post-meniscectomy pain. *The Clinical Journal of Pain*, 31, 265–272.

Travell, J., & Simons, D. (1992). *Myofascial pain and dysfunction: the trigger point manual, volume 2*. Philadelphia: Lippincott Williams and Wilkins.

Vaarbakken, K., Steen, H., Samuelsen, G., Dahl, H. A., Leergaard, T. B., & Stuge, B. (2015). Primary functions of the quadratus femoris and obturator externus muscles indicated from lengths and moment arms measured in mobilized cadavers. *Clinical Biomechanics*, 30, 231–237.

van Wingerden, J. P., Vleeming, A., Snijders, C. J., & Stoeckart, R. (1993). A functional-anatomical approach to the spine-pelvis mechanism: interaction between the biceps femoris muscle and the sacrotuberous ligament. *European Spine Journal*, 2, 140–144.

Velázquez-Saornil, J., Ruíz-Ruíz, B., Rodríguez-Sanz, D., Romero-Morales, C., López-López, D., & Calvo-Lobo, C. (2017). Efficacy of quadriceps vastus medialis dry needling in a rehabilitation protocol after surgical reconstruction of complete anterior cruciate ligament rupture. *Medicine, 96,* e6726.

Vercellini, P., Somigliana, E., Viganò, P., Abbiati, A., Barbara, G., & Fedele, L. (2009). Chronic pelvic pain in women: etiology, pathogenesis and diagnostic approach. *Gynecological Endocrinology, 25,* 149–158.

Vleeming, A., Alpert, H., Ostgaard, H., Sturesson, B., & Stuge, B. (2008). European guidelines for the diagnosis and treatment of pelvic girdle pain. *European Spine Journal, 17,* 794–819.

Vleeming, A., Stoeckart, R., & Snijders, C. J. (1989). The sacrotuberous ligament: a conceptual approach to its dynamic role in stabilizing the sacroiliac joint. *Clinical Biomechanics, 4,* 201–203.

Weiss, J. M. (2001). Pelvic floor myofascial trigger points: manual therapy for interstitial cystitis and the urgency-frequency syndrome. *The Journal of Urology, 166,* 2226–2231.

Wente, K., & Spitznagle, T. (2017). Movement-related urinary urgency: a theoretical framework and retrospective, cross-sectional study. *Journal of Women's Health Physical Therapy, 41,* 83–90.

Wesselmann, U. (2001). Interstitial cystitis: a chronic visceral pain syndrome. *Urology, 57,* 32–39.

Yüksela, Ö.H., Memetoglu, Ö.G., Ürkmeza, A., Î, A., & Verit, A. (2015). The role of physical activity in the treatment of erectile dysfunction. *Revista Internacional de Andrología, 13*(4), 115–119.

Zermann, D. H., Ishigooka, M., Doggweiler-Wiygul, R., Schubert, J., & Schmidt, R. A. (2001). The male chronic pelvic pain syndrome. *World Journal of Urology, 19,* 155–224.

Zondervan, K. T., Yudkin, P. L., Vessey, M. P., Jenkinson, C. P., Dawes, M. G., Barlow, D. H., et al. (2001). The community presence of chronic pelvic pain in in women and associated illness behavior. *The British Journal of General Practice, 51,* 541–547.

CHAPTER 12

Deep Dry Needling of the Leg and Foot Muscles

ORLANDO MAYORAL DEL MORAL • MARÍA TORRES LACOMBA • JAN DOMMERHOLT

INTRODUCTION

Muscles in the foot and leg are at a challenging cross-roads location as they are included in the referral patterns of multiple proximal muscles such as the gluteus minimus, medius and maximus muscles, the piriformis, tensor fasciae latae, adductors longus and brevis, vastus lateralis, sartorius, semitendinosus and semimembranosus, and biceps femoris muscles (Travell & Simons, 1992; Dejung et al., 2001). The links between proximal and distal muscles may have a predominant sensory pattern, whereby secondary hyperalgesia from proximal trigger points (TrPs) may be present in the leg and foot but may also be predominantly mechanical in nature. TrPs in the gluteal medius muscle, for example, may cause an altered gait pattern leading to overuse of the gastrocnemius muscle. Pain and dysfunction caused by TrPs in foot and calf muscles induce gait alterations that overload muscles higher in the lower limbs and in the spine (Lewit, 2010). For example, subjects with a lowered arch had significantly more TrPs in the flexor digitorum longus, tibialis posterior, and vastus medialis muscles compared with controls (Zuil-Escobar et al., 2015).

Often, patients experience mixed patterns combining biomechanical and sensory aspects. Cuccia (2011) described a direct link between dental occlusion and the plantar arch. Such correlations are not limited to the lower leg and foot. Several studies found correlations between mouth opening, TrP sensitivity, and stretching of the hamstring muscles (Bretischwerdt et al., 2010; Rodriguez-Blanco et al., 2015; Espejo-Antúnez et al., 2016). Even more intriguing is the finding that treating suboccipital muscles can increase hamstrings flexibility (Aparicio et al., 2009; Cho et al., 2015).

The muscles in the foot and leg are the first line of defense of any anatomical or biomechanical problems occurring in the foot and, consequently, become easily overloaded by these issues leading to development and activation of TrPs (Travell & Simons, 1992; Saggini

et al., 1996). Joint dysfunctions and inappropriate shoes can also either cause or add to these problems. In other words, the treatment of TrPs in the leg and foot muscles is necessary but usually insufficient to fully solve our patients' problems because proximal muscles, as well as several other perpetuating factors, must be addressed for a complete and long-lasting relief of the symptoms. A multimodal approach including dry needling (DN) is recommended over single modality treatment approaches (Segura-Perez et al., 2017).

The reliability of identifying TrPs in the lower leg has been confirmed by Sanz and colleagues (2016), who were able to reach acceptable pairwise interrater agreement for the presence or absence of TrPs and local twitch responses in the tibialis anterior muscle and for taut bands, referred pain, and the jump sign with the extensor digitorum longus muscle. The percent agreement for the fibularis brevis muscle varied. Latent TrPs are commonly found in asymptomatic individuals. The finding of a taut band and tender spot were the most reliable diagnostic criteria (Zuil-Escobar et al., 2016). Note that in the US nomenclature, the peroneal muscles are now referred to as the fibularis muscles. In this chapter, we use the US term.

CLINICAL RELEVANCE OF TRIGGER POINTS IN LEG AND FOOT PAIN SYNDROMES

Pain syndromes in the leg and foot span from simple delayed onset muscle soreness to plantar fasciitis, including calf cramps, shin splints, Morton's neuroma, tendinopathy of the Achilles tendon and other tendons, posterior tibial nerve or deep fibularis nerve entrapments, compartment syndromes, ankle or foot sprains, instability, complex regional pain syndrome type I (CRPS I), intermittent claudication, and metatarsalgia, among others. The contributions of TrPs in the leg and foot muscles to these conditions can be highly variable, but scientific evidence and clinical impressions support that TrPs often play an important role. Professional soccer players with ankle pain presented commonly with TrPs particularly in the tibialis anterior and fibularis muscles (Pérez Costa & Torres-Lacomba, 2016). Salom-Moreno and colleagues (2015) confirmed that TrPs in the fibularis muscles play a significant role in ankle instability. Adding DN of TrPs in the fibularis muscles to a proprioceptive and strengthening exercise program improved outcomes in pain and function even 1 month after therapy had been concluded. A case report of a patient with postsurgical knee pain mentioned that the combination of ultrasonography-guided pulsed radiofrequency, physiotherapy, medication, and DN of TrPs in the quadriceps, hamstrings, adductors, sartorius, gracilis, gastrocnemius, and popliteus, successfully resolved the patient's pain for at least 6 months (Vas et al., 2014). A study of patients with a variety of foot problems, such as plantar fasciitis, metatarsalgia, hallux valgus and hallux rigidus, Morton's neuroma, and longitudinal arch pain, among others, compared manual TrP treatments and customised orthotics with a treatment protocol with only soft prefabricated insoles. The combination of customised orthotics and TrP compression yielded significantly better results as assessed by the Foot Function Index and the Patients' Perceived Improvement Score (Hains et al., 2015).

Moghtaderi and colleagues (2014) observed that the application of extracorporeal shock wave therapy for plantar fasciitis was more effective when TrPs in the gastrocnemius and soleus muscles were included in the therapy. In addition, clinical experience shows that symptoms arising from TrPs often mimic many of these conditions, inducing incorrect diagnoses that lead to erroneous and ineffective treatments. A combination of TrPs in the tibialis posterior, the soleus, and gastrocnemius muscles, for example, may mimic an Achilles tendinopathy. TrPs in the third dorsal interosseous muscle may reproduce the symptoms of a Morton's neuroma, whereas TrPs in the fibularis muscles may imitate the pain of an ankle sprain, and so on.

Although many different possible aetiologies are proposed for calf cramps, TrPs in the calf muscles, particularly in the gastrocnemius, seem to be important contributors (Travell & Simons, 1992; Ge et al., 2008; Xu et al., 2010). A clinical trial with a small sample of 24 subjects showed that xylocaine injections of TrPs in the gastrocnemius muscle induced a significantly better long-term efficacy on calf cramps compared with oral quinine (Prateepavanich et al., 1999). TrPs in the gastrocnemius and soleus muscles were successfully treated with a multimodal approach consisting of TrP pressure release, TrP self-release, and a home stretching program (Grieve et al., 2013a). In another study, Grieve and colleagues (2013b) found that a single application of manual compression of TrPs in the gastrocnemius and soleus muscles combined with stretching improved ankle range of motion in 22 recreational runners with a clinically meaningful increase.

Plantar heel pain, often diagnosed as plantar fasciitis, is commonly due to TrPs in the calf and foot musculature. Several reports have shown this close relationship and proven that conservative treatment of TrPs in calf muscles is useful in the treatment of plantar heel pain and plantar fasciitis (Nguyen, 2010; Renan-Ordine et al., 2011). Ajimsha and colleagues (2014) found that myofascial release was helpful in reducing plantar heel pain. DN and injections of TrPs in the calf and foot muscles may be helpful in the management of this condition (Imamura et al., 1998; Kushner & Ferguson, 2005; Cotchett et al., 2010; Sconfienza et al., 2011; Akhbari et al., 2014). Cotchett and colleagues (2014) reported that DN significantly reduced plantar heel pain, although the level of minimally important difference was insufficient. Eftekharsadat and colleagues (2016) confirmed that TrP DN significantly reduced the pain of plantar fasciitis, but it had no significant effect on ankle dorsiflexion and eversion. A recent meta-analysis of seven randomised controlled trials has shown that TrP DN effectively reduced the pain associated with plantar fasciitis (He & Ma, 2017).

An older study attributed medial tibial stress syndrome (shin splints) to overload of the attachments of the soleus muscle (Michael & Holder, 1985). One study showed that tension in the soleus, tibialis posterior, and flexor digitorum longus muscles caused a tenting effect that exerted a force on the distal tibial fascia directed to its tibial crest insertion (Bouche & Johnson, 2007). Another study demonstrated that the plantar flexors of the ankle were significantly weaker in medial tibial stress syndrome (Madeley et al., 2007). Increased tension and weakness are two cardinal features of muscles affected by TrPs. Nevertheless, the possible involvement of TrPs in these muscles in medial tibial stress syndrome has not yet been established unequivocally, and no clinical trial to date has proven that TrP treatment can be of help in the management of this condition.

Although Travell and Simons (1992) suggested that there was a 'a strong possibility that, in muscles prone to developing a compartment syndrome, TrPs may make a significant contribution', there is no

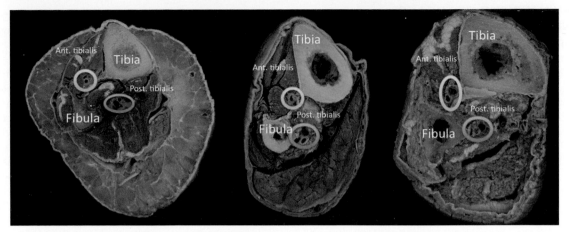

FIG. 12.1 Anatomical differences between specimens of the neurovascular bundles in the leg. (Photos courtesy of Willard/Carreiro Anatomy Collection.)

actual evidence in the literature. The safety of using DN, which could potentially cause some bleeding in the muscle, has also not been established in patients with compartment syndrome; hence, more aggressive DN approaches such as Hong's fast-in and fast-out technique, screwed-in/out techniques, or DN with thick needles may be considered possible contraindications. The risk of bleeding is increased when patients take anticoagulants, but this is not an absolute contraindication to DN (Muñoz et al., in press). Yet there is some question as to whether needling of deeper muscles, such as the tibialis posterior muscle or the lateral pterygoid muscle, can be performed safely without ultrasound guidance considering their close proximity to major arteries. On the one hand, clinicians have been needling the posterior tibialis muscle without any evidence of injury, but it is at least conceivable that, in some individuals, there may be an increased risk of bleeding. A recent case report describing a 41-year-old female with a vertebral artery dissection after receiving acupuncture to the neck demonstrated that small filiform needles are able to damage blood vessels (Hong et al., 2017). As the location of the neurovascular bundles in the leg can vary substantially (Fig. 12.1), a clinician may never know the exact location; however, it is unknown what the actual risk is of damage to these deeper blood vessels. Upon review of other needling procedures, such as venipuncture, electromyography, and botulinum toxin injections, Muñoz and colleagues concluded that DN does not pose a severe risk, but some caution is nevertheless warranted (Muñoz et al., in press).

Allen and colleagues (1999) reported that 42% of patients with complex regional pain syndrome (CRPS) in the lower extremities presented with active TrPs in their proximal muscles. In this study, only the lumbar paraspinous and gluteal musculature were examined, which raises the question as to what percentage of active TrPs would have been found if other lower extremity muscles had been included in the examination (Allen et al., 1999). Early treatment of TrPs is usually recommended in patients with CRPS I to decrease their pain intensity and disability (Dommerholt, 2004). Although the use of DN has not yet been reported for CRPS, a recent report of two cases of upper limb CRPS I showed promising results with treatment of proximal TrPs with botulinum toxin injections (Safarpour & Jabbari, 2010). Chang (2017) described using TrP injections in several cases with CRPS.

TrPs in the popliteus, plantaris, and gastrocnemius can also contribute to posterior knee pain, which is more commonly attributed to knee joint problems. TrPs in the proximal part of the gastrocnemius muscle can be responsible for posterior knee pain in patients before (Mayoral et al., 2013) and after (Aceituno, 2003) total knee replacement surgery and after knee arthroscopy (Rodríguez et al., 2005). DN is used increasingly in the treatment of tendinopathies such as Achilles tendinopathy (see Chapter 3). Chaudhry (2017) suggested to combine ultrasound-guided, high volume, image-guided injections with DN for Achilles tendinopathy, but acknowledged the limited research.

Further research is needed to elucidate the possible contribution of TrPs to the previously mentioned conditions or to other structural problems such as hammer toes (Travell & Simons, 1992) or hallux valgus, or to different leg and foot nerve entrapments (Crotti et al., 2005; Saggini et al., 2007).

DRY NEEDLING OF THE LEG AND FOOT MUSCLES

Popliteus Muscle

- *Anatomy:* The popliteus muscle is an obtuse triangle in shape. Laterally and proximally, it attaches to the lateral condyle of the femur, to the posterior capsule of the knee joint, to the lateral meniscus, and to the head of the fibula. Medially and distally, it attaches to the posteromedial surface of the tibia.
- *Function:* The function of the popliteus muscle is medial rotation of the tibia in an open kinetic chain and lateral rotation of the femur in a closed kinetic chain. The muscle also assists marginally with knee flexion.
- *Innervation:* Tibial nerve fibres from L4, L5, and S1 spinal nerves.
- *Referred Pain:* Typically, the popliteus muscle refers to the back of the knee and to the medial and anteromedial side of the proximal leg (Mayoral del Moral et al., 2017).
- *Needling technique:* The patient lies on the side of the involved extremity with the hip and knee flexed to approximately 90 degrees. The muscle is palpated right behind the proximal third of the tibia, and the needle is inserted towards the TrP in a lateral direction with a slight anterior superior orientation (Fig. 12.2), keeping the needle close to the posterior aspect of the tibia or even touching the bone with the tip of the needle as a reference.
- *Precautions:* The neurovascular bundle is in the midline of the leg, resting on the popliteus muscle, and must be avoided by keeping the needle close to the posterior aspect of the tibia. Branches of the saphenous nerve run superficial in the region where the needle is inserted. If the needle touches any of these branches, the patient will feel a superficial electrical sensation over the medial part of the leg. Should this happen during the first millimeters of needle penetration through the skin, the needle should be withdrawn and reinserted a few millimeters away.

Gastrocnemius Muscle

- *Anatomy:* The gastrocnemius muscle is divided into a lateral and a medial head. Proximally, each head anchors to the corresponding condyle of the femur and to the capsule of the knee joint. Distally, both heads insert into the Achilles tendon, which attaches to the posterior surface of the calcaneus bone.
- *Function:* The function of the gastrocnemius muscle is plantar flexion and supination of the foot with limited contribution to knee flexion (with the knee extended) and to knee stabilisation. In a closed kinetic chain, the gastrocnemius muscle contributes to knee and ankle stability.
- *Innervation:* Tibial nerve by fibres from S1 and S2.
- *Referred pain:* Most TrPs in the gastrocnemius muscle refer pain locally. TrPs in the belly of the medial head tend to refer pain to the instep of the foot, sometimes spreading to the lower posterior thigh, the back of the knee, and the posteromedial aspect of leg and ankle. The muscle also refers to the Achilles tendon (Mayoral del Moral et al., 2017), and, exceptionally, to the posterior thigh (Kellgren, 1938), with pain and increased tension in the hamstring muscles (Mayoral del Moral et al., 2017).
- *Needling technique:* The patient lies in the prone position with the knee slightly flexed and the leg supported by a pillow. For TrPs in the central part of the medial head, a pincer palpation is used to locate and fix the taut band and the TrP. The needle is angled medially, towards the thumb or fingers (Fig. 12.3). For TrPs in the central part of the lateral head, a flat

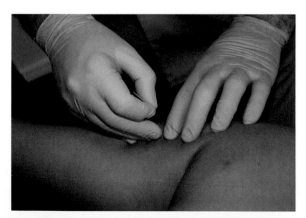

FIG. 12.2 Dry needling of the popliteus muscle.

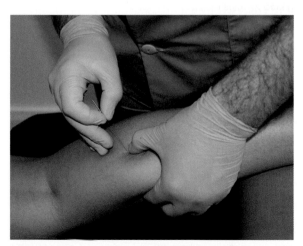

FIG. 12.3 Dry needling of the medial head of the gastrocnemius muscle.

palpation is more commonly used to locate and fix the taut band and the TrPs. The needle is directed perpendicular to the skin, aiming towards the TrP in a posteroanterior direction with a slightly lateral angulation (Fig. 12.4). For TrPs in the proximal part of any of both heads, flat palpation is used to locate and fix the TrPs. The needle is directed towards the TrP in a posteroanterior orientation (Fig. 12.5).

• *Precautions:* The sciatic nerve usually splits into the tibial and peroneal nerves in the lower third of the thigh. The tibial nerve, together with the popliteal vessels, runs along the popliteal fossa between the proximal parts of both heads of the gastrocnemius muscle. The fibularis nerve runs downward close to the biceps femoris muscle tendon. This means that the proximal part of the medial head of the gastrocnemius muscle lies between the tibial nerve along with the popliteal vessels and the tendons of the semitendinosus and semimembranosus muscles.

The proximal portion of the lateral head of gastrocnemius muscle and its TrPs are between the fibularis nerve and the tibial nerve. If needling of these proximal gastrocnemius TrPs is indicated, the popliteal fossa must be palpated thoroughly before the needling procedure to locate the nerves and tendons. Anatomical variations such as a premature split of the two divisions of the common fibularis nerve at the popliteal level may be identified, and needling TrPs in the proximal part of the lateral head of the gastrocnemius muscle or into the plantaris muscle would not be indicated. The recommended position to palpate this region is shown in Fig. 12.6. Clinicians should identify the available safe needling space between the semitendinosus muscle tendon and the tibialis nerve, and the space between the fibularis and tibialis nerves and their relationship with the biceps femoris muscle tendon. In the prone position, only the tendons are palpable (especially when the patient slightly contracts the knee flexors), and by using the tendons as landmark, the needle can be directed towards the safe spaces.

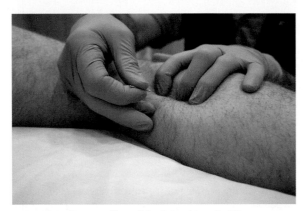

FIG. 12.4 Dry needling of the lateral head of the gastrocnemius muscle.

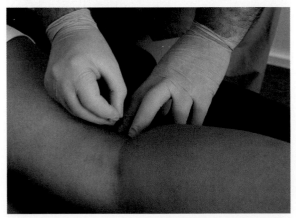

FIG. 12.5 Dry needling of the proximal part of the lateral head of the gastrocnemius muscle.

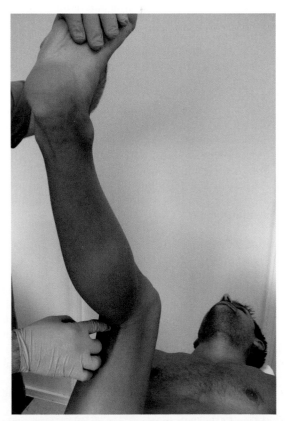

FIG. 12.6 Palpation of the posterior-lateral aspect of the knee (biceps femoris).

When needling the proximal portions of the gastrocnemius muscle, it is conceivable that the needle may touch the back part of the capsule of the knee joint, but there is no scientific evidence that this would increase the risk of infection. Nevertheless, Ernst and colleagues (2011) did mention several cases of septic arthritis in a review of adverse events of acupuncture, which suggests that disinfection of the skin should be considered.

- The medial sural cutaneous nerve descends between the two heads of the gastrocnemius muscle. When needling the central bellies of both heads of the gastrocnemius muscles, the midline must be avoided by angulating the needle laterally when needling the lateral head and medially when needling the medial head.

Plantaris Muscle

- *Anatomy:* Proximally, the plantaris muscle attaches to the upper part of the lateral condyle of the femur. Distally, its long tendon anchors to the medial aspect of the calcaneus, blending with the fibres of the Achilles tendon.
- *Function:* The main function of the plantaris muscle is plantar flexion and inversion of the foot. In a closed kinetic chain, it assists in knee flexion.
- *Innervation:* Tibial nerve through a branch containing fibres from L5, S1, and S2.
- *Referred pain:* The referred pain pattern of the plantaris muscle is to the back of the knee, sometimes reaching midcalf level.
- *Needling technique:* Because the plantaris muscle is partially covered by the upper part of the lateral head of gastrocnemius muscle, the needling technique is similar to the approach for the gastrocnemius muscle and shown in Fig. 12.5.
- *Precautions:* The tibial and fibularis nerves and popliteal vessels must be avoided similar to the gastrocnemius muscle.

Soleus Muscle

- *Anatomy:* The soleus muscle originates in the posterior aspect of the head and proximal third of the fibula, in the popliteal line of the tibia and in the tendinous arch between both bones. The soleus fibres attach distally to a superficial tendinous sheet, which continues directly to the Achilles tendon that in turn attaches to the posterior part of the calcaneus.
- *Function:* The function of the soleus muscle is plantar flexion and inversion of the foot.
- *Innervation:* A branch of the tibial nerve containing fibres from L5, S1, and S2.
- *Referred pain:* TrPs in the soleus muscle refer mostly to the distal part of the Achilles tendon, to the posterior and plantar surfaces of the heel, to the upper half of the calf, and, very rarely, to the ipsilateral sacroiliac joint. Simons and colleagues mentioned an exceptional referral pattern to the ipsilateral jaw area (Simons, et al., 1999).

- *Needling technique:* For distal medial or lateral TrPs, the muscle can be held in a pincer between the thumb and two fingers, with the patient either in prone (Fig. 12.7) or in a sidelying position. The needle is directed towards the opposite finger or thumb. In some patients the TrPs can also be needled with a flat palpation. Proximal TrPs can be needled towards the fibula with the patient lying on the uninvolved side (Fig. 12.8).
- *Precautions:* When needling the medial part of the muscle, care must be taken to avoid needling the tibial nerve.

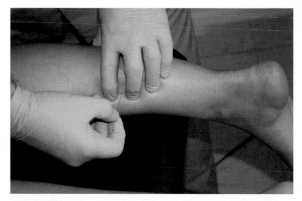

FIG. 12.7 Dry needling of the soleus muscle with pincer palpation.

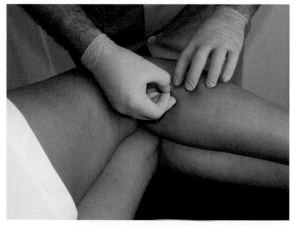

FIG. 12.8 Dry needling of the proximal part of soleus muscle.

Flexor Digitorum Longus Muscle

- *Anatomy:* Proximally, the flexor digitorum longus muscle attaches to the posterior aspect of the tibia and to the deep layer of the fascia cruris, which is the intermuscular septum shared with the tibialis posterior muscle. Distally, its four tendons attach to the base of the distal phalanx of the second, third, fourth, and fifth toes, respectively.
- *Function:* The function of the flexor digitorum longus muscle includes plantar flexion, inversion, and adduction of the foot, as well as flexion of the distal phalanx of each of the four lesser toes.
- *Innervation:* A branch of the tibial nerve containing fibres from L5 and S1.
- *Referred pain:* The flexor digitorum longus muscle refers mainly to the middle of the plantar forefoot. Sometimes the pain referral includes the medial side of the ankle and calf.
- *Needling technique:* With the patient lying on the involved side with the hip and knee flexed to about 90 degrees, TrPs are palpated with a flat technique right behind the posterior surface of the tibia. The needle is inserted towards the tibia, mainly in a lateral direction with a slightly anterior orientation (Fig. 12.9), keeping the needle close to the

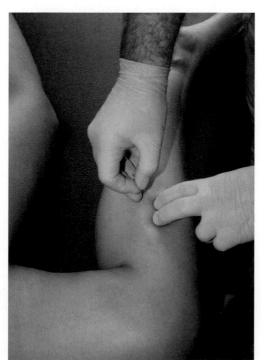

FIG. 12.9 Dry needling of the flexor digitorum longus muscle.

posterior aspect of the tibia or even touching the bone with the tip of the needle as a reference.
- *Precautions:* The tibial nerve and the posterior tibial vessels lie right behind the muscle. Keeping the needle close to the bone helps to avoid contact with the neurovascular bundle.

Tibialis Posterior Muscle

- *Anatomy:* Proximally, the tibialis posterior muscle originates on the inner posterior borders of the tibia and fibula and on the interosseous membrane. Distally, its tendon attaches to the bases of the second, third, and fourth metatarsals, the three cuneiforms, the cuboid, the tuberosity of the navicular, and the sustentaculum tali of the calcaneus.
- *Function:* Functions of the tibialis posterior muscle include supination and plantar flexion of the foot; it also contributes to stabilisation of the foot during weight-bearing activities.
- *Innervation:* Posterior tibial nerve, arising from the sciatic nerve and containing fibres from L5 and S1.
- *Referred pain:* The tibialis posterior muscle refers mainly to the Achilles tendon but often also refers to the sole of the foot and, less often, to the midcalf and heel.
- *Needling technique:* The recommended needling technique is similar to the approach described previously for the flexor digitorum longus muscle (see Fig. 12.9), with the only difference that the needle must be inserted deeper to reach the tibialis posterior muscle (see Fig. 12.1). Due to the deep location of the tibialis posterior muscle, palpation of TrPs in the muscle is not possible. Therefore to determine the site of the TrP, deep posteroanterior pressure is applied through the calf muscles in order to elicit deep tenderness that could possibly be attributed to the tibialis posterior muscle. The needle is used both as a therapeutic and as a diagnostic tool when the presence of the TrP is confirmed. In an alternate approach, the needle is inserted in an anterior to posterior direction through the tibialis anterior muscle, keeping the needle close to the tibia (Fig. 12.10).
- *Precautions:* In general, the needle is kept close to the tibia bone to avoid touching the neurovascular bundles, including the posterior tibial vessels and tibial nerve in the recommended technique and the anterior tibial vessels and deep peroneal nerve in the alternate technique. In the recommended approach, if the needle is inserted too deep, it will pierce the interosseous membrane and could touch the deep peroneal nerve, which the patient will experience as an electrical shooting pain towards the ankle and foot.

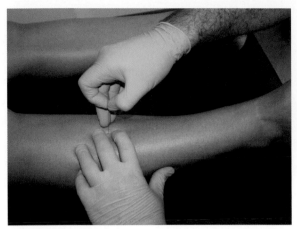

FIG. 12.10 Dry needling of the tibialis posterior muscle with an anterior approach.

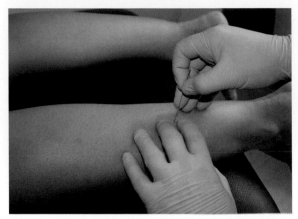

FIG. 12.11 Dry needling of the flexor hallucis longus muscle.

Considering the close proximity to major arteries and the wide anatomical variances, ultrasound guidance potentially increases the accuracy and decreases the risk when needling the tibialis posterior muscle.

Flexor Hallucis Longus Muscle

- *Anatomy:* The flexor hallucis longus muscle originates in the lower two-thirds of the posterior surface of the fibula and in the interosseous membrane. Its tendon anchors to the base of the distal phalanx of the great toe.
- *Function:* The function of the flexor hallucis longus muscle includes plantar flexion and inversion of the foot and flexion of the distal phalanx of the first toe.
- *Innervation:* A branch of the tibial nerve that contains fibres from L5, S1, and S2.
- *Referred pain:* The flexor hallucis longus muscle refers pain to the plantar surface of the first toe, including the head of the first metatarsal.
- *Needling technique:* With the patient in prone position, the muscle is palpated using a flat palpation technique for tenderness, applying deep anterior pressure just lateral to the midline against the fibula through the soleus muscle, gastrocnemius muscles, and the aponeurosis, which at a lower level will become the Achilles tendon. If tenderness is found, the needle will both confirm and treat the TrP with an anterior and slightly lateral needling direction (Fig. 12.11). The posterior aspect of the fibula is used as an anatomical landmark to assure the proper position of the needle and a sufficient depth of penetration.
- *Precautions:* Directing the needle laterally towards the fibula decreases the possibility of touching the peroneal vessels.

Fibularis Longus and Brevis Muscles

- *Anatomy:* The fibularis longus muscle arises from the head and upper two-thirds of the lateral surface of the body of the fibula and also from the intermuscular septa between it and the adjacent muscles. It inserts in the ventral and lateral sides of the base of the first metatarsal bone and of the medial cuneiform. The fibularis brevis muscle originates in the lower two-thirds of the lateral aspect of the body of the fibula and in the adjacent intermuscular septa and is partially covered by the fibularis longus muscle. It inserts into the tuberosity at the lateral side of the base of the fifth metatarsal bone.
- *Function:* The function of the fibularis muscles is stabilisation of the leg upon the foot and plantar flexion and eversion of the foot.
- *Innervation:* Superficial fibularis nerve through branches containing fibres from L4, L5, and S1.
- *Referred pain:* The muscles refer pain chiefly above, behind, and below the lateral malleolus of the ankle and a short distance along the lateral surface of the foot. TrPs in the fibularis longus muscle may also refer pain to the lateral aspect of the leg.
- *Needling technique:* With the patient lying on the uninvolved side with hips and knees flexed to approximately 90 degrees, the muscle is palpated with a flat technique, and the needle is inserted perpendicular to the skin in a lateral to medial direction, towards the fibula (Fig. 12.12). As an alternative, the needle can also be inserted a short distance away from the TrP and directed in a gradually deeper fashion towards the TrP, which helps in avoiding needling the common fibularis nerve.
- *Precautions:* In the proximal third of the fibularis longus muscle, care must be taken to avoid needling

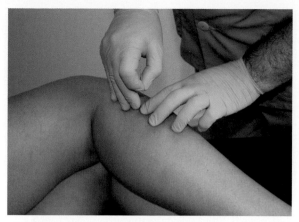

FIG. 12.12 Dry needling of the fibularis longus muscle.

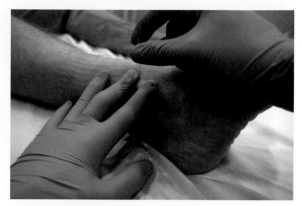

FIG. 12.13 Dry needling of the fibularis tertius muscle.

the common fibularis nerve, which lies deep to the muscle. The superficial fibularis nerve runs between the fibularis brevis and tertius muscles. When needling the fibularis brevis muscle, clinicians must avoid needling into an anterior direction and, as a rule, needle away from the nerve.

Fibularis Tertius Muscle

- *Anatomy:* The fibularis tertius muscle originates in the lower half of the anterior aspect of the fibula and in the crural intermuscular septum between it and the fibularis brevis muscle. It inserts in the mediodorsal surface of the base of the metatarsal bone of the fifth digit and in the base of the fourth metatarsal.
- *Function:* The function of the fibularis tertius muscle includes eversion and dorsiflexion of the foot.
- *Innervation:* Deep fibularis nerve with fibres coming from L5 and S1.
- *Referred pain:* The fibularis tertius muscle refers pain primarily to the anterolateral side of the ankle and, sometimes, to the lateral side of the heel.
- *Needling technique:* With the patient lying in supine position, TrPs are located by flat palpation. The needle is aimed in an anteroposterior direction against the fibula (Fig. 12.13).
- *Precautions:* Directing the needle laterally passed the fibula must be avoided to steer clear of the superficial fibularis nerve, which runs between both the fibularis brevis and tertius muscles.

Tibialis Anterior Muscle

- *Anatomy:* The tibialis anterior muscle originates in the upper two-thirds of the lateral surface of the tibia and inserts into the medial and plantar aspects of the medial cuneiform bone and into the medial surface of the base of the first metatarsal bone.
- *Function:* The function of the tibialis anterior muscle includes dorsiflexion and supination of the foot.
- *Innervation:* Deep fibularis nerve with fibres coming from L4, L5, and S1.
- *Referred pain:* The tibialis anterior muscle refers to the anteromedial aspect of the ankle and over the great toe. Sometimes, its TrPs also refer to the shin and to the anteromedial surface of the foot.
- *Needling technique:* With the patient in the supine position, the TrP is located with a flat palpation technique, and the needle is directed with a slightly medial direction towards the tibia (Fig. 12.14A). As an alternative, the needle can also be inserted a short distance away from the TrP and directed in a gradually deeper fashion towards the TrP, which helps in avoiding needling the underlying neurovascular structures (Fig. 12.14B).
- *Precautions:* The neurovascular bundle, formed by the anterior tibial artery and vein and the deep fibularis nerve, runs right behind the lateral part of the tibialis anterior muscle. Directing the needle into a medial direction towards the tibia avoids contacting with these structures.

Extensor Digitorum Longus Muscle

- *Anatomy:* The extensor digitorum longus muscle originates from the lateral condyle of the tibia, from the upper three-fourths of the anterior surface of the body of the fibula, from the upper part of the interosseous membrane, and from the intermuscular septa between it and the tibialis anterior muscle on the medial side and the peroneal muscles on the lateral side. Distally, its tendon divides into four slips that insert in the second and third phalanges of the four lesser toes.

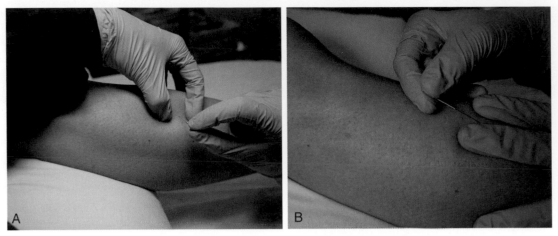

FIG. 12.14 Dry needling of the tibialis anterior muscle.

- *Function:* The functions of the extensor digitorum longus muscle include dorsiflexion and eversion of the foot and extension of the four lesser toes.
- *Innervation:* Branches of the deep fibularis nerve containing fibres from L4, L5, and S1.
- *Referred pain:* The extensor digitorum longus muscle refers to the dorsum of the foot and toes.
- *Needling technique:* With the patient supine, TrPs are located by flat palpation, and the needle is inserted close to the border of the tibialis anterior muscle in an anteroposterior direction towards the fibula (Fig. 12.15).
- *Precautions:* Care must be taken to avoid touching the deep fibularis nerve, which, in the proximal part of the muscle, lies deep underneath the muscle. Directing the needle towards the fibula avoids contact with the neurovascular bundle.

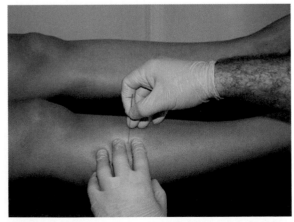

FIG. 12.15 Dry needling of the extensor digitorum longus muscle.

Extensor Hallucis Longus Muscle

- *Anatomy:* The extensor hallucis longus muscle originates from the middle two-fourths of the anteromedial surface of the fibula medial to the origin of the extensor digitorum longus muscle and also from the interosseous membrane. Its tendon attaches distally to the base of the distal phalanx of the great toe, and through an expansion of the tendon, it also attaches usually to the base of the proximal phalanx.
- *Function:* The functions of the extensor hallucis longus muscle include dorsiflexion and inversion of the foot and extension of the great toe.
- *Innervation:* Branches of the deep fibularis nerve containing fibres from L4, L5, and S1.
- *Referred pain:* The extensor hallucis longus muscle refers to the distal aspect of the dorsum of the first metatarsal, sometimes spreading distally to the tip of the great toe.
- *Needling technique:* The patient is in the supine position. The TrP is located with a flat palpation technique, and the needle is inserted close to the lateral border of the tibialis anterior muscle in an anteroposterior direction with a lateral angulation towards the fibula (Fig. 12.16).
- *Precautions:* The deep fibularis nerve and the anterior tibial vessels are covered by the tibialis anterior muscle and by the medial part of the extensor hallucis longus muscle. Directing the needle laterally towards the fibula helps to avoid contact with the neurovascular bundle.

Extensor Digitorum Brevis and Extensor Hallucis Brevis Muscles

- *Anatomy:* The extensor digitorum brevis and extensor hallucis brevis muscles anchor proximally to the

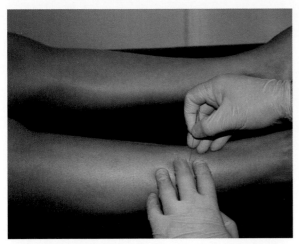

FIG. 12.16 Dry needling of the extensor hallucis longus muscle.

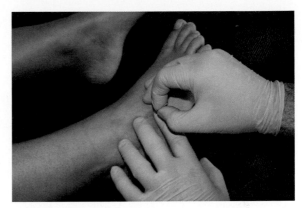

FIG. 12.17 Dry needling of the extensor digitorum brevis and extensor hallucis brevis muscles.

superior aspect of the calcaneus, to the lateral talocalcaneal ligament, and to the cruciate crural ligament. Distally, the extensor hallucis brevis muscle inserts at the dorsal surface of the base of the first phalanx of the great toe, and the extensor digitorum brevis muscle ends in three tendons, which insert into the lateral sides of the tendons of the extensor digitorum longus muscle of the second, third, and fourth toes.

- *Function:* The extensor digitorum brevis muscle extends the second, third, and fourth toes. The oblique direction of its traction counteracts the obliquity given to the toes by the long extensor, which produces an even extension when both muscles contract. The extensor hallucis brevis extends the proximal phalanx of the great toe.
- *Innervation:* Deep fibularis nerve with fibres from L5 and S1.
- *Referred pain:* The extensor digitorum brevis and extensor hallucis brevis muscles refer to the dorsum of the foot.
- *Needling technique:* The patient is in the supine position. The taut band and the TrPs are located with a flat palpation technique. The needle is directed perpendicular to the skin towards the TrPs. Most of the times the needle will make contact with the underlying bone (Fig. 12.17).
- *Precautions:* The deep fibularis nerve and the dorsal vessels of the foot run medial to the extensor hallucis brevis muscle; consequently, when needling this muscle directing the needle medially must be avoided.

Abductor Hallucis Muscle

- *Anatomy:* Proximally, the abductor hallucis muscle attaches to the medial process of the tuberosity of

the calcaneus, to the laciniate ligament (flexor retinaculum of the foot), to the plantar aponeurosis, and to the intermuscular septum between it and the flexor digitorum brevis muscle. Distally, its tendon inserts together with the medial tendon of the flexor hallucis brevis muscle into the medial or the plantar side of the base of the first phalanx of the great toe.

- *Function:* The functions of the abductor hallucis muscle include flexion and abduction of the first phalanx of the great toe.
- *Innervation:* Medial plantar nerve that carries fibres from L5 and S1.
- *Referred pain:* The abductor hallucis muscle refers primarily to the medial side of the heel, occasionally including the instep.
- *Needling technique:* The patient is lying on the involved side. The therapist sits by the table, facing the feet of the patient. The arm of the therapist passes over the patient's involved leg and holds it firmly on the table to avoid unexpected movements of the extremity. TrPs are located using a flat palpation technique and the needle is inserted perpendicular to the skin, in a lateral direction, towards the underlying bone (Fig. 12.18).
- *Precautions:* The neurovascular bundle, formed by the tibialis posterior vessels and the medial and lateral plantar nerves, passes deep to the proximal third of this muscle. Ideally, these structures are avoided when needling this part of the muscle, but it is often not possible to identify the plantar nerves.

Abductor Digiti Minimi Muscle

- *Anatomy:* Proximally, the abductor digiti minimi muscle attaches to the lateral process of the tuberosity of the calcaneus, to the inferior surface of the calcaneus

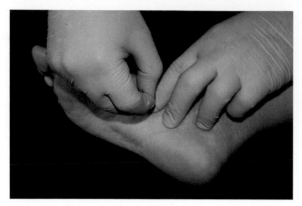

FIG. 12.18 Dry needling of the abductor hallucis muscle.

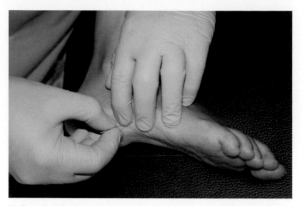

FIG. 12.19 Dry needling of the abductor digiti minimi muscle.

between the two processes of the tuberosity, to the front part of the medial process, to the plantar aponeurosis, and to the intermuscular septum between it and the flexor digitorum brevis. Distally, its tendon inserts with the flexor digiti minimi brevis into the fibular side of the base of the first phalanx of the fifth toe.

- *Function:* The functions of the abductor digiti minimi muscle include abduction and flexion of the proximal phalanx of the fifth toe.
- *Innervation:* Lateral plantar nerve through fibres from S1 and S2.
- *Referred pain:* The abductor digiti minimi muscle refers mainly to the plantar side of the fifth metatarsal head.
- *Needling technique:* With the patient lying on the uninvolved side, the therapist sits by the table, facing the feet of the patient. The arm of the therapist passes over the patient's involved leg and holds it firmly on the table to avoid unexpected movements of the extremity. TrPs are located either by flat or by pincer palpation. In both ways the needle is directed in a medial and dorsal direction towards the underlying bone (Fig. 12.19). Because the fifth toe is free to move, the local twitch responses can be seen as minor abduction and flexion movements.
- *Precautions:* The medial margin of the muscle is close to the lateral plantar vessels and nerves. Directing the needle towards the bone avoids touching these neurovascular structures. It is often not possible to identify the plantar nerves.

Flexor Digitorum Brevis Muscle

- *Anatomy:* Proximally, the flexor digitorum brevis muscle arises from the medial process of the tuberosity of the calcaneus, from the plantar fascia, and

from the adjacent intermuscular septa. Distally, it divides into four tendons, one for each of the four lesser toes. At the base of the first phalanx, each tendon divides into two slips to allow passage of the corresponding tendon of the flexor digitorum longus. The two portions of the tendon then reunite; finally, it splits a second time and is inserted into both sides of the second phalanx.

- *Function:* The function of the flexor digitorum brevis muscle is flexion of the second phalanx of each of the four lesser toes.
- *Innervation:* Medial plantar nerve by fibres coming from L5 and S1.
- *Referred pain:* The flexor digitorum brevis muscle refers mainly to the sole over the heads of the second through fourth metatarsals. Sporadically, pain spills over into the head of the fifth metatarsal.
- *Needling technique:* With the patient in the prone position, the therapist sits by the table, facing the feet of the patient. The arm of the therapist passes over the patient's involved leg and holds it firmly on the table to avoid unexpected movements of the extremity. TrPs are palpated with a flat palpation technique. It is sometimes difficult to distinguish tenderness due to strain of the plantar fascia, to TrPs in the flexor digitorum brevis muscle, to TrPs in quadratus plantaris muscle, or to any combination of the three. DN is a viable treatment for any of these conditions. The needle is directed towards the palpated tender area in a plantar to dorsal direction (Fig. 12.20) until the tip reaches the bone, which suggests that the three possibly involved structures have been addressed.
- *Precautions:* The lateral plantar vessels and nerve and, to a lesser extent, the medial plantar nerve lie between the flexor digitorum brevis muscle and

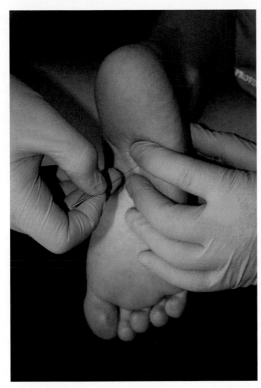

FIG. 12.20 Dry needling of the flexor digitorum brevis and quadratus plantae muscle.

quadratus plantaris muscle. The needle must be handled carefully to avoid touching these structures, although it may not be possible to identify the plantar nerves.

Quadratus Plantaris/Flexor Accessorius Muscle

- *Anatomy:* The quadratus plantaris muscle has two heads, which are separated from each other by the long plantar ligament. The medial and larger head originates in the medial concave surface of the calcaneus. The lateral head, flat and tendinous, arises from the lateral border of the calcaneus and from the long plantar ligament. Both heads join at an acute angle and end in a flattened band, which inserts into the lateral margin and upper and under surfaces of the tendon of the flexor digitorum longus. Note that in the US nomenclature, the quadratus plantaris muscle is now referred to as the flexor accessorius muscle.
- *Function:* The quadratus plantaris muscle assists the flexor digitorum longus in flexion of the four lesser toes, offsetting the oblique pull of this muscle.

- *Innervation:* Lateral plantar nerve by fibres from S2 and S3.
- *Referred pain:* The quadratus plantaris muscle refers to the plantar surface of the heel.
- *Needling technique:* The recommended technique is the same as described previously for the flexor digitorum brevis muscle (see Fig. 12.20). For the quadratus plantaris muscle, the needle can also be inserted through the instep, in a medial to lateral direction, right below the bone. This technique is better tolerated by some patients and may be safer considering the neurovascular bundle; however, in our experience, this approach is much less effective and should be reserved for patients with a low pain threshold.
- *Precautions:* The lateral plantar vessels and nerve and, to a lesser extent, the medial plantar nerve lie between the flexor digitorum brevis muscle and quadratus plantaris muscle. The needle must be handled carefully to avoid touching these structures, although it may not be possible to identify the plantar nerves.

Flexor Hallucis Brevis Muscle

- *Anatomy:* Proximally, the flexor hallucis brevis muscle anchors to the medial part of the under surface of the cuboid bone, to the contiguous portion of the third cuneiform, and to the prolongation of the tendon of the tibialis posterior muscle, which is attached to that bone. It then divides into two portions, which insert distally into the medial and lateral aspects of the base of the first phalanx of the great toe. A sesamoid bone is present in each tendon at its insertion.
- *Function:* The function of the flexor hallucis brevis muscle includes flexion of the first phalanx of the great toe at the metatarsophalangeal joint. The medial head abducts the first phalanx, and the lateral head adducts the first phalanx.
- *Innervation:* Medial plantar nerve containing fibres from L5 and S1.
- *Referred pain:* The flexor hallucis brevis muscle refers primarily to the plantar and medial aspects of the head of the first metatarsal with occasional spillover into the entire great toe and a good part of the second toe.
- *Needling technique:* The patient lies on the involved side. The arm of the therapist passes over the patient's involved leg and holds it firmly on the table to avoid unexpected movements of the extremity. TrPs are palpated with a flat palpation technique. The needle is inserted from the medial side of the foot, right below the first metatarsal bone (Fig. 12.21). When the needle hits the TrP, local twitch responses

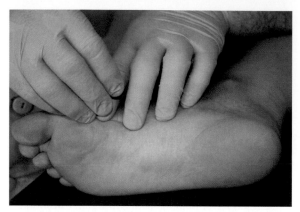

FIG. 12.21 Dry needling of the flexor hallucis brevis and adductor hallucis muscles.

may produce abrupt flexion movements of the first phalanx of the great toe.

- *Precautions:* The proper digital nerve runs adjacent to the plantar surface of the medial head of this muscle. The needle must be handled carefully and stay close to the bone to avoid touching the nerve.

Adductor Hallucis Muscle

- *Anatomy:* The adductor hallucis muscle has two heads. The oblique head arises from the bases of the second, third, and fourth metatarsal bones and from the sheath of the tendon of the fibularis longus muscle. Distally, it inserts together with the lateral head of the flexor hallucis brevis muscle into the lateral side of the base of the first phalanx of the great toe. The transverse head arises from the plantar metatarsophalangeal ligaments of the third, fourth, and fifth toes and from the transverse ligament of the metatarsus. It inserts into the lateral side of the base of the first phalanx of the great toe, blending with the tendon of insertion of the oblique head.
- *Function:* The functions of the adductor hallucis muscle include adduction of the great toe and flexion of the proximal phalanx of the great toe.
- *Innervation:* Lateral plantar nerve by fibres from S2 and S3.
- *Referred pain:* The adductor hallucis muscle refers to the sole of the foot in the area of the first through fourth metatarsal heads.
- *Needling technique:* Because the oblique head of the muscle is practically in the same plane as the flexor hallucis brevis, side by side with its lateral head, the needling technique for the oblique head of the adductor hallucis muscle is the same described previously for the flexor hallucis brevis muscle

(see Fig. 12.21), although to reach the oblique head of the adductor hallucis muscle the needle needs to be advanced further. Local twitch responses may move the great toe towards the second toe, which confirms that a TrP was needled. TrPs in the oblique head of the adductor hallucis muscle can also be needled directly from the sole of the foot. The transverse head is better approached from the dorsum of the foot. The arm of the therapist passes over the patient's involved leg and holds it firmly on the table to avoid unexpected movements of the extremity. TrPs are palpated with a flat palpation technique at the sole of the foot just proximal to the metatarsal heads. When a TrP is located the finger of the therapist stays pointing to the TrP, and the needle is inserted in the dorsum of the foot, aiming at the therapist's finger, through the interosseous space which better allows the TrP to be reached (Figs. 12.22 and 12.23). In a way, this is a modified pincer needling technique.

- *Precautions:* The precautions for the oblique head of the adductor hallucis muscle are the same as for the flexor hallucis brevis muscle. For the transverse head, depending on which interosseous space is being needled, the needle could possibly contact the medial or the lateral branches of the superficial fibular nerve, the terminal medial branch of the deep fibular nerve, the common plantar digital nerves, or the medial plantar nerve. Considering the small diameter of these branches, it is unlikely that a needle would cause any significant injury; however,

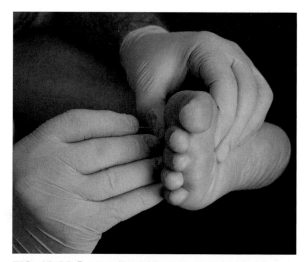

FIG. 12.22 Dry needling of the transverse head of the adductor hallucis muscle and of the dorsal and plantar interossei muscles.

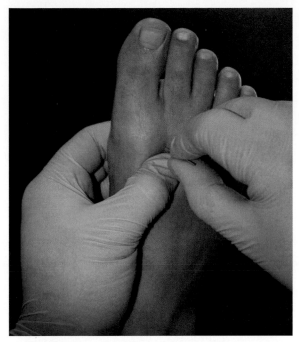

FIG. 12.23 Dry needling of the transverse head of the adductor hallucis muscle and of the dorsal and plantar interossei muscles.

clinicians should be aware of the potential risk (Mayoral del Moral et al., 2017).

Dorsal and Plantar Interossei Muscles

- *Anatomy:* There are four dorsal interossei and three plantar interossei in the foot. Proximally, each dorsal interosseous muscle originates in the proximal half of the two adjacent metatarsal bones and inserts distally at the base of the first phalanx and at the aponeurosis of the tendon of the extensor digitorum longus. Thus the first dorsal interosseous inserts into the medial side of the second toe and the other three insert into the lateral sides of the second, third, and fourth toes. Proximally, each plantar interosseous attaches to the base and medial half of the third, fourth, or fifth metatarsal and anchors distally to the medial side of the base of the first phalanx of the same digit and usually to the dorsal aponeurosis of the extensor digitorum longus tendon.
- *Function:* The dorsal interossei abduct the second, third, and fourth toes, flex the first phalanges, and extend the second and the third phalanges of these toes. The plantar interossei adduct the third, fourth, and fifth toes, flex the

first phalanges, and extend the third phalanges of these same toes.
- *Innervation:* All interossei are innervated by the lateral plantar nerve by fibres from S2 and S3.
- *Referred pain:* The interossei muscles refer to the side of the digit to which the tendon anchors, to the dorsum, and to the sole of the foot along the distal part of the corresponding metatarsal.
- *Needling technique:* With the patient supine, the arm of the therapist passes over the patient's involved leg to hold it firmly on the table to avoid unexpected movements of the extremity. The clinician assesses the muscles for spot tenderness using a flat palpation technique. As an alternative, the eraser part of a wooden pencil can be used, which allows getting in between the metatarsal bones. The needle is inserted from the dorsal aspect towards the tender spot and the opposing finger using a modified pincer palpation. The needle must probe in both lateral and medial directions to explore both heads of the dorsal interosseous and also the corresponding plantar interosseous (see Fig. 12.23). Movement of the toes should not be restricted by the palpating hand because abduction or adduction movements produced by local twitch responses will indicate which interosseous muscle was treated.
- *Precautions:* The same precautions as described for the transverse head of the adductor hallucis muscle apply to the interossei muscles.

REFERENCES

Aceituno, J. (2003). Dolor persistente en hueco poplíteo tras prótesis total de rodilla: incidencia y tratamiento del punto gatillo 3 del gastrocnemio. *Fisioterapia, 25,* 209–214.

Ajimsha, M. S., Binsu, D., & Chithra, S. (2014). Effectiveness of myofascial release in the management of plantar heel pain: a randomized controlled trial. *The Foot, 24*(2), 66–71.

Akhbari, B., Salavati, M., Ezzati, K., & Mohammadian, S. (2014). The use of dry needling and myofascial meridians in a case of plantar fasciitis. *Journal of Chiropractic Medicine, 13,* 43–48.

Allen, G., Galer, B. S., & Schwartz, L. (1999). Epidemiology of complex regional pain syndrome: a retrospective chart review of 134 patients. *Pain, 80,* 539–544.

Aparicio, E. Q., Quirante, L. B., Blanco, C. R., & Sendin, F. A. (2009). Immediate effects of the suboccipital muscle inhibition technique in subjects with short hamstring syndrome. *Journal of Manipulative and Physiological Therapeutics, 32*(4), 262–269.

Bretischwerdt, C., Rivas-Cano, L., Palomeque-del-Cerro, L., Fernández-de-las-Peñas, C., & Alburquerque-Sendin, F.

(2010). Immediate effects of hamstring muscle stretching on pressure pain sensitivity and active mouth opening in healthy subjects. *Journal of Manipulative and Physiological Therapeutics, 33*(1), 42–47.

Bouche, R. T., & Johnson, C. H. (2007). Medial tibial stress syndrome (tibial fasciitis): a proposed pathomechanical model involving fascial traction. *Journal of the American Podiatric Medical Association, 97*, 31–36.

Chang, S. H. (2017). Complex regional pain syndrome is a manifestation of the worsened myofascial pain syndrome: case review. *Journal of Pain Research, 6*(4), 1000294.

Cho, S. H., Kim, S. H., & Park, D. J. (2015). The comparison of the immediate effects of application of the suboccipital muscle inhibition and self-myofascial release techniques in the suboccipital region on short hamstring. *Journal of Physical Therapy Science, 27*(1), 195–197.

Chaudhry, F. A. (2017). Effectiveness of dry needling and high-volume image-guided injection in the management of chronic mid-portion Achilles tendinopathy in adult population: a literature review. *European Journal of Orthopaedic Surgery and Traumatology, 27*(4), 441–448.

Cotchett, M. P., Landorf, K. B., & Munteanu, S. E. (2010). Effectiveness of dry needling and injections of myofascial trigger points associated with plantar heel pain: a systematic review. *Journal of Foot and Ankle Research, 3*, 18.

Cotchett, M. P., Munteanu, S. E., & Landorf, K. B. (2014). Effectiveness of trigger point dry needling for plantar heel pain: a randomized controlled trial. *Physical Therapy, 94*(8), 1083–1094.

Crotti, F. M., Carai, A., Carai, M., Sgaramella, E., & Sias, W. (2005). Entrapment of crural branches of the common peroneal nerve. *Acta Neurochirurgica Supplement, 92*, 69–70.

Cuccia, A. M. (2011). Interrelationships between dental occlusion and plantar arch. *Journal of Bodywork and Movement Therapies, 15*(2), 242–250.

Dejung, B., Gröbli, C., Colla, F., & Weissmann, R. (2001). *Triggerpunkt-Therapie. Die Behandlung akuter und chronischer Schmerzen im Bewegungsapparat mit manueller Triggerpunkt-Therapie und Dry Needling.* Bern: Verlag Hans Huber.

Dommerholt, J. (2004). Complex regional pain syndrome 2: physical therapy management. *Journal of Bodywork and Movement Therapies, 8*, 241–248.

Eftekharsadat, B., Babaei-Ghazani, A., & Zeinolabedinzadeh, V. (2016). Dry needling in patients with chronic heel pain due to plantar fasciitis: a single-blinded randomized clinical trial. *Medical Journal of the Islamic Republic of Iran, 30*, 401.

Ernst, E., Lee, M. S., & Choi, T. Y. (2011). Acupuncture: does it alleviate pain and are there serious risks? A review of reviews. *Pain, 152*(4), 755–764.

Espejo-Antúnez, L., Castro-Valenzuela, E., Ribeiro, F., Albornoz-Cabello, M., Silva, A., & Rodriguez-Mansilla, J. (2016). Immediate effects of hamstring stretching alone or combined with ischemic compression of the masseter muscle on hamstrings extensibility, active mouth opening and pain in athletes with temporomandibular dysfunction. *Journal of Bodywork and Movement Therapies, 20*(3), 579–587.

Ge, H. Y., Zhang, Y., Boudreau, S., Yue, S. W., & Arendt-Nielsen, L. (2008). Induction of muscle cramps by nociceptive stimulation of latent myofascial trigger points. *Experimental Brain Research, 187*, 623–629.

Grieve, R., Barnett, S., Coghill, N., & Cramp, F. (2013a). Myofascial trigger point therapy for triceps surae dysfunction: a case series. *Manual Therapy, 18*(6), 519–525.

Grieve, R., Cranston, A., Henderson, A., John, R., Malone, G., & Mayall, C. (2013b). The immediate effect of triceps surae myofascial trigger point therapy on restricted active ankle joint dorsiflexion in recreational runners: a crossover randomised controlled trial. *Journal of Bodywork and Movement Therapies, 17*(4), 453–461.

Hains, G., Boucher, P. B., & Lamy, A. M. (2015). Ischemic compression and joint mobilisation for the treatment of nonspecific myofascial foot pain: findings from two quasi-experimental before-and-after studies. *Journal of the Canadian Chiropractic Association, 59*(1), 72–83.

He, C., & Ma, H. (2017). Effectiveness of trigger point dry needling for plantar heel pain: a meta-analysis of seven randomized controlled trials. *Journal of Pain Research, 10*, 1933–1942.

Hong, S., Park, Y., & Lateral, Lee C. N. (2017). Medullary infarction caused by Oriental acupuncture. *European Neurology, 79*(1-2), 63.

Imamura, M., Fischer, A. A., Imamura, S. T., Kaziyama, H. S., Carvalho, A. E., & Salomao, O. (1998). Treatment of myofascial pain components in plantar fasciitis speeds up recovery: documentation by algometry. *Journal of Musculoskeletal Pain, 6*, 91–110.

Kellgren, J. H. (1938). Observations on referred pain arising from muscle. *Clinical Science, 3*, 175–190.

Kushner, R. M., & Ferguson, L. W. (2005). Heel and arch pain. In L. W. Ferguson & R. D. Gerwin (Eds.), *Clinical mastery in the treatment of myofascial pain* (pp. 391–413). Baltimore: Lippincot Williams & Wilkins.

Lewit, K. (2010). *Manipulative therapy. Musculoskeletal medicine.* Edinburgh: Churchill Livingstone-Elsevier.

Madeley, L. T., Munteanu, S. E., & Bonanno, D. R. (2007). Endurance of the ankle joint plantar flexor muscles in athletes with medial tibial stress syndrome: a case-control study. *Journal of Science and Medicine in Sport, 10*, 356–362.

Mayoral, O., Salvat, I., Martin, M. T., Martin, S., Santiago, J., Cotarelo, J., & Rodriguez, C. (2013). Efficacy of myofascial trigger point dry needling in the prevention of pain after total knee arthroplasty: a randomized, double-blinded, placebo-controlled trial. *Evidence-based Complementary and Alternative Medicine. 2013*: 694941.

Mayoral del Moral, O., Torres Lacomba, I., & Sánchez Méndez, Ó. (2017). Punción seca de músculos y otras estructuras de la pierna y el pie. In O. Mayoral del Moral & I. Salvat Salvat (Eds.), *Fisioterapia invasiva del síndrome de dolor miofascial. Manual de punción seca de puntos gatillo.* Editorial Médica Panamericana: Madrid.

Michael, R. H., & Holder, L. E. (1985). The soleus syndrome. A cause of medial tibial stress (shin splints). *The American Journal of Sports Medicine, 13*, 87–94.

Moghtaderi, A., Khosrawi, S., & Dehghan, F. (2014). Extracorporeal shock wave therapy of gastroc-soleus trigger points in patients with plantar fasciitis: a randomized, placebo-controlled trial. *Advanced Biomedical Research, 3,* 99.

Muñoz, M., Calvo, S., Dommerholt, J., & Herrero, P. (2018). Dry needling and anti-thrombotic drugs; what do we know so far and what are the clinical implications for dry needling. *Acupuncture in Medicine.* In press.

Nguyen, B. M. (2010). Trigger point therapy and plantar heel pain: a case report. *The Foot, 20,* 158–162.

Pérez Costa, E., & Torres-Lacomba, M. (2016). Presencia de puntos gatillo miofasciales en futbolistas de competición con dolor de tobillo: estudio piloto transversal. *Fisioterapia, 38*(6), 280–285.

Prateepavanich, P., Kupniratsaikul, V., & Charoensak, T. (1999). The relationship between myofascial trigger points of gastrocnemius muscle and nocturnal calf cramps. *Journal of the Medical Association of Thailand, 82,* 451–459.

Renan-Ordine, R., Alburquerque-Sendin, F., de Souza, D. P., Cleland, J. A., & Fernández-de-las-Peñas, C. (2011). Effectiveness of myofascial trigger point manual therapy combined with a self-stretching protocol for the management of plantar heel pain: a randomized controlled trial. *The Journal of Orthopaedic and Sports Physical Therapy, 41,* 43–50.

Rodriguez-Blanco, C., Cocera-Morata, F. M., Heredia-Rizo, A. M., Ricard, F., Almazan-Campos, G., & Oliva-Pascual-Vaca, A. (2015). Immediate effects of combining local techniques in the craniomandibular area and hamstring muscle stretching in subjects with temporomandibular disorders: a randomized controlled study. *Journal of Alternative and Complementary Medicine, 21*(8), 451–459.

Rodríguez Fernández, A. L., Bartolomé Martín, J. L., Martínez Cepa, C. B., Coronel del Río, L. A., & Pérez-Caballer Pérez, A. (2005). Dolor miofascial tras la artroscopia de rodilla: estudio de la prevalencia y de los posibles factores de activación. *Fisioterapia, 27,* 201–209.

Safarpour, D., & Jabbari, B. (2010). Botulinum toxin A (Botox) for treatment of proximal myofascial pain in complex regional pain syndrome: two cases. *Pain Medicine, 11,* 1415–1418.

Saggini, R., Bellomo, R. G., Affaitati, G., Lapenna, D., & Giamberardino, M. A. (2007). Sensory and biomechanical characterization of two painful syndromes in the heel. *The Journal of Pain, 8*(3), 215–222.

Saggini, R., Giamberardino, M. A., Gatteschi, L., & Vecchiet, L. (1996). Myofascial pain syndrome of the peroneus longus: biomechanical approach. *The Clinical Journal of Pain, 12,* 30–37.

Salom-Moreno, J., Ayuso-Casado, B., Tamaral-Costa, B., Sánchez-Milá, Z., Fernández-de-las-Peñas, C., & Alburquerque-Sendi, F. (2015). Trigger point dry needling and proprioceptive exercises for the management of chronic ankle instability: a randomized clinical trial. *Evidence-based complementary and alternative medicine: eCAM.* 2015.

Sanz, D. R., Lobo, C. C., Lopez, D. L., Morales, C. R., Marin, C. S., & Corbalan, I. S. (2016). Interrater reliability in the clinical evaluation of myofascial trigger points in three ankle muscles. *Journal of Manipulative and Physiological Therapeutics, 39*(9), 623–634.

Sconfienza, L. M., Lacelli, F., Bandirali, M., Perrone, N., Serafini, G., & Silvestri, E. (2011). Long-term survey of three different ultrasound guided percutaneous treatments of plantar fasciitis: results of a randomized controlled trial [abstract]. *Ultraschall in der Medizin, 32,* 99–100.

Segura-Perez, M., Hernandez-Criado, M. T., Calvo-Lobo, C., Vega-Piris, L., Fernandez-Martin, R., & Rodriguez-Sanz, D. A. (2017). Multimodal approach for myofascial pain syndrome: a prospective study. *Journal of Manipulative and Physiological Therapeutics, 40*(6), 397–403.

Simons, D. G., Travell, J. G., & Simons, L. S. (1999). *Myofascial pain and dysfunction. The trigger point manual. Upper half of body* (2 ed.). Baltimore: Williams & Wilkins.

Travell, J. G., & Simons, D. G. (1992). *Myofascial pain and dysfunction. The trigger point manual. The lower extremities.* Baltimore: Williams & Wilkins.

Vas, L., Khandagale, N., & Pai, R. (2014). Successful management of chronic postsurgical pain following total knee replacement. *Pain Medicine, 15*(10), 1781–1785.

Xu, Y. M., Ge, H. Y., & Arendt-Nielsen, L. (2010). Sustained nociceptive mechanical stimulation of latent myofascial trigger point induces central sensitization in healthy subjects. *The Journal of Pain, 11,* 1348–1355.

Zuil-Escobar, J. C., Martinez-Cepa, C. B., Martin-Urrialde, J. A., & Gomez-Conesa, A. (2015). Prevalence of myofascial trigger points and diagnostic criteria of different muscles in function of the medial longitudinal arch. *Archives of Physical Medicine and Rehabilitation, 96*(6), 1123–1130.

Zuil-Escobar, J. C., Martinez-Cepa, C. B., Martin-Urrialde, J. A., & Gomez-Conesa, A. (2016). The prevalence of latent trigger points in lower limb muscles in asymptomatic subjects. *PM & R: The Journal of Injury, Function, and Rehabilitation, 8*(11), 1055–1064.

CHAPTER 13

Superficial Dry Needling

PETER BALDRY (1920–2016)

INTRODUCTION

After a long and distinguished career with many contributions to a broad range of medical applications, not the least the field of dry needling, Dr. Peter Baldry has passed away. In honor and recognition of his many contributions, we have not altered this chapter from the first publication.

In the treatment of myofascial trigger point (TrP) pain, the Czech physician Karel Lewit was one of the first to advocate the insertion of a needle deep into the muscle in order to penetrate the TrP itself. Lewit (1979) stated 'that the effectiveness of deep dry needling (DDN) is related to the intensity of pain produced at the trigger zone and to the precision with which the site of maximum tenderness is located by the needle'. Chan Gunn, a Canadian physician, has also written extensively in support of a technique denominated 'intramuscular stimulation' (Gunn, 1996). This involves inserting a needle deep into the muscle at a TrP site, but, unlike Lewit, Gunn is of the opinion that it is not necessary to penetrate the TrP itself. Nevertheless, it can be a somewhat distressing procedure because, as Gunn has stated, when a needle is inserted into a tightly contracted band of a muscle, the patient may experience a peculiar cramplike sensation as the needle is grasped, which at times can be excruciatingly painful. Furthermore, because the spasm is frequently prolonged and, due to this, the needle is so firmly grasped, it may take 10 to 30 minutes before it can be released. Gunn's contributions are described in detail in Chapter 15 of this book.

Another advocate of DDN is Jennifer Chu, an American physician who is strongly influenced by Gunn. She reserved DDN specifically for the alleviation of TrP pain that occurs as a secondary event after the development of either a cervical or lumbar radiculopathy (Chu, 1997, 1999). Although the focus of this book is mostly on DDN, this chapter aims to describe an alternate needling approach to the management of patients with myofascial pain and TrPs.

SUPERFICIAL DRY NEEDLING

When starting to deactivate TrPs myself in the 1970s, it was initially my practice to employ Lewit's deep dry needling technique. However, when in the early 1980s a patient was referred to me with pain down the arm from a TrP in the anterior scalene muscle, it seemed to me unduly hazardous to push the needle into the muscle itself because of the proximity to the apex of the lung. Thus I inserted it only into the subcutaneous tissues, immediately overlying the TrP. This proved to be all that was necessary; for after leaving the needle there for about 30 seconds, on taking it out, not only had the exquisite tenderness at the TrP site disappeared, but also the pain in the arm had been alleviated. This superficial dry needling (SDN) technique was then employed to deactivate TrPs present in deeper lying muscles in various parts of the body and found to be equally efficacious.

Macdonald and colleagues (1983), at Charing Cross Hospital in London, have provided evidence for the efficacy of SDN in a trial carried out on patients with pain arising from TrPs in the lower back. In their study, 17 patients with chronic myofascial pain in the lumbar region were divided into two groups. The treatment group had needles inserted to a depth of 4 mm at TrP sites. The control group had electrodes applied to the skin overlying TrPs with noncurrent carrying wires attached to a specially impressively adapted transcutaneous electrical nerve stimulation machine replete with flashing lights, dials, and a cooling system that made a 'whirring' sound! The results of this trial showed that the effectiveness of SDN is significantly greater than that of a placebo.

VARIABLE REACTIVITY TO NEEDLE-EVOKED NERVE STIMULATION

Felix Mann, a medical acupuncturist in London, was one of the first to stress that the responsiveness of individuals to needle-evoked nerve stimulation is widely variable with a minority being either particularly strong or weak reactors (Mann, 1992). There are now grounds for believing that the latter group of people has a genetically determined ability to secrete excessive amounts of endorphin antagonists (Peets & Pomeranz, 1978; Han, 1995, 2001).

PROCEDURE RECOMMENDED FOR THE CARRYING OUT OF SUPERFICIAL DRY NEEDLING

In view of the above considerations, it is the authors' practice (Baldry, 1995, 1998, 2001, 2002a, 2002b, 2005) when using SDN at a TrP site to initially insert a needle (0.3 mm in diameter and 30 mm long) into the tissues overlying the TrP to a depth of about 5 to 10 mm, thus allowing it to be self-standing and then leaving it in place initially for about 30 seconds. An active TrP is of such exquisite tenderness that the application of firm pressure to it gives rise to a flexion withdrawal reaction (the jump sign) and often to the utterance of an expletive ('shout' sign). On withdrawing the needle, pressure equal to that initially employed is reapplied to the TrP site to assess whether these two reactions have been abolished. This is usually the case, but if not, the needle is reinserted and left in the tissues for 2 to 3 minutes. Occasionally, in a particularly weak reactor, it is found necessary to stimulate even more strongly by reinserting the needle and not only leaving it there for an even longer period but also by intermittently twirling it. The reason for determining each patient's responsiveness in this way is because exceeding a patient's optimum needle stimulation requirement is liable to cause a temporary but nevertheless distressing exacerbation of pain. This having been said, it must be remembered that there is a small group of patients that are such very strong reactors that leaving a needle in situ for even 30 seconds is more than is required. In such cases, all that is necessary is to insert the needle into the tissues and to then immediately withdraw it.

THE INITIAL CONSULTATION

In view of all this, before SDN is embarked upon, it is necessary to inform the patient that any pain relief initially obtained may only last for 1 to 2 days and that conversely, but rarely, due to the particular technique adopted, there may be a temporary exacerbation of it. The patient should also be told that needling is initially carried out once a week and that after a time, when necessary, at increasingly long intervals. It also has to be explained that the number of treatment sessions, the length of time between each one and the period for which they have to be given is dependent on whether an individual is a strong, average, or weak responder, and on the length of time the pain has been present before treatment being started.

SYSTEMATIC SEARCH FOR TRIGGER POINTS

As it is essential for needling to be carried out at every TrP, it is clearly important for the search for them to be done in a systematic manner. Then, after treatment, it is necessary to palpate the muscles in the affected region again to ensure that no TrP has been overlooked.

It is necessary at the first treatment session to deactivate only one TrP at a time, as by this means it is possible to assess whether or not the patient is a strong, weak, or average responder. Then on subsequent occasions, in everyone but strong reactors, all TrPs may be deactivated simultaneously.

MUSCLE STRETCHING EXERCISES

After each SDN, the patient should be encouraged to regularly stretch muscles that have become shortened as a result of the TrP activity. Any exercises designed to strengthen the muscles should, however, be avoided as these are liable to cause muscle overloading and the consequent reactivation of the TrP.

MEASURES TO BE TAKEN TO PREVENT TRIGGER POINT REACTIVATION

Clearly any pain relief obtained by the carrying out of SDN at TrP sites will not be maintained unless any underlying postural, anatomical, and biochemical disorders contributing to the initial development of TrP activity are recognised and corrected.

Postural Disorders

After treatment of TrP pain in the neck, the patient should be told to avoid postures that cause the cervical muscles to become persistently kinked, flexed, or hyperextended. Examples include overloading as a result of lying in bed reading a book for a prolonged period by the light of a bedside lamp, keeping the neck muscles persistently elevated such as when sitting at a computer for any length of time, and causing them to become kinked for a long period as result of sleeping with the head on either too few or too many pillows.

During the initial physical examination, note should be taken as to whether one shoulder is higher than the other. If so, this may be due to a C-shaped scoliosis caused by unequal leg length, with one leg being 6 mm or less shorter than the other with, as a consequence, sagging of the shoulder on the side opposite to that of the short leg. Alternatively, if due to an S-shaped scoliosis, the leg length difference should be 1.3 cm or more with sagging of the shoulder on the same side as the short leg. In order to assess whether or not there is lower leg length inequality, the patient should stand with the legs straight and the feet together so that the relative heights of both greater trochanter and iliac crests can be compared. Alternatively, lower leg length inequality may be established by radiological examination (Travell & Simons, 1992). However, although this is clearly a more accurate investigation, it is in the authors' experience not one that is always necessary.

Whenever a lower leg length inequality is found, it is necessary to decide whether this is a true one requiring the heel on the shorter side to be raised by increasing the thickness of the heel of the shoe or if it is an apparent one due to shortening of the quadratus lumborum muscle as a consequence of TrP activity in it and therefore correctable by treating this.

Management of Stress

Persistent stress may not only be a cause of TrP activity developing, but it also may cause it to persist (McNulty et al., 1994). Banks and colleagues (1998) have found that TrP electromyography (EMG) activity increases dramatically in response to emotional stress. It therefore often follows that treatment directed to reducing this is essential. The authors' preferred method in such a case is to employ hypnotherapy and to teach the patient to carry out autohypnosis on a regular basis in a manner similar to that employed by Hilgard and Hilgard (1994).

Biochemical Disorders

Gerwin (1992, 1995) has drawn attention to the importance of those with TrP activity of excluding various biochemical disorders that are liable to cause this to persist. These include lack of vitamin B12, hypothyroidism, low serum folic acid levels, and iron deficiency. With respect to the latter, Gerwin and Dommerholt (2002) reported that 'of women with a chronic sense of coldness and chronic myofascial pain, 65% had a low normal or below normal serum ferritin due to an iron intake insufficient to replace their menstrual iron loss'.

SUMMARY

In this chapter the treatment of TrP pain with superficial dry needling has been advocated. It has been stressed that patients may be either strong, average, or weak reactors. This is why initially needling should only be carried out at one TrP site at a time in order to avoid giving a strong reactor a greater stimulus than required and, by so doing, exacerbating the pain. It is necessary to explain to patients with this disorder that treatment is initially given once a week and that in those with a short history of pain, this is usually all that is required. In cases, however, in which pain has been present for some considerable time, it should be made clear that treatment is likely to be necessary at gradually increasing intervals for a much longer period. It has also been emphasised that in addition to the carrying out of SDN, it is necessary to diagnose and treat any underlying disorder that may contribute to the development of TrP activity such as skeletal deformities, stress, and biochemical deficiencies.

REFERENCES

Baldry, P. E. (1995). Superficial dry needling at myofascial trigger point sites. *Journal of Musculoskeletal Pain, 3*, 117–126.

Baldry, P. E. (1998). Trigger point acupuncture. In J. Filshie & A. White (Eds.), *Medical acupuncture: a Western scientific approach*. Edinburgh: Churchill Livingstone.

Baldry, P. E. (2001). *Myofascial pain and fibromyalgia syndromes: a clinical guide to diagnosis and management*. Edinburgh: Churchill Livingstone.

Baldry, P. E. (2002a). Management of myofascial trigger point pain. *Acupuncture in Medicine, 20*, 2–10.

Baldry, P. E. (2002b). Superficial versus deep dry needling. *Acupuncture in Medicine, 20*, 78–81.

Baldry, P. E. (2005). *Acupuncture, trigger points and musculoskeletal pain* (3rd ed.). Churchill Livingstone, Edinburgh: Elsevier.

Banks, S. L., Jacobs, D. W., Gevirtz, R., & Hubbard, D. R. (1998). Effects of autogenic relaxation training on electromyographic activity in active myofascial trigger points. *Journal of Musculoskeletal Pain, 6*, 23–32.

Chu, J. (1997). Twitch-obtaining intramuscular stimulation (TOIMS): effectiveness for long-term treatment of myofascial pain related to cervical radiculopathy. *Archives of Physical Medicine and Rehabilitation, 78*, 1042.

Chu, J. (1999). Twitch-obtaining intramuscular stimulation. Observations in the management of radiculopathic chronic low back pain. *Journal of Musculoskeletal Pain, 7*(4), 131–146.

Gerwin, R. D. (1992). The clinical assessment of myofascial pain. In D. C. Turk & R. Melzack (Eds.), *Handbook of pain assessment*. New York: Guildford Press.

Gerwin, R. D. (1995). A study of 96 subjects examined both for fibromyalgia and myofascial pain. *Journal of Musculoskeletal Pain, 3*(Suppl. 1), 121.

Gerwin, R. D., & Dommerholt, J. (2002). Treatment of myofascial pain syndromes. In R. Weiner (Ed.), *Pain management: a practical guide for physicians*. (pp. 235–249). Boca Raton: CRC Press.

Gunn, C. C. (1996). *The Gunn approach to the treatment of chronic pain*. Edinburgh: Churchill Livingstone.

Han, J. S. (1995). Cholecystokinin octapeptide (CCK-8): a negative feedback control mechanism for opioid analgesia. *Progress in Brain Research, 105,* 263–271.

Han, J. S. (2001). Opioid and antiopiod peptides: a model of yin-yang balance in acupuncture mechanism of pain modulation. In G. Stux & R. Hammersclag (Eds.), *Clinical acupuncture, scientific basis.* Berlin: Springer-Verlag.

Hilgard, E. R., & Hilgard, J. R. (1994). *Hypnosis in the relief of pain.* New York: Brunner-Mazel.

Lewit, K. (1979). The needle effect in the relief of myofascial pain. *Pain, 6,* 83–90.

Macdonald, A. J. R., Macrae, K. D., Master, B. R., & Rubin, A. P. (1983). Superficial acupuncture in the relief of chronic low-back pain. *Annals of The Royal College of Surgeons of England, 65,* 44–46.

Mann, F. (1992). *Reinventing acupuncture.* Oxford: Butterworth-Heinemann.

McNulty, W. H., Gervitz, R. N., Hubbard, D. R., et al. (1994). Needle electromyographic evaluation of trigger point response to a psychological stress. *Psychophysiology, 31,* 313–316.

Peets, J., & Pomeranz, B. (1978). CXBX mice deficient in opiate receptors show poor electro-acupuncture analgesia. *Nature, 273,* 675–676.

Travell, J. G., & Simons, D. G. (1992). *Myofascial pain and dysfunction: the trigger point manual.* Baltimore: Williams & Wilkins.

CHAPTER 14

Dry Needling from a Western Medical Acupuncture Perspective

MIKE CUMMINGS

INTRODUCTION AND HISTORICAL DEVELOPMENT

Dry Needling—A Historical Perspective

Fossil evidence of trepanning suggests that man has used high threshold physical techniques in the treatment of disease since Neolithic times (Martin, 2000; Parry, 1936). Bone etchings from China dating back to 1600 BC are said to provide some of the earliest evidence of acupuncture techniques. Older still are the sharpened stones called *Bian shi,* although it is questioned whether or not these were actually instruments of acupuncture (Bai & Baron, 2001). Harder evidence—in a softer format—comes from the silk scrolls found in Han Tomb No. 3 (dated to 168 BC) at Mawangdui, Changsha, China, in the early 1970s. These manuscripts describe an early meridian system with 11 rather than 12 paired meridians and the use of moxibustion, which is a treatment involving the application of heat by burning the herb *Artemisia vulgaris.* The pericardium meridian is missing (Chen, 1997) from these early manuscripts. There is also an emphasis on information derived from tactile examination of the living body (Hsu, 2005) rather than from dissection postmortem. However, there is no description of acupuncture needling in these manuscripts (Bai & Baron, 2001). The discovery of Ötzi, the Tyrolean iceman frozen from 3200 BC, suggests the use of a therapeutic needling technique with a needle made from bone, which may have developed in Europe (Dorfer et al., 1999). It seems clear that acupuncture-like therapies have developed independently in different civilisations around the world; this is probably due to late evolutionary features in the mammalian nervous system, combined with intelligence, and the consequent use of tools in humans.

Children learn at a very early age to rub energetically directly over the site of acute pain to reduce the noxious sensation. In the case of a more chronic discomfort from aching, 'knotted' muscle, we tend to massage the local tissues more deeply and vigorously even though doing so may temporarily exacerbate the discomfort. This is likely to be conditioned behaviour resulting from the analgaesic effect of somatic sensory stimulation. With the development of stone tools, it is easy to hypothesise a progression of therapeutic techniques that resulted ultimately in piercing the skin and muscle at a site of chronic pain. It may be that successful treatment of myofascial pain by piercing the body at the site of tenderness not only encouraged the practice, but also lead to the recognition of areas of the body that were most likely to harbour these tender points. In some parts of the world, people developed superficial techniques of scratching or cauterising the skin, whereas in the Far and Middle East the technique of acupuncture developed (Cummings, 2004).

Traditional Acupuncture

The development of acupuncture points probably resulted from clinical observation that certain places in the body were more likely to harbour tender points than others and that treating these points by pressure or piercing could relieve pain and various other nonpainful symptoms. Early physicians would have also noted that careful examination of the body surface revealed tender points in healthy subjects. Consistent patterns of pain referral from myofascial trigger points and the relief resulting from needling these and other muscle points would have lead them to make links between some of the points. Radiation patterns of painful medical conditions such as sciatica, other radiculopathies, and possibly the consistent rashes of herpes zoster would have added to the impression that the established points were connected. These hypotheses do not explain the location of all acupuncture points, nor the paths of all the meridians, but there is clearly considerable overlap between myofascial trigger points and acupuncture points (Melzack et al., 1977) and between the pain referral patterns of the former and meridians (Dorsher, 2009). Although these potential correlations have caused great debate, the theoretical backgrounds of these concepts are clearly distinct.

The Chinese and others probably used acupuncture pragmatically for centuries before it became systematised within a documented form of medicine some 2000 years ago (Veith, 1972). The theories developed were influenced by rational observations imposed upon a limited clinical knowledge base and in the philosophical framework of Taoism. The tendency towards syncretism resulted in the adoption and inclusion of many different theories; over the centuries this has resulted in the development of a complex system of medicine. Traditional Chinese medicine can be initially unpalatable to the skeptical Western scientist. However, on closer inspection it reveals that it is built on a series of logical assumptions, and, although some of these are clearly wrong, many may still represent valid clinical observations.

Western Medical Acupuncture

Western medical acupuncture is a term with a variety of potential meanings. The most literal interpretation invokes thoughts of geographical boundaries, but the term was probably introduced to distinguish a developing system of needle therapy with a basis in Western medical science from its traditional philosophical roots that happened to be in the East. Filshie and Cummings (1999) interpret 'Western medical acupuncture' as the scientific application of acupuncture as a therapy after orthodox clinical diagnosis. It is important to note that the scientific evaluation of acupuncture is not restricted to the West (Han & Terenius, 1982) and therefore adherence to a geographical definition is inappropriate. Probably a more accurate description of 'Western medical acupuncture' (WMA) is a modern scientific approach to therapy involving dry needling of tissues that has been developed from the introduction and evaluation of traditional Chinese acupuncture techniques in the West (Cummings, 2004).

More recently the definition of WMA has been reconsidered and redefined (White, 2009): 'Western medical acupuncture is a therapeutic modality involving the insertion of fine needles; it is an adaptation of Chinese acupuncture using current knowledge of anatomy, physiology, and pathology, and the principles of evidence based medicine'.

Galileo established the modern scientific method in the 17th century when he introduced systematic verification through planned experiments to the existing ancient methods of reasoning and deduction (MacLachlan, 1999). This system was adopted by the scientific community throughout the globe, and, with the addition of statistical analysis, it remains established practice today. The ethical practice of medicine requires the practitioner to understand and use scientific method; however, there is great debate over the use of certain methods of testing efficacy when applied to potentially complex interventions such as acupuncture.

NEUROPHYSIOLOGICAL MECHANISMS OF THE TECHNIQUE
Neurophysiology of Acupuncture Needling

The therapeutic effects of acupuncture needling are mediated through stimulation of the peripheral nervous system and so can be abolished by local anaesthetic (Chiang et al., 1973; Dundee & Ghaly, 1991). In particular, stimulation of Aδ or type III afferent nerve fibres has been implicated as the key component in producing analgesia (Chung et al., 1984). The therapeutic effects of needling can be divided into three categories based on the area influenced: local, segmental, and general.

Local effects

Local effects are mediated through antidromic stimulation of high threshold afferent nerves in the same way as the 'triple response' first described by Professor Sir Thomas Lewis (Lewis, 1927; Rous & Gilding, 1930). Release of trophic and vasoactive neuropeptides, including neuropeptide Y (NPY), calcitonin-gene-related-peptide (CGRP), and vasoactive-intestinal-peptide (VIP), has been demonstrated after acupuncture in patients with xerostomia (Dawidson et al., 1998a, 1998b). It is likely that the release of CGRP and VIP from peripheral nerves stimulated by needling results in enhanced circulation and wound healing in rats (Jansen et al., 1989a, 1989b); equivalent sensory stimulation has proved effective in human patients (Lundeberg et al., 1988).

Increased circulation resulting from nerve stimulation is probably one of the most important local effects of acupuncture; in rats it appears to be principally mediated by the release of CGRP (Sato et al., 2000). The effect of acupuncture on muscle blood flow, however, may not rely solely on nerve stimulation (Shinbara et al., 2008). Under normal circumstances in healthy human subjects, blood flow in muscle and skin is increased by needling local muscle points and less affected by needling skin (Sandberg et al., 2003). But this situation may be reversed if the subject is very sensitive, for example, in patients with fibromyalgia (Sandberg et al., 2004). The increase in muscle and skin blood flow after local needling of muscle in patients with work-related trapezius myalgia appears to be lower than in healthy subjects, and this may reflect the degree of sympathetic activation and hypersensitivity of these patients (Sandberg et al., 2005).

In 2010, Goldman and colleagues (2010) published a very detailed paper, including data from multiple experiments in rodent models of inflammatory and neuropathic pain, demonstrating a unilateral distal antinociceptive effect of acupuncture needling with manual stimulation via release of adenosine. Moré and colleagues (2013) went on to show that a similar antinociceptive effect could be abolished by high levels of caffeine consumption in a rodent model.

Segmental effects

Through stimulation of high threshold ergoreceptors in muscle, needling can have a profound influence on sensory modulation within the dorsal horn at the relevant segmental level. C fibre pain transmission is inhibited via enkephalinergic interneurons in lamina II, the substantia gelatinosa. Bowsher (1998) reviews the basic science literature, which supports this mechanism, and White (1999) appraises experimental and clinical evidence. Segmental stimulation appears to have a more powerful effect than an equivalent stimulus from a distant segment in modulating pain (Chapman et al., 1977; Lundeberg et al., 1989; Zhao, 2008), local autonomic activity (Sato et al., 1993), and itch (Lundeberg et al., 1987). Aδ or type III afferent nerve fibres can be stimulated by superficial needling as well as by needling deeper tissues, but it seems that segmental stimuli from the latter (usually muscle) have a more powerful effect (Lundeberg et al., 1987; Lundeberg et al., 1989; Ceccherelli et al., 1998; Zhao, 2008).

When treating somatic pain, including muscle pain, in the clinical setting, it is difficult to differentiate between local and segmental effects of treatment because local needling can mediate both effects. Segmental effects are easier to illustrate when local needling is not possible, for example, in visceral complaints. Segmental electroacupuncture under the name percutaneous tibial nerve stimulation has been shown to affect bladder function in patients with overactive bladder symptoms (Van Balken et al., 2001, 2003; Macdiarmid et al., 2010; Peters et al., 2010).

Visceral blood flow after acupuncture has also been studied. Although segmental effects appear to dominate (Stener-Victorin et al., 1996, 2003, 2004, 2006), nonsegmental mechanisms are also apparent (Uchida & Hotta, 2008).

Heterosegmental effects

Although segmental stimulation appears to be the more powerful effect, needling anywhere in the body can influence afferent processing throughout the spinal cord. The needle stimulus travels from the segment of origin to the ventral posterior lateral nucleus of the thalamus and projects from there to the sensory cortex. Collaterals in the midbrain synapse in the periaqueductal grey (PAG), from where inhibitory fibres descend, via the nucleus raphe magnus, to influence afferent processing in the dorsal horn at every level of the spinal cord. Serotonin is the prominent neurotransmitter in the caudal stages of this descending pain pathway, and the fibres synapse with the enkephalinergic interneurons in lamina II. A second descending system from the PAG travels via the nucleus raphe gigantocellularis; its fibres are noradrenergic, and their influence is mediated directly on lamina II cells rather than via enkephalinergic interneurons. Diffuse noxious inhibitory control (DNIC) is the term introduced by Le Bars and colleagues to define a third analgaesic system, which is induced by a noxious stimulus anywhere in the body (Le Bars et al., 1979). Heterosegmental needling exerts influence through all three mechanisms to different degrees (Bowsher, 1998; White, 1999) and possibly through others as yet undefined.

General effects

General effects are more difficult to define, and there is clearly some overlap with heterosegmental effects. The latter term is used here to denote effects mediated at every segment of the spinal cord, as opposed to effects mediated by humeral means or by influence on higher centres in the CNS controlling general responses. Acupuncture needling has proven efficacy in the treatment of nausea and vomiting (Vickers, 1996; Lee & Done, 2004; Lee & Fan, 2009), and this effect is likely to be mediated centrally. There is a substantial body of work that indicates the importance of β-endorphin and other endogenous opioids in acupuncture analgesia (Han & Terenius, 1982; Han, 2004, 2010; Zhao, 2008), and correlations have been identified between the endorphin releasing effect of acupuncture and that of prolonged exercise (Thoren et al., 1990). Further correlations in terms of neuropeptide release have been noted (Bucinskaite et al., 1996); it has also been suggested that chronic activation of opioid systems by exercise, or potentially by acupuncture, may mediate enhanced immunity, with decreased upper respiratory infections and protection against some forms of cancer (Jonsdottir, 1999).

Functional magnetic resonance imaging (fMRI) studies indicate general effects on limbic structures (Hui et al., 2000) and indicate the importance of the nature of the needle stimulus in achieving this effect (Hui et al., 2007, 2009, 2010). Such effects may be important in pain as well as other conditions that affect general wellbeing.

In 2014, a team led by Luis Ulloa from Rochester, New Jersey (Torres-Rosas et al., 2014), demonstrated a remarkable effect of 10 minutes stimulation of tibialis anterior with electroacupuncture in a rodent model of septic shock. This brief stimulation resulted in survival of the majority of animals, compared with 100% mortality in the controls. This effect was derived through stimulation of small afferent nerves in muscle, increased vagal tone, and dopamine release from the adrenal gland.

Although target-directed expectation (Benedetti et al., 1999) may theoretically play a role in the mechanism of acupuncture under some circumstances, the effects of acupuncture do not appear to be explained entirely by expectation (Kong et al., 2009b, 2009a). In clinical practice, context driven effects are considered important (Finniss et al., 2010), but in this environment it is challenging to untangle the direct effects of acupuncture needling on central nervous system structures from the indirect effects related to the context of treatment.

Trigger Point Needling

The mechanism of action of direct needling in the deactivation of trigger points is undetermined. Despite the fact that a causal relationship has not been established between direct needling of trigger points and improvement in symptoms, a discussion of the potential mechanisms involved may still be useful in developing future research questions. Simons and colleagues (1999) commented on the results of two trials that compare direct dry and direct wet needling of trigger points (Skootsky et al., 1989; Hong, 1994) and conclude that the critical therapeutic factor in both techniques is mechanical disruption by the needle. The common factor is certainly needle insertion into the trigger point; however, Hong (1994) highlighted the importance of stimulating a local twitch response in achieving an immediate effect and, with Simons, cites evidence that the local twitch response is mediated by a segmental spinal reflex (Hong & Simons, 1998). Fine and colleagues (1988) performed a rigorous experimental study in which trigger points were subject to direct wet needling and clearly demonstrated that an opioid mechanism was involved in trigger point pain relief. In light of this evidence it seems likely that the needle works more often through sensory stimulation than through mechanical disruption; this would be consistent with the mechanism of action of acupuncture analgesia (Han & Terenius, 1982; Han, 2004;

Zhao, 2008; Han 2010). Having said that, techniques vary considerably, and it is possible that the more vigorous and fast insertion trigger point needling has a direct mechanical effect on endplates, muscle spindles, or fibres themselves. Readers are referred to Chapter 2 of the current textbook for physiological mechanisms of trigger point dry needling.

CLINICAL RESEARCH
Methodological Difficulties of Clinical Acupuncture Research

The principal methodological difficulties in clinical trials that study the efficacy of acupuncture are concerned with controls and blinding (Lewith & Vincent, 1998; White et al., 2001b; Cummings & White, 2016). For a placebo control to be credible the subjects receiving it must believe that they have had an active treatment, identical to, or at least equivalent in potency to, the active intervention. Ideally, for any needling therapy the control should involve an inactive form of needling, but it seems clear that a needle placed anywhere in the body is likely to have some neurophysiological effect (Lewith & Machin, 1983)—perhaps as a result of the noxious stimulus (Le Bars et al., 1979) of a needle piercing skin, or perhaps related to context-driven and interactional effects including target-directed expectation (Benedetti et al., 1999) and complex conditioned responses (Lundeberg & Lund, 2008).

An innovation in needle design (Streitberger & Kleinhenz, 1998; Kleinhenz et al., 1999) appeared at first to overcome the problem of needle penetration of skin by using a blunt needle that slid up into the coiled metal of the handle. This device was credible to the subject, but in order to simulate needle retention in the body, it needed to be attached to the skin. This was done by inserting it through an adhesive plaster dressing over a small plastic ring placed over the point. In practice, however, the blunt needles pushed with enough force to get through the plaster and also occasionally penetrated the skin surface (Konrad Streitberger: personal communication, 2001). The Park sham device, which consists of a plastic guide tube of adjustable height with a sticky base, was developed as an alternative method of holding the sham needle in place (Park et al., 2002); however, the subject could be unmasked if a needle fell out of the device. A convincing control procedure should result in blinding of the subject, but it is almost impossible to blind an experienced therapist who is performing both real and sham needling techniques. A common way of reducing bias in this situation is to use a blind assessor. A nonpenetrating needle device that blinds the practitioner as well as the subject has been developed and validated (Takakura & Yajima, 2007, 2008). However, it seems that simple nonpenetrating sham acupuncture procedures such as blunted cocktail sticks tapped on the skin can be highly effective in clinical trials (Cherkin et al., 2009), and so the measured efficacy of true acupuncture over sham techniques in clinical trials is often small and not statistically significant.

Evidence for Acupuncture Needling in Chronic Pain Conditions

Chronic low back pain

A Cochrane review on acupuncture and dry needling for low back pain, which included 35 RCTs, concluded that (Furlan et al., 2005) 'for chronic low back pain, acupuncture is more effective for pain relief and functional improvement than no treatment or sham treatment immediately after treatment and in the short term only'.

A systematic review published in the same year also found acupuncture to be significantly more effective than sham acupuncture in chronic low back pain (Manheimer et al., 2005). More recent systematic reviews have not included meta-analysis. The Cochrane review (including meta-analysis) is being updated and the pooled results are not expected to change substantially (Andrea Furlan: personal communication, 2010).

In the UK, 2009 guidelines from the National Institute for Health and Clinical Excellence (NICE, 2009) for early management of persistent nonspecific low back pain between 6 months and 1 year included consideration of 12 sessions of acupuncture over 3 months. This recommendation was overturned in a subsequent guideline (NICE, 2016), which caused considerable controversy, as the evidence for acupuncture appeared to exceed that of more conventional interventions that were recommended in NG59.

The most robust statistical data comes from the Acupuncture Trialists Collaboration (ATC) lead by Andrew Vickers (Vickers et al., 2012). They performed an individual patient data (IPD) meta-analysis with data from the highest quality RCTs of acupuncture in chronic pain conditions (19 trials, 17,922 patients). Highly statistically significant benefits were measured over sham and usual care controls, but the effect size over sham was small. Subsequent network meta-analysis with the same data indicates that sham acupuncture has clear benefits over usual care controls in terms of health-related quality of life, suggesting real effects of sham acupuncture, which is already recognised

to be superior to most other placebo controls (Meissner et al., 2013).

Chronic headache

The first Cochrane review on acupuncture for idiopathic chronic headache was tentatively positive (Melchart et al., 2001) but criticised for including trials on both migraine prophylaxis and chronic tension type headache. In 2009 the Cochrane review was updated and split into acupuncture for migraine prophylaxis (Linde et al., 2009a) and acupuncture for tension-type headache (Linde et al., 2009b). The latter recorded an effect of acupuncture over sham. This was not the case for migraine prophylaxis; however, acupuncture was marginally superior to drug prophylaxis. In the 2016 update of the reviews with more data (including IPD summary figures from Vickers et al., 2012), acupuncture proved to be marginally superior to sham as well as drug prophylaxis in migraine (Linde et al., 2016a), and it continued to be superior to sham in tension-type headache (Linde et al., 2016b).

NICE (2012) did recommend acupuncture, but concluded that the drug topiramate was twice as good from a very limited network meta-analysis (NMA). This is explained by the exclusion of data from direct comparisons between acupuncture and drug prophylaxis, along with the large differences in responder rates to sham acupuncture compared with drug placebos (White & Cummings, 2012).

Osteoarthritis

A systematic review included 13 RCTs (White et al., 2007). The results from the five high quality trials (n = 1334) were pooled in meta-analysis for the primary outcome and demonstrated a significant effect of acupuncture versus sham in short term pain. A subsequent review by Manheimer and colleagues found very similar results in their meta-analysis (Manheimer et al., 2007), although their interpretation of the clinical relevance of the results differed entirely. The recent Cochrane review of acupuncture for peripheral joint osteoarthritis (OA) (Manheimer et al., 2010) included 16 trials and 3498 participants. Twelve trials were on OA knee, three on OA hip, and one included both. The authors concluded:

> 'Sham-controlled trials show statistically significant benefits; however, these benefits are small, do not meet our predefined thresholds for clinical relevance, and are probably due at least partially to placebo effects from incomplete blinding. Waiting list-controlled trials of acupuncture for peripheral joint osteoarthritis suggest statistically significant and clinically relevant benefits, much of which may be due to expectation or placebo effects.'

White and Cummings (2009) argue that you only test the biological plausibility of acupuncture against sham acupuncture, not its clinical relevance.

The IPD meta-analysis by Vickers and colleagues (2012) confirms a clear statistical benefit of acupuncture over sham and a clinically relevant benefit over usual care controls. Despite this and an NMA suggesting that acupuncture is one of the best nonpharmacological therapies (Corbett et al., 2013), it has not been recommended for osteoarthritis by NICE in the UK (NICE, 2014).

Shoulder pain

The Cochrane review on acupuncture for shoulder pain in 2005 was inconclusive but suggested that there may be a short-term benefit on pain and function (Green et al., 2005). Since then there have been two interesting trials. Vas and colleagues (2008) demonstrated the advantage of manual acupuncture to a single point (ST38) versus sham (mock TENS) along with physical therapy rehabilitation for shoulder pain in 425 subjects. The GRASP trial (German Randomised Acupuncture trial for chronic Shoulder Pain) tested acupuncture against a distant superficial off-point sham and conventional orthopaedic care in 424 subjects with chronic shoulder pain (Molsberger et al., 2010). Acupuncture proved to be superior to sham and conventional orthopaedic care, although the dropout rate in the sham group was rather high at 45%.

Similar to the other pain categories discussed previously, the IPD meta-analysis by Vickers and colleagues (2012) confirms a clear statistical benefit of acupuncture over sham, but unlike spinal pain (back & neck pain data combined), osteoarthritis, and headache, the effect size over sham exceeded what would be considered by NICE to be a minimal important clinical difference.

Evidence for Needling in Myofascial Pain

A systematic review published in 2001 of 23 randomised controlled trials conclusively shows that, when treating myofascial pain with trigger point injection, the nature of the injected substance makes no difference to the outcome and that there is no therapeutic benefit in wet over dry needling (Cummings & White, 2001). These conclusions were supported by all the high quality trials in the review. The review did not find any rigorous evidence that needling therapies have a specific effect in myofascial pain, as authors Cummings and White (2001) concluded:

'The hypothesis that needling therapies have specific efficacy in the treatment of myofascial pain is not supported by the research to date, but this review suggests that any

effect derived from these therapies is likely to be derived from the needle, rather than from either, an injection of liquid in general, or any substance in particular. All groups in the review in whom trigger points were directly needled showed marked improvement in their symptoms; therefore further research is urgently needed to establish the specific effect of trigger point needling, with emphasis on the use of an adequate control for the needle'.

This review has not been formally updated, but from the author's knowledge of the literature published since 2001, there would be no substantial change to the conclusions. A further review with meta-analysis including only trials of dry needling was inconclusive, although the results were compatible with a treatment effect of dry needling on myofascial trigger point pain (Tough et al., 2009). Another review including meta-analysis with an anatomically limited focus (upper quadrant) was positive for dry needling (Kietrys et al., 2013).

CLINICAL APPLICATION OF THE TECHNIQUE
Safety Aspects

Acupuncture involves the insertion of needles (usually stainless steel) into the body. Although it is often perceived by the general public as 'natural' and 'safe', along with many complementary therapies, it is neither natural nor completely safe. As with any needling therapy, the serious risks are associated with the transmission of blood-borne infection and direct trauma. Rampes and Peuker categorise adverse events associated with acupuncture as follows (Rampes & Peuker, 1999):

1. Delayed or missed diagnosis
2. Deterioration of disorder under treatment
3. Pain
4. Vegetative (autonomic) reactions
5. Viral or bacterial infections
6. Trauma of tissues and organs
7. Miscellaneous

If acupuncture is performed as a therapy by a regulated healthcare professional within his or her sphere of competence, the first two categories will be avoided.

Persistent pain attributed to acupuncture treatment is rare, but temporary exacerbation of the presenting complaint for a day or so is common (MacPherson et al., 2001a, 2001b; White et al., 2001a). Pain lasting up to 180 days after needling has been reported in a prospective study of over 2 million treatment sessions, apparently due to nerve damage (Witt et al., 2009). The author has heard verbal reports of persistent neuropathic pain around needle insertion points after acupuncture; however, these events are likely to be very rare because filiform acupuncture needles do not have a cutting edge. Although in the past nerves were directly targeted at some acupuncture points, contemporary practice in the West tends to avoid direct needling of nerves (White et al., 2008b).

Autonomic reactions include syncope and sedation. Syncope can be largely avoided by treating patients while lying on an examination couch; however, very occasionally a profound sinus bradycardia will result in loss of consciousness of a patient who is lying down. Sedation is relatively common and occurs in perhaps 20% of patients after their first two treatments. In maybe 5% of patients there is always some degree of sedation associated with acupuncture treatment. Sedation is rarely seen as adverse event by the patients and is only of concern in terms of driving home or operating machinery after treatment.

Infections associated with acupuncture treatment are rare but can be serious (White, 2004). Worldwide, hepatitis B would be the most common infection related to acupuncture, but this is now very rare in the West as a result of the use of sterile disposable needles and clean techniques.

Traumatic complications of acupuncture needling are avoidable, but on occasion they have been fatal. The most frequent of the serious traumatic adverse effects is pneumothorax, which is estimated (from prospective studies) to occur between 1:200,000 (White, 2004) and 1:1 million (Witt et al., 2009) treatment sessions. The drawback with these estimates is that they include all acupuncture session, not just those in which there has been needling over the thorax.

Point Selection

The two main themes in Western medical acupuncture are dry needling of trigger points and segmental acupuncture (Cummings, 2016). The latter is defined as the technique of needling an area of the soma innervated by the same spinal segment as the disordered structure under treatment (Filshie & Cummings, 1999). Based on neurophysiological and clinical evidence (Chapman et al., 1977; Lundeberg et al., 1987, 1989; Sato et al., 1993; Bowsher, 1998; Ceccherelli et al., 1998; White, 1999), the main principle in point selection is to stimulate the soma as close as is practical to the seat of the pathology or at least within the same segment. Local trigger points, tender points, or acupuncture points are chosen, and often these will overlap so that the key point to stimulate is a trigger point, which is tender by definition, at the site of an acupuncture point. The figures in this chapter illustrate commonly used acupuncture points and trigger points represented by body region (Figs. 14.1–14.10 and Tables 14.1–14.5). If the key element of the somatic pathology is a myofascial trigger point, this is arguably the only point that it is necessary to treat. In most other cases the analgesia afforded by local needling may be enhanced by using one or more points at a distance from the pathology in addition to the relevant local points. Distant points are chosen because they stimulate the appropriate segment or because they are conveniently located and known to generate strong needling sensation (heterosegmental acupuncture). In individual cases, point selection may be modified by the need to avoid local conditions (e.g., skin infection, ulceration, moles and tumours, varicosities) or to avoid regional conditions such as hydrostatic oedema, lymphedema, anaesthetic or hyperaesthetic areas, or ischaemia. As a general rule, therapeutic needling should be performed in healthy tissue.

Needle Technique

Sterile, single-use, disposable needles should always be used. In most cases acupuncture needling involves stimulation of muscle tissue. Needling of muscle and possibly fascial planes between muscle tissues produces a characteristic sensation, often described as a dull, diffuse ache, pressure, swelling, or numbness, which can be referred some distance from the point of stimulation. Needling of other tissues of the soma such as skin, ligament, tendon, periosteum, and the fascial covering of muscle produces relatively localised and often sharp sensations, although there appear to be differences with age, particularly with periosteal needling. If the aim is to stimulate a point in muscle, a rapid insertion through the skin and superficial layers minimises discomfort for the patient. Practitioners who are learning the technique find that the use of an introducer facilitates a rapid, often painless insertion. If an introducer is not used, the practitioner will stretch the skin over the point during insertion. Once through the skin, the needle should be rapidly advanced to the desired position or muscle layer and begin stimulation by rotation back and forth combined with a varying degree of 'lift and thrust' (slight withdrawal and reinsertion) until the desired sensation is achieved. If constant stimulation of the needle is required, an electrical stimulator can be used. For the latter technique, usually a minimum of two needles are inserted, and a specially designed electroacupuncture device is used to deliver the electrical stimulus.

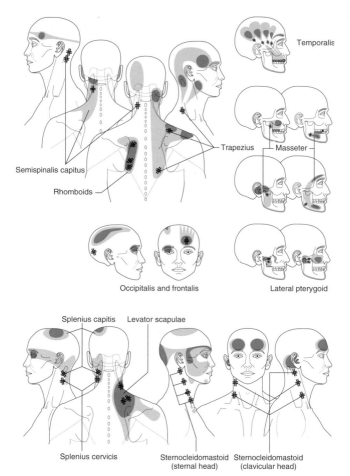

FIG. 14.1 Head, face, and neck: myofascial trigger points and pain reference zones. (Reprinted with permission from: White A, Cummings M, Filshie J (2008). An introduction to Western medical acupuncture. London: Churchill Livingstone.)

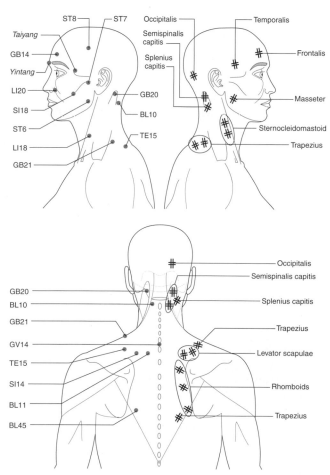

FIG. 14.2 Head, face, and neck: classical acupuncture points and trigger points. (Reprinted with permission from: White A, Cummings M, Filshie J (2008). An introduction to Western medical acupuncture. London: Churchill Livingstone.)

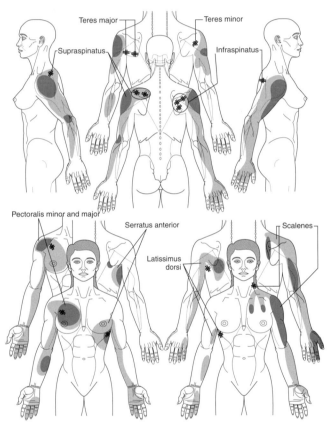

FIG. 14.3 Shoulder and arm: myofascial trigger points and pain reference zones. (Reprinted with permission from: White A, Cummings M, Filshie J (2008). An introduction to Western medical acupuncture. London: Churchill Livingstone.)

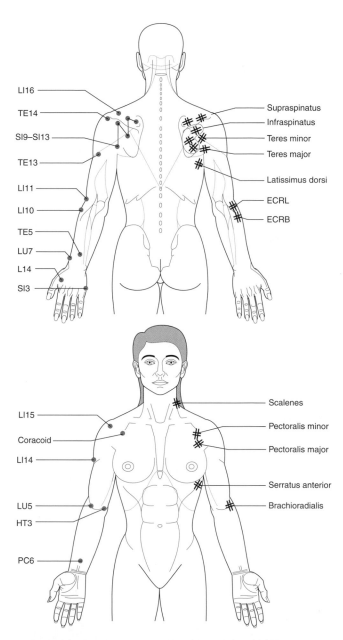

FIG. 14.4 Shoulder and arm: classical acupuncture points and trigger points. (Reprinted with permission from: White A, Cummings M, Filshie J (2008). An introduction to Western medical acupuncture. London: Churchill Livingstone.)

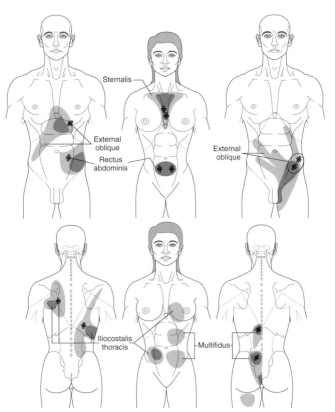

FIG. 14.5 Thorax and abdomen: myofascial trigger points and pain reference zones. (Reprinted with permission from: White A, Cummings M, Filshie J (2008). An introduction to Western medical acupuncture. London: Churchill Livingstone.)

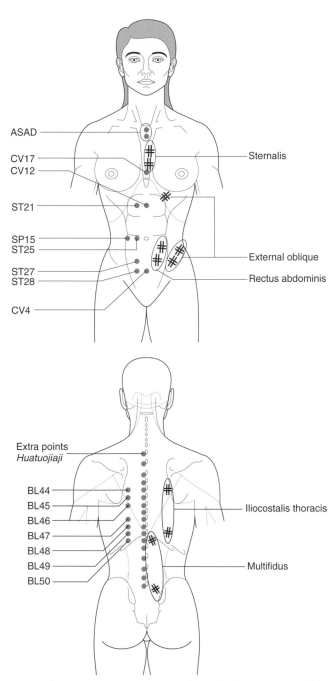

FIG. 14.6 Thorax, abdomen, and spine: classical acupuncture points and trigger points. (Reprinted with permission from: White A, Cummings M, Filshie J (2008). An introduction to Western medical acupuncture. London: Churchill Livingstone.)

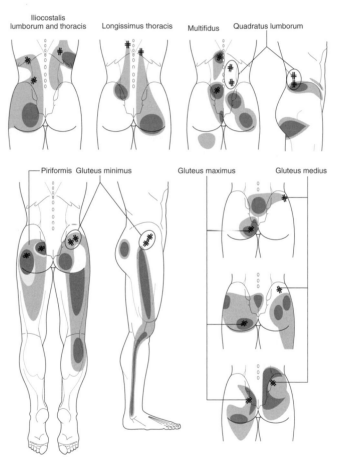

FIG. 14.7 Low back and hip girdle: classical acupuncture points and trigger points. (Reprinted with permission from: White A, Cummings M, Filshie J (2008). An introduction to Western medical acupuncture. London: Churchill Livingstone.)

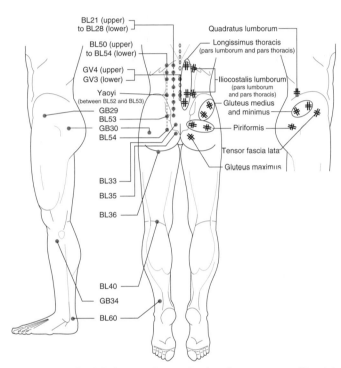

FIG. 14.8 Low back and hip girdle: myofascial trigger points and pain reference zones. (Reprinted with permission from: White A, Cummings M, Filshie J (2008). An introduction to Western medical acupuncture. London: Churchill Livingstone.)

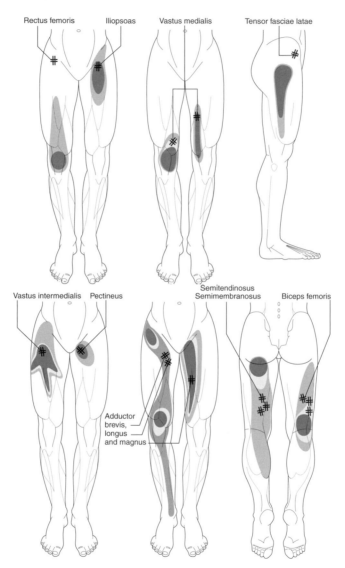

FIG. 14.9 Lower limb: myofascial trigger points and pain reference zones. (Reprinted with permission from: White A, Cummings M, Filshie J (2008). An introduction to Western medical acupuncture. London: Churchill Livingstone.)

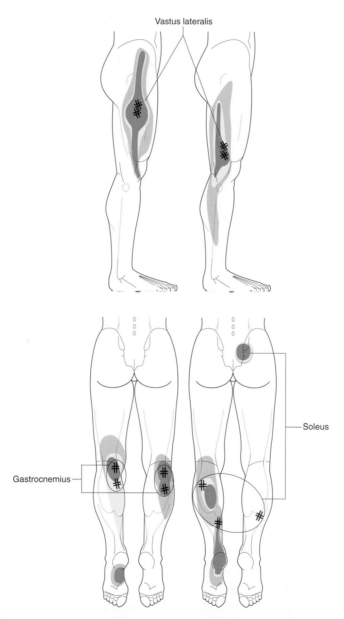

FIG. 14.10 Lower limb: classical acupuncture points and trigger points. (Reprinted with permission from: White A, Cummings M, Filshie J (2008). An introduction to Western medical acupuncture. London: Churchill Livingstone.)

TABLE 14.1
Face, Head, and Neck

Face		
Yintang	Midpoint between the eyebrows	D Vi
	Angulation: oblique inferior　　　　**Target:** procerus or periosteum	M VII
	Headache, hayfever, relaxation	S Vi
Taiyang	1 *cun* posterior to the midpoint between the lateral end of the eyebrow and the lateral canthus of the eye	D Vii
	Angulation: perpendicular　　　　**Target:** temporalis	M Viii
	Headache, eye symptoms	S Vii
GB14	1 *cun* above the middle of the eyebrow, directly above the pupil when the eyes are looking straight ahead	D Vi
	Angulation: oblique inferio　　　　**Target:** frontalis	M VII
	Headache, eye symptoms	S Vi
LI 20	In the nasolabial groove, level with the widest part of the ala nasi	D Vii
	Angulation: superiorly along groove　　　　**Target:** facial muscles	M VII
	Hayfever, nasal symptoms	S Vii
ST6	1 fingerbreadth anterior and superior to the angle of the jaw, on the prominence of masseter	D C2/C3
	Angulation: perpendicular　　　　**Target:** masseter	M Viii
	Dental pain, facial pain	S Viii
ST7	In the depression anterior to the temporomandibular joint and below the zygomatic arch	D Viii
	Angulation: perpendicular　　　　**Target:** lateral pterygoid	M Viii
	Dental pain, facial pain	S Viii
ST8	0.5 *cun* superior to the upper line of origin of the temporalis muscle, directly above ST7 and ST6 on a vertical line 0.5 *cun* posterior to Taiyang	D Vi/Vii
	Angulation: perpendicular　　　　**Target:** epicranial tissues	M Viii/VIIS Vi/Vii
	Headache	
SI18	Directly below the lateral canthus of the eye in the depression at the lower border of the zygomatic bone, just anterior to the attachment of masseter	D Vii
	Angulation: slightly superior　　　　**Target:** connective tissue space	M Viii/S Vii
	Facial pain, trigeminal neuralgia	
LI18	Between the sternal and clavicular heads of sternocleidomastoid (SCM), level with the laryngeal prominence (the tip of the Adam's apple)	D C2/C3
	Angulation: posterior　　　　**Target:** fascial plane in SCM	M XI/C2/C3 S n/a
	Pain from sternocleidomastoid—headache or facial pain **CAUTION: note the proximity of the carotid artery**	
Head and Neck		
GB20	Below the occipital bone, in the depression between trapezius and sternocleidomastoid and above splenius capitis	D C2/C3
	Angulation: towards opposite eyebrow　　　　**Target:** semispinalis capitis	M C1/C2
	Headache, neck pain, and stiffness **CAUTION: note the position of the vertebral artery**	S C1/C2

(Continued)

TABLE 14.1 Face, Head and Neck—cont'd		
Head and Neck		
BL10	1.3 *cun* lateral to the spinous process of C2, between C1 and C2	D C3 M C1 to C5 S C2/C3
	Angulation: towards lamina of C2 **Target:** obliquus inferior	
	Neck pain and stiffness **CAUTION: note the position and depth of the spinal cord and vertebral artery**	
GB21	Midway between GV14 and tip of the acromion at the highest point of trapezius	D C3 M C3/C4S n/a
	Angulation: tangential to ribs, posteriorly **Target:** upper trapezius	
	Headache, neck pain and stiffness, anxiety **CAUTION: note the proximity of the pleura between the 1st and 2nd ribs**	
TE15	Midway between the points GB21 and SI13 at the superior angle of the Scapula (SI13—tender depression superior to medial end of scapular spine)	D C3 M C3/C4 S n/a
	Angulation: perpendicular **Target:** trapezius	
	Shoulder pain, neck pain and stiffness **CAUTION: note the proximity of the pleura in slim patients**	
GV14	Between spinous processes C7 and T1	D C4/C5/T1 M C8S C8
	Angulation: transverse **Target:** interspinous ligament	
	Spinal neck pain, headache of cervical origin	
SI14	3 *cun* lateral to spinous process of T1	D C3/C4 M C3/C4/C5 S C5
	Angulation: tangential towards scapula **Target:** levator scapulae	
	Shoulder pain, neck pain and stiffness **CAUTION: do not needle deeply unless confident of angulation relative to scapula**	
BL11	1.5 *cun* lateral to the lower border of the spinous process of T1	D C4/T1 M C4/C5 S T1/T2
	Angulation: oblique towards spine **Target:** rhomboid minor	
	Neck pain and stiffness, dyspnoea **CAUTION: do not needle deeply unless confident of angulation relative to pleura**	
BL45	3 *cun* lateral to the lower border of the spinous process of T6	D T5/T6 M T6/T7 S T6/T7
	Angulation: oblique towards spine **Target:** iliocostalis thoracis	
	Dorsal back pain, dyspnoea **CAUTION: do not needle deeply unless confident of angulation relative to pleura**	

D = dermatome; i = ophthalmic; ii = maxillary; iii = mandibular divisions; M = myotome; n/a = not applicable; S = sclerotome; V = trigeminal nerve; VII = facial nerve; XI = accessory nerve.

TABLE 14.2
Shoulder and Arm

Posterior Aspect

LI16	In the depression medial to the acromion and between the lateral extremities of the clavicle and scapular spine	D C3 M C3 to C6 S C5/C6
	Angulation: perpendicular **Target:** supraspinatus	
	Shoulder and arm pain	
TE14	Posterolateral and inferior to the posterior tip of the acromion, in the depression between the middle and posterior fibres of deltoid	D C3/C4 M C5/C6 S C6
	Angulation: perpendicular **Target:** infraspinatus insertion	
	Shoulder and arm pain	
SI9	1 *cun* superior to the posterior axillary crease when the arm hangs by the side of the body	D T3/T4 M C5/C6/C7 S C7
	Angulation: perpendicular **Target:** teres major	
	Shoulder and arm pain	
SI10	In the depression below the spine of the scapula, directly superior to the posterior axillary crease when the arm hangs by the side of the body	D C3/C4 M C5/C6 S C6
	Angulation: perpendicular **Target:** infraspinatus	
	Shoulder and arm pain	
SI11	One-third down a line from the midpoint of the scapular spine to the inferior angle of the scapula	D C4/T1/T2 M C5/C6 S C5/C6
	Angulation: perpendicular **Target:** infraspinatus	
	Shoulder and arm pain	
SI12	Directly above SI11 in the middle of the suprascapular fossa, about 1 *cun* above the middle of the superior border of the scapular spine	D C3/C4 M C3 to C6 S C5
	Angulation: towards suprascapular fossa **Target:** supraspinatus	
	Shoulder and arm pain **CAUTION: do not needle deeply unless confident of position relative to scapula**	
SI13	In the tender depression superior to the medial end of the scapular spine	D C4/T1 M C3 to C6 S C5
	Angulation: towards suprascapular fossa **Target:** supraspinatus	
	Shoulder and arm pain **CAUTION: do not needle deeply unless confident of position relative to scapula**	
TE13	On the line connecting the olecranon and TE14, 3 *cun* distal to TE14 on the posterior border of deltoid, 2 *cun* lateral to the posterior axillary fold	D C5 M C6/C7/C8 S C6/C7
	Angulation: perpendicular **Target:** lateral head of triceps	
	Shoulder and arm pain **CAUTION: note the proximity of the radial nerve**	
LI11	At the radial end of the antecubital crease, halfway between the biceps tendon and the lateral epicondyle	D C5/C6 M C5/C6 S C6/C7
	Angulation: perpendicular **Target:** extensor carpi radialis longus	
	Lateral epicondylalgia, forearm pain, immunomodulation	
LI10	2 *cun* distal to LI11, on the line connecting LI11 with LI5 (the centre of the anatomical snuff box)	D C5/C6 M C5/C6/C7 S C6/C7
	Angulation: perpendicular **Target:** extensor carpi radialis longus or supinator	
	Lateral epicondylalgia, forearm pain	

(Continued)

TABLE 14.2
Shoulder and Arm—cont'd

Posterior Aspect		
TE5	On the dorsal surface of forearm, 2 *cun* proximal to wrist joint, between radius and ulna, and between extensor indicis and extensor pollicis longus	D C6 to C8 M C7/C8 S C7/C8
	Angulation: perpendicular　　**Target:** connective tissue plane	
	Local pain, wrist and forearm, major point for central effects	
LU7	On the radial aspect of the radial styloid, 1.5 *cun* from the wrist crease, between the tendons of abductor pollicis longus and brachioradialis	D C6 M C7/C8 S C6
	Angulation: proximal oblique　　**Target:** connective tissue space	
	Wrist and forearm pain	
LI4	On the dorsal aspect of the hand, in the middle of the 1st web space, halfway along the second metacarpal bone	D C6/C7 M T1 S n/a
	Angulation: perpendicular　　**Target:** 1st dorsal interosseous	
	General point for pain; major point for central effects **CAUTION: the radial artery is at the apex of the 1st web space**	
SI3	On the palmar aspect of the neck of the 5th metacarpal, in the tissue plane between the metacarpal neck and the hypothenar muscles	D C8 M T1 S C8
	Angulation: perpendicular　　**Target:** connective tissue plane	
	Hand pain; also used for pain elsewhere especially spinal pain	
Anterior Aspect		
LI15	Anterolateral and inferior to the anterior tip of the acromion, in the groove between the anterior and middle fibres of deltoid	D C4 M C5 S C5
	Angulation: perpendicular　　**Target:** supraspinatus insertion	
	Shoulder and arm pain	
Coracoid	Anterior to the glenohumeral joint, between the fibres of deltoid and pectoralis major	D C4 M C5/C6 S C5
	Angulation: perpendicular　　**Target:** coracoid	
	Shoulder and arm pain	
LI14	Between the distal attachment of deltoid and the long head of biceps, in a tender depression, three-fifths of the distance on a line from LI11 to LI15	D C5/C6 M C5/C6 S C5/C6
	Angulation: perpendicular　　**Target:** connective tissue plane	
	Shoulder and arm pain	
LU5	On the cubital crease of the elbow, in the depression on the radial side of the biceps tendon	D C5/C6 M C5/C6 S C5/C6
	Angulation: perpendicular　　**Target:** brachioradialis	
	Elbow or forearm pain	
HT3	At the medial end of the antecubital crease when the elbow is fully flexed	D T1 M C5 to T1 S C7
	Angulation: perpendicular　　**Target:** pronator teres	
	Medial epicondylalgia, forearm pain **CAUTION: note the proximity of the brachial artery**	
PC6	2 *cun* proximal to the distal wrist crease, between the tendons of flexor carpi radialis and palmaris longus	D C6/C8/T1 M C7/C8 S n/a
	Angulation: oblique proximal　　**Target:** flexor digitorum superficialis	
	Nausea and vomiting, carpal tunnel syndrome **CAUTION: note the position of the median nerve directly below**	

D = dermatome; M = myotome; S = sclerotome; n/a = not applicable.

TABLE 14.3
Thorax and Abdomen

Anterior Aspect		
ASAD	Two points in the midline just below the sternal notch over the manubrium **Angulation:** perpendicular **Target:** periosteum of manubrium *Anxiety, sickness, and dyspnoea*	D C4/T2 M C5/C6 S T1
CV17	In the centre of the sternum at the 4th intercostal space (level with nipples in a man) **Angulation:** cranial oblique at 30 degrees to the sternum **Target:** periosteum of the sternum or sternalis *Chest pain, respiratory conditions* **CAUTION: a sternal foramen occurs at this point in 10% of men and 4% of women; never needle perpendicularly**	D T5 M C8, T1 S T1
CV12	On the midline of the upper abdomen, midway between the umbilicus and the lower border of the body of the sternum **Angulation:** perpendicular **Target:** linea alba *Upper gastrointestinal disorders, including nausea and vomiting* **CAUTION: avoid needling through the abdominal wall**	D T8 M T8 S n/a
CV4	On the midline of the lower abdomen, 3 *cun* inferior to the umbilicus, and 2 *cun* superior to the pubic symphysis **Angulation:** perpendicular **Target:** linea alba *Lower gastrointestinal, urological, and gynaecological symptoms* **CAUTION: avoid needling through the abdominal wall**	D T11/T12 M T11/T12 S n/a
SP15	At the lateral border of rectus abdominis level with the umbilicus **Angulation:** perpendicular **Target:** linea semilunaris *Abdominal pain* **CAUTION: avoid needling through the abdominal wall**	D T10/T11 M T10/T11 S n/a
Kidney and stomach meridians run parallel with CV with points over the abdomen at most segments—any tender point can be treated.		
ST21	2 *cun* lateral to CV12 **Angulation:** medial oblique (nonclassical) **Target:** rectus abdominis *Upper abdominal pain; gastroenterological symptoms* **CAUTION: avoid needling through the abdominal wall**	D T7/T8 M T7/T8 S n/a
ST25	2 *cun* lateral to the umbilicus, halfway between the umbilicus and the linea semilunaris (SP15) **Angulation:** perpendicular **Target:** rectus abdominis *Abdominal pain; gastroenterological symptoms* **CAUTION: avoid needling through the abdominal wall**	D T10 M T10 S n/a
ST27	2 *cun* lateral to the midline and 2 *cun* inferior to the umbilicus **Angulation:** medial oblique (nonclassical) **Target:** rectus abdominis *Abdominal pain; lower gastrointestinal, urological and gynaecological symptoms* **CAUTION: avoid needling through the abdominal wall**	D T11/T12 M T11/T12 S n/a

(Continued)

TABLE 14.3
Thorax and Abdomen—cont'd

Anterior Aspect		
ST28	2 *cun* lateral to the midline and 3 *cun* inferior to the umbilicus	D T12/L1 M T12/L1 S n/a
	Angulation: medial oblique (nonclassical) **Target:** rectus abdominis	
	Abdominal pain; lower gastrointestinal, urological, and gynaecological symptoms **CAUTION: avoid needling through the abdominal wall**	

Posterior Aspect		
Huatuojiaji	A series of 17 extra points, 0.5 *cun* lateral to the lower border of the spinous processes of T1 to L5	D T1 to L1 M T1 to L5 S T1 to L5
	Angulation: oblique towards spine **Target:** multifidus	
	Spinal pain; segmental acupuncture	
Bladder line—outer	3 *cun* lateral to the midline, on a vertical line joining the medial edge of the scapula and the outer border of the lumbar erector spinae	D T5 to T9 M T6 to T12 S T6 to T12—rib level
	Angulation: oblique towards spine **Target:** iliocostalis thoracis	
	Dorsal back pain, ventral pain **CAUTION: do not needle deeply unless confident of angulation relative to pleura**	
BL44	Level with the lower border of T5	
BL45	Level with the lower border of T6	
BL46	Level with the lower border of T7	
BL47	Level with the lower border of T9	
BL48	Level with the lower border of T10	
BL49	Level with the lower border of T11	
BL50	Level with the lower border of T12	

D = dermatome; M = myotome; n/a = not applicable; S = sclerotome.

TABLE 14.4 Back and Hip Girdle		
Lateral Aspect		
GB29	Midway between the anterior superior iliac spine and the greater trochanter	D L2/L3
	Angulation: perpendicular **Target:** tensor fasciae latae	M L5/S1/S2
	Hip girdle pain	S L4/L5/S1
	CAUTION: deep needling may penetrate the capsule of the hip joint	
GB30	One-third of the way from the highest point of the greater trochanter to the sacral hiatus	D L2/L3
	Angulation: towards symphysis pubis **Target:** tensor fasciae latae	M L5/S1/S2
	Hip girdle pain, back pain, leg pain, sciatica	S L4/L5/S1
	CAUTION: avoid direct needling of the sciatic nerve	
GB34	In the depression just anterior and inferior to the head of the fibula	D L5
	Angulation: perpendicular **Target:** fibularis longus	M L5/S1
	Leg pain, general point for musculoskeletal pain	S L5
	CAUTION: avoid needling the common fibular nerve	
BL60	In the depression midway between the lateral malleolus and the Achilles tendon	D L5/S1
	Angulation: perpendicular **Target:** connective tissue	M L5/S1
	Leg pain, Achilles tendon pain	S S1/S2
Posterior Aspect		
GV4	Between spinous processes L2 and L3	D T9/T10
	Angulation: transverse **Target:** interspinous ligament	M L2
	Spinal pain	S L2
GV3	Between spinous processes L4 and L5	D T11/T12
	Angulation: transverse **Target:** interspinous ligament	M L4
	Spinal pain	S L4
BL line—inner	1.5 *cun* lateral to the midline, halfway between the outer bladder line and the spine	D T9 to S2
	Angulation: oblique towards spine **Target:** erector spinae	S T12 to S2
	Back pain	
BL21	Level with the lower border of T12	M T10/T11
BL22	Level with the lower border of L1	M T11/T12
BL23	Level with the lower border of L2	M T12/L1
BL24	Level with the lower border of L3	M L1/L2
BL25	Level with the lower border of L4	M L2/L3
BL26	Level with the lower border of L5	M L3/L4
BL27	Level with the S1 posterior foramen, or upper aspect of the posterior superior iliac spine	M L4
		S S1
	Angulation: perpendicular **Target:** erector spinae or multifidus	
BL28	Level with the S2 posterior foramen, or the lower aspect of the posterior superior iliac spine	M L5
		S S2
	Angulation: perpendicular **Target:** erector spinae or multifidus	

(Continued)

TABLE 14.4
Back and Hip Girdle—cont'd

Posterior Aspect			
BL33	Over the S3 posterior foramen		D S2/S3 M L5 S S3
	Angulation: perpendicular	**Target:** S3 posterior foramen	
	Local pain,disturbance of pelvic organs, e.g., detrusor instability		
BL35	0.5 *cun* lateral to the tip of the coccyx		D S3/S4 M L5/S1/S2 S S4/coccygeal
	Angulation: perpendicular	**Target:** sacrotuberous ligament	
	Coccydinia		
BL36	In the transverse gluteal crease, in a depression between the hamstring muscles		D S2/S3 M L5/S1/S2 S L5
	Angulation: perpendicular	**Target:** hamstring attachment	
	Local pain, hamstring pain, sciatica		
BL40	On the popliteal crease midway between the tendons of biceps femoris and semitendinosus		D S1/S2 M S1/S2 S n/a
	Angulation: perpendicular	**Target:** connective tissue	
	Local pain, sciatica		
BL line—outer	3 *cun* lateral to the midline, on a vertical line joining the medial edge of the scapula and the outer border of the lumbar erector spinae		D T9 to S2 S n/a mostly
	Angulation: oblique towards spine unless stated otherwise later in this table		
	Back pain		
BL50	Level with the lower border of T12		M T10/T11
BL51	Level with the lower border of L1		M T11/T12
BL52	Level with the lower border of L2		M T12/L1
Yaoyi	Level with the lower border of L4		M L2/L3
BL53	Level with the S2 posterior foramen, or the lower aspect of the posterior superior iliac spine		D L2/S3 M L4 to S2 S L5
	Angulation: perpendicular	**Target:** gluteus medius	
	Hip girdle pain, back pain		
BL54	Level with the S4 posterior foramen in the sciatic notch		D S2/S3 M L5 to S2 S S2/S3
	Angulation: perpendicular	**Target:** piriformis	
	Hip girdle pain, back pain, leg pain, sciatica **CAUTION: avoid needling the sciatic nerve**		
BL60	At the level of the most prominent part of the lateral malleolus, halfway between it and the Achilles tendon		D L5/S1 M L5/S1 S n/a
	Angulation: perpendicular toward K13	**Target:** connective tissue space	
	Painful conditions, especially of spine, distant point in sciatica		

D = dermatome; M = myotome; n/a = not applicable; S = sclerotome.

TABLE 14.5
Lower Limb

Thigh and Lower Leg: Anterior Aspect

ST31	In a depression just lateral to sartorius, at the junction of a vertical line through the anterior superior iliac spine and a horizontal line at the level of the lower border of the pubic symphysis	D L2 M L2/L3/L4 S L3/L4
	Angulation: perpendicular **Target:** rectus femoris	
	Thigh pain, anterior knee pain (rectus femoris)	
ST32	6 *cun* superior to the upper lateral margin of the patella on a line that joins the lateral border of the patella to the anterior superior iliac spine	D L2 M L3/L4 S L3
	Angulation: perpendicular **Target:** vastus lateralis	
	Thigh pain	
ST33	3 *cun* superior to the upper lateral margin of the patella on a line that joins the lateral border of the patella to the anterior superior iliac spine	D L2/L3 M L3/L4 S L3
	Angulation: perpendicular **Target:** vastus lateralis	
	Thigh and knee pain	
ST34	2 *cun* superior to the upper lateral margin of the patella on a line that joins the lateral border of the patella to the anterior superior iliac spine	D L2/L3 M L3/L4 S L3
	Angulation: perpendicular **Target:** vastus lateralis	
	Knee pain	
ST35	In the hollow on the lateral aspect of the patella tendon directly over the joint line	D L3/L4/L5 M L3/L4 S L3/L4/L5
	Angulation: towards the patella tendon (nonclassical) **Target:** knee capsule	
	Knee pain **CAUTION: avoid needling into the knee joint**	
Xiyan	In the hollows on either side of the patella tendon directly over the joint line	D L3/L4/L5 M L3/L4 S L3/L4/L5
	Angulation: towards the patella tendon (nonclassical) **Target:** knee capsule	
	Knee pain **CAUTION: avoid needling into the knee joint**	
ST36	3 *cun* inferior to the knee joint, 1 fingerbreadth lateral to the lower border of the tibial tuberosity, in the middle of the upper third of the tibialis anterior	D L4/L5 M L4/L5 S L4/L5
	Angulation: perpendicular **Target:** tibialis anterior	
	Knee pain, abdominal problems, major combination for central effects	
Zongping	1 *cun* inferior to ST36	D L4/L5 M L4/L5 S L4/L5
	Angulation: perpendicular **Target:** tibialis anterior	
	Used with ST36 for EA— major combination for central effects	
ST40	On the anterolateral aspect of the lower leg, midway between the tibiofemoral joint line and the lateral malleolus, 2 fingerbreadths lateral to the anterior crest of the tibia	D L5 M L5/S1 S L5/S1
	Angulation: perpendicular **Target:** extensor hallucis longus	
	Local pain, a variety of traditional indications **CAUTION: avoid needling to the depth of the anterior tibial artery**	
SP11	6 *cun* superior to SP10 on a line connecting SP10 with SP12	D L3 M L2/L3/L4 S L3
	Angulation: perpendicular **Target:** vastus medialis	
	Thigh and knee pain (vastus medialis) **CAUTION: note the position of the femoral artery**	

(Continued)

TABLE 14.5
Lower Limb—cont'd

Thigh and Lower Leg: Anterior Aspect

SP10	2 *cun* proximal to the superiomedial border of the patella, in the centre of vastus medialis	D L3 M L2/L3/L4 S L3
	Angulation: perpendicular **Target:** vastus medialis	
	Knee pain (vastus medialis)	
SP9	In a depression inferior to the medial condyle of the tibia and posterior to the medial border of the tibia, at the same level as GB34	D L3 M L2/L3/L4 S L3
	Angulation: perpendicular **Target:** connective tissue space	
	Knee pain, gynaecological and urological problems	
SP6	3 *cun* superior to the most prominent part of the medial malleolus, on the medial border of the tibia	D L4/S1/S2 M S1/S2 S L4/L5
	Angulation: perpendicular **Target:** flexor digitorum longus	
	Gynaecological problems, major point for central effects	
LR4	Anterior to the medial malleolus, in the depression just medial to the tendon of tibialis anterior	D L4/L5 M L4/L5 S L4/L5
	Angulation: perpendicular **Target:** connective tissue space	
	Ankle pain **CAUTION: avoid needling into the ankle joint**	
LR3	On the dorsum of the foot, in the 1st metatarsal space, in a depression distal to the junction of the bases of the 1st and 2nd metatarsals	D L4/L5 M S2/S3 S L5/S1
	Angulation: perpendicular **Target:** 1st dorsal interosseous	
	Local pain, headache, abdominal problems, major point for central effects **CAUTION: the dorsalis pedis artery is at the apex of the 1st metatarsal space**	

Thigh and Lower Leg: Lateral Aspect

GB29	On the lateral aspect of the hip midway between the anterior superior iliac spine and the greater trochanter	D L2 M L4/L5/S1 S L3/L4/L5
	Angulation: perpendicular **Target:** tensor fasciae latae or glutei	
	Hip girdle pain **CAUTION: deep needling may penetrate the capsule of the hip joint**	
GB30	One-third of the way to the sacral hiatus from the most prominent part of the greater trochanter	D L2/L3/S2 M L5/S1/S2 S L4/L5/S1
	Angulation: perpendicular **Target:** lateral piriformis	
	Low back pain, hip girdle pain, sciatica **CAUTION: avoid needling the sciatic nerve**	
GB31	7 *cun* above the popliteal crease in the palpable furrow just posterior to the iliotibial tract	D L2 M L3/L4 S L3
	Angulation: perpendicular **Target:** vastus lateralis or intermedius	
	Thigh and knee pain	
GB32	In the palpable furrow just posterior to the iliotibial tract, 2 *cun* below GB32	D L2 M L3/L4 S L3
	Angulation: perpendicular **Target:** vastus lateralis or intermedius	
	Thigh and knee pain	

TABLE 14.5
Lower Limb—cont'd

Thigh and Lower Leg: Lateral Aspect		
GB33	On the lateral aspect of the knee 3 *cun* superior to GB34, in a depression between the femur and the tendon of biceps femoris	D L2/L3/S2 M L4 to S2 S L3/L4
	Angulation: perpendicular **Target:** connective tissue space	
	Knee pain **CAUTION: if the knee is flexed this point is close to the posterior joint margin**	
GB34	In the depression about 1 *cun* anterior and inferior to the head of the fibula	D L5 M L5/S1 S L5
	Angulation: perpendicular **Target:** fibularis longus	
	Knee pain **CAUTION: avoid deep needling because the anterior tibial artery and common fibular nerve are deep to this point**	
GB39	3 *cun* superior to the lateral malleolus, between the fibular shaft and the tendon of fibularis longus (use digital pressure to form a groove between the tendon and the fibula)	D L5/S1 M L5/S1 S L5/S1
	Angulation: perpendicular **Target:** fibularis brevis	
	Lower leg and ankle pain **CAUTION: avoid forceful ankle movement when a needle is placed in this point**	
GB40	In the depression anterior and inferior to the lateral malleolus	D L5/S1 M L5/S1 S S1/S2
	Angulation: perpendicular **Target:** connective tissue space	
	Ankle pain CAUTION: avoid needling into the ankle joint	
GB41	In the depression distal to the junction of the 4th and 5th metatarsals, lateral to the tendon of extensor digitorum longus that passes to the 5th toe	D L5/S1 M S1/S2 S S2
	Angulation: perpendicular **Target:** 4th dorsal interosseous	
	Forefoot pain	
Thigh and Lower Leg: Posterior Aspect		
BL36	In the transverse gluteal crease, in a depression between the hamstring muscles	D S2/S3 M L5/S1/S2 S L5
	Angulation: perpendicular **Target:** hamstring attachment	
	Local pain, hamstring pain, sciatica	
BL40	On the popliteal crease midway between the tendons of biceps femoris and semitendinosus, in the connective tissue space between the heads of gastrocnemius	D S1/S2 M S1/S2 S n/a
	Angulation: perpendicular **Target:** connective tissue space	
	Local pain, sciatica **CAUTION: note the popliteal artery and tibial nerve are deep to this point**	
BL55	2 *cun* inferior to BL40, on the line connecting BL40 and BL57, between the two heads of gastrocnemius	D S1/S2 M S1/S2 S n/a
	Angulation: perpendicular **Target:** fascial plane	
	Calf pain	
BL56	In the fascial plane between the heads of gastrocnemius, 5 *cun* below BL40, midway between BL55 and BL57	D S1/S2 M S1/S2 S n/a
	Angulation: perpendicular **Target:** fascial plane	
	Calf pain	

(Continued)

TABLE 14.5 Lower Limb—cont'd		
Thigh and Lower Leg: Posterior Aspect		
BL57	In the depression formed below the bellies of the gastrocnemius muscle when the muscle is flexed, midway between BL40 and BL60	D S1/S2 M S1/S2 S n/a
	Angulation: perpendicular **Target:** musculotendinous junction	
	Calf pain	
BL58	7 *cun* directly superior to BL60, lateral to and approximately 1 *cun* inferior to BL57, at the musculotendinous junction of the lateral head of gastrocnemius	D L5/S1/S2 M S1/S2 S n/a
	Angulation: perpendicular **Target:** musculotendinous junction	
	Calf pain	
BL60	At the level of the most prominent part of the lateral malleolus, halfway between it and the Achilles tendon	D L5/S1 M L5/S1 S n/a
	Angulation: perpendicular toward KI3 **Target:** connective tissue space	
	Painful conditions especially of spine, distant point in sciatica	
KI3	At the level of the most prominent part of the medial malleolus, halfway between it and the Achilles tendon	D L4/S2 M S2 S n/a
	Angulation: perpendicular toward BL60 **Target:** connective tissue space	
	Ankle problems, urogenital problems, major point for central effects	

D = dermatome; M = myotome; n/a = not applicable; S = sclerotome.

Dry needling of trigger points involves a very similar procedure, although the practitioner will often lift and thrust the needle to a greater degree and with a variation in needle direction, aiming to hit the trigger point precisely. When the needle directly impinges on the trigger point, a local twitch is often seen or felt in the associated band of muscle, and the symptoms derived from that point are reproduced.

In clinical practice a wide variety of needling techniques have been described. These range from superficial needling to periosteal needling, with a variety of intermediate depths in muscle. Superficial needling of acupuncture points is common in Japanese forms of acupuncture, and Baldry (2005) described a superficial needling technique exclusively over trigger points (Chapter 13). Periosteal needling was first described by Mann (1998), although he, as most Western practitioners who came after him, uses a variety of techniques (Mann, 2000). As suggested previously, muscle is the most common site of stimulation. Depth and strength of needling in this tissue ranges from brief, superficial stimulation of the muscle surface to deep, repetitive intramuscular stimulation. The latter is not uncommon in Chinese acupuncture, but is also promoted by some practitioners in the West, in particular by Gunn (1989, 1998), who targets motor points and paraspinal muscles (Chapter 15).

Clinical Aspects

There is a range of different responses to acupuncture treatment, from no effect in 5% or 10% of the population at one end to profound analgesia and improved well-being, in a similar proportion, at the other end. Empirical observation suggests that about 70% of the population have a useful response. Patient selection will clearly influence success: a healthy patient with a short-lived myofascial pain syndrome is much more likely to have a beneficial outcome than a debilitated patient with a chronic, ill-defined, and complex problem.

It is difficult to define a 'dose' for acupuncture treatment (White et al., 2008a) because on many occasions a judicious single needle insertion may have the same effect as 10 or more needles left in place for 20 minutes; in addition, similar strength, sequential treatments often have increasing potency in the early stages of a course of treatment. Experimental work does appear to support a type of dose-response relationship for sensory stimulation (Lundeberg, personal communication, 1997), but it is unlikely to be linear. There is probably a stepwise increase in potency down the following list:
1. Superficial, heterosegmental needling with minimal sensation
2. Superficial, segmental needling with minimal sensation

3. Deep, heterosegmental needling with strong sensation
4. Deep, segmental needling with strong sensation
5. Deep, segmental needling with electrical stimulation sufficient to cause muscle contraction

Although acupuncture is likely to do more than simply offer pain relief, the standard pattern of effect from treatment is most easily appreciated in terms of analgesia. There may be little or no effect after the first session, as the practitioner will usually start with gentle treatment. This is to avoid aggravating the complaint in those most sensitive to needling. The initial response is seen within the first 72 hours after treatment, and its onset is often not perceived until the day after needling. Repeat treatments are performed either biweekly or weekly, and the interval can be lengthened with the response. Typically, there is a progressive increase in the quality and duration of the effect after repeated sessions; in chronic pain states, symptom control can be maintained for some patients with relatively infrequent treatments, perhaps every 4 to 6 weeks.

Prognosis

As there is limited evidence from controlled trials of the specific efficacy of needling techniques, simple audit and experience of practitioners must often be called upon as a guide in clinical practice. Myofascial pain syndromes appear to respond very well to direct needling of the relevant trigger points, with a successful outcome reported in 90% or more of cases (Cummings, 1996) in a military primary care population. Musculoskeletal pain in general is helped by acupuncture in 70% of cases, but in some of the more difficult enthesopathies, response rates may be only 40% to 60%; in many such cases adequate advice and rehabilitation is as important as the symptomatic treatment mediated through the needle. In chronic pain conditions with or without elements of myofascial pain, there is now evidence from very large cohort studies to guide prognosis in clinical practice. In general we see that about 50% of subjects improve to a substantial degree, for example, a 50% reduction in headache frequency (Cummings, 2009).

SUMMARY

Needling therapies have been applied to the treatment of pain for thousands of years, and the techniques used today probably do not differ dramatically from those applied to Ötzi in 3200 BC. Empirical evidence suggests that direct needling of trigger points is probably the most valuable needling technique, but definitive research to establish the specific action of the needle is still sought. All practitioners who treat musculoskeletal dysfunction would find the technique of needling trigger points or local acupuncture points useful, but adequate knowledge of anatomy and infection control procedures is essential.

REFERENCES

Bai, X., & Baron, R. (2001). *Acupuncture: visible holism.* Butterworth-Heinemann.

Baldry, P. E. (2005). *Acupuncture, trigger points & musculoskeletal pain* (3rd ed.). Edinburgh: Churchill Livingstone.

Benedetti, F., Arduino, C., & Amanzio, M. (1999). Somatotopic activation of opioid systems by target-directed expectations of analgesia. *The Journal of Neuroscience, 19,* 3639–3648.

Bowsher, D. (1998). Mechanisms of acupuncture. In J. Filshie & A. White (Eds.), *Medical acupuncture — a Western scientific approach* (1st ed., pp. 69–82). Edinburgh: Churchill Livingstone.

Bucinskaite, V., Theodorsson, E., Crumpton, K., et al. (1996). Effects of repeated sensory stimulation (electroacupuncture) and physical exercise (running) on openfield behaviour and concentrations of neuropeptides in the hippocampus in WKY and SHR rats. *The European Journal of Neuroscience, 8,* 382–387.

Ceccherelli, F., Gagliardi, G., Visentin, R., & Giron, G. (1998). Effects of deep vs. superficial stimulation of acupuncture on capsaicin-induced edema. A blind controlled study in rats. *Acupuncture & Electro-Therapeutics Research, 23,* 125–134.

Chapman, C. R., Chen, A. C., & Bonica, J. J. (1977). Effects of intrasegmental electrical acupuncture on dental pain: evaluation by threshold estimation and sensory decision theory. *Pain, 3,* 213–227.

Chen, Y. (1997). Silk scrolls: earliest literature of meridian doctrine in ancient China. *Acupuncture & Electro-Therapeutics Research, 22,* 175–189.

Cherkin, D. C., Sherman, K. J., Avins, A. L., et al. (2009). A randomized trial comparing acupuncture, simulated acupuncture, and usual care for chronic low back pain. *Archives of Internal Medicine, 169,* 858–866.

Chiang, C. Y., Chang, C. T., Chu, H. L., & Yang, L. F. (1973). Peripheral afferent pathway for acupuncture analgesia. *Scientia Sinica, 16,* 210–217.

Chung, J. M., Fang, Z. R., Hori, Y., Lee, K. H., & Willis, W. D. (1984). Prolonged inhibition of primate spinothalamic tract cells by peripheral nerve stimulation. *Pain, 19,* 259–275.

Corbett, M. S., Rice, S. J. C., Madurasinghe, V., et al. (2013). Acupuncture and other physical treatments for the relief of pain due to osteoarthritis of the knee: network meta-analysis. *Osteoarthritis and Cartilage, 21,* 1290–1298.

Cummings, M. (2004). Acupuncture and trigger point needling. In B. Hazelman, G. Riley, & C. Speed (Eds.), *Soft tissue rheumatology* (pp. 275–282). Cambridge: Oxford University Press.

Cummings, M. (2009). Modellvorhaben Akupunktur — a summary of the ART, ARC and GERAC trials. *Acupuncture in Medicine, 27,* 26–30.

Cummings, M. (2016). Western medical acupuncture — the approach to treatment. In J. Filshie, A. White, & M. Cummings (Eds.), *Medical acupuncture — a Western scientific approach* (pp. 100–124). London: Elsevier.

Cummings, M., & White, A. (2016). A critical approach to randomised controlled trials of acupuncture. In J. Filshie, A. White, & M. Cummings (Eds.), *Medical acupuncture — a Western scientific approach* (pp. 279–297). London: Elsevier.

Cummings, T. M. (1996). A computerised audit of acupuncture in two populations: civilian and forces. *Acupuncture in Medicine, 14*, 37–39.

Cummings, T. M., & White, A. R. (2001). Needling therapies in the management of myofascial trigger point pain: a systematic review. *Archives of Physical Medicine and Rehabilitation, 82*, 986–992.

Dawidson, I., Angmar-Mansson, B., Blom, M., Theodorsson, E., & Lundeberg, T. (1998a). Sensory stimulation (acupuncture) increases the release of vasoactive intestinal polypeptide in the saliva of xerostomia sufferers. *Neuropeptides, 32*, 543–548.

Dawidson, I., Angmar-Mansson, B., Blom, M., Theodorsson, E., & Lundeberg, T. (1998b). The influence of sensory stimulation (acupuncture) on the release of neuropeptides in the saliva of healthy subjects. *Life Sciences, 63*, 659–674.

Dorfer, L., Moser, M., Bahr, F., et al. (1999). A medical report from the stone age? *Lancet, 354*, 1023–1025.

Dorsher, P. T. (2009). Myofascial referred-pain data provide physiologic evidence of acupuncture meridians. *The Journal of Pain, 10*, 723–731.

Dundee, J. W., & Ghaly, G. (1991). Local anesthesia blocks the antiemetic action of P6 acupuncture. *Clinical Pharmacology and Therapeutics, 50*, 78–80.

Filshie, J., & Cummings, T. M. (1999). Western medical acupuncture. In E. Ernst & A. White (Eds.), *Acupuncture: a scientific appraisal* (pp. 31–59). Oxford: Butterworth Heinemann.

Fine, P. G., Milano, R., & Hare, B. D. (1988). The effects of myofascial trigger point injections are naloxone reversible. *Pain, 32*, 15–20.

Finniss, D. G., Kaptchuk, T. J., Miller, F., & Benedetti, F. (2010). Biological, clinical, and ethical advances of placebo effects. *Lancet, 375*, 686–695.

Furlan, A. D., van Tulder, M. W., Cherkin, D. C., et al. (2005). Acupuncture and dry-needling for low back pain. *Cochrane Database of Systematic Reviews*, CD001351.

Goldman, N., Chen, M., Fujita, T., et al. (2010). Adenosine A1 receptors mediate local anti-nociceptive effects of acupuncture. *Nature Neuroscience, 13*, 883–888. https://doi.org/10.1038/nn.2562.

Green, S., Buchbinder, R., & Hetrick, S. (2005). Acupuncture for shoulder pain. *Cochrane Database of Systematic Reviews*, CD005319.

Gunn, C. (1989). *Treating myofascial pain, intramuscular stimulation (IMS) for myofascial pain syndromes of neuropathic origin*. Seattle: University of Washington.

Gunn, C. C. (1998). Acupuncture and the peripheral nervous system. In J. Filshie & A. White (Eds.), *Medical acupuncture — a Western scientific approach* (1st ed., pp. 137–150). Edinburgh: Churchill Livingstone.

Han, J. S. (2004). Acupuncture and endorphins. *Neuroscience Letters, 361*, 258–261.

Han, J. S. (2011). Acupuncture analgesia: Areas of consensus and controversy. *Pain. 152*(3 Suppl), S41–48.

Han, J. S., & Terenius, L. (1982). Neurochemical basis of acupuncture analgesia. *Annual Review of Pharmacology and Toxicology, 22*, 193–220.

Hong, C. Z. (1994). Lidocaine injection versus dry needling to myofascial trigger point. The importance of the local twitch response. *American Journal of Physical Medicine & Rehabilitation, 73*, 256–263.

Hong, C. Z., & Simons, D. G. (1998). Pathophysiologic and electrophysiologic mechanisms of myofascial trigger points. *Archives of Physical Medicine and Rehabilitation, 79*, 863–872.

Hsu, E. (2005). Tactility and the body in early Chinese medicine. *Science in Context, 18*, 7–34.

Hui, K. K., Liu, J., Makris, N., et al. (2000). Acupuncture modulates the limbic system and subcortical gray structures of the human brain: evidence from fMRI studies in normal subjects. *Human Brain Mapping, 9*, 13–25.

Hui, K. K., Marina, O., Claunch, J. D., et al. (2009). Acupuncture mobilizes the brain's default mode and its anti-correlated network in healthy subjects. *Brain Research, 1287*, 84–103.

Hui, K. K., Marina, O., Liu, J., Rosen, B. R., & Kwong, K. K. (2010). Acupuncture, the limbic system, and the anticorrelated networks of the brain. *Autonomic Neuroscience, 157*, 81–90.

Hui, K. K., Nixon, E. E., Vangel, M. G., et al. (2007). Characterization of the "deqi" response in acupuncture. *BMC Complementary and Alternative Medicine, 7*, 33.

Jansen, G., Lundeberg, T., Kjartansson, J., & Samuelson, U. E. (1989a). Acupuncture and sensory neuropeptides increase cutaneous blood flow in rats. *Neuroscience Letters, 97*, 305–309.

Jansen, G., Lundeberg, T., Samuelson, U. E., & Thomas, M. (1989b). Increased survival of ischaemic musculocutaneous flaps in rats after acupuncture. *Acta Physiologica Scandinavica, 135*, 555–558.

Jonsdottir, I. H. (1999). Physical exercise, acupuncture and immune function. *Acupuncture in Medicine, 17*, 50–53.

Kietrys, D. M., Palombaro, K. M., Azzaretto, E., et al. (2013). Effectiveness of dry needling for upper quarter myofascial pain: a systematic review and meta-analysis. *The Journal of Orthopaedic and Sports Physical Therapy, 43*, 620–634.

Kleinhenz, J., Streitberger, K., Windeler, J., et al. (1999). Randomised clinical trial comparing the effects of acupuncture and a newly designed placebo needle in rotator cuff tendinitis. *Pain, 83*, 235–241.

Kong, J., Kaptchuk, T. J., Polich, G., et al. (2009a). Expectancy and treatment interactions: a dissociation between acupuncture analgesia and expectancy evoked placebo analgesia. *NeuroImage, 45*, 940–949.

Kong, J., Kaptchuk, T. J., Polich, G., et al. (2009b). An fMRI study on the interaction and dissociation between expectation of pain relief and acupuncture treatment. *NeuroImage, 47*, 1066–1076.

Le Bars, D., Dickenson, A. H., & Besson, J. M. (1979). Diffuse noxious inhibitory controls (DNIC). I. Effects on dorsal horn convergent neurones in the rat; II. Lack of effect on non-convergent neurones, supraspinal involvement and theoretical implications. *Pain, 6*, 305–327.

Lee, A., & Done, M. L. (2004). Stimulation of the wrist acupuncture point P6 for preventing postoperative nausea and vomiting. *Cochrane Database of Systematic Reviews*, CD003281.

Lee, A., & Fan, L. T. (2009). Stimulation of the wrist acupuncture point P6 for preventing postoperative nausea and vomiting. *Cochrane Database of Systematic Reviews*, CD003281.

Lewis, T. (1927). *The blood vessels of the human skin and their responses*. London: Shaw.

Lewith, G. T., & Machin, D. (1983). On the evaluation of the clinical effects of acupuncture. *Pain, 16*, 111–127.

Lewith, G. T., & Vincent, C. A. (1998). The clinical evaluation of acupuncture. In J. Filshie & A. White (Eds.), *Medical acupuncture — a Western scientific approach* (1st ed., pp. 205–224). Edinburgh: Churchill Livingstone.

Linde, K., Allais, G., Brinkhaus, B., et al. (2009a). Acupuncture for migraine prophylaxis. *Cochrane Database of Systematic Reviews*, CD001218.

Linde, K., Allais, G., Brinkhaus, B., et al. (2016a). Acupuncture for the prevention of episodic migraine. *Cochrane Database of Systematic Reviews*, CD001218.

Linde, K., Allais, G., Brinkhaus, B., et al. (2009b). Acupuncture for tension-type headache. *Cochrane Database of Systematic Reviews*, CD007587.

Linde, K., Allais, G., Brinkhaus, B., et al. (2016b). Acupuncture for tension-type headache. *Cochrane Database of Systematic Reviews*, CD007587.

Lundeberg, T., Bondesson, L., & Thomas, M. (1987). Effect of acupuncture on experimentally induced itch. *The British Journal of Dermatology, 117*, 771–777.

Lundeberg, T., Eriksson, S., Lundeberg, S., & Thomas, M. (1989). Acupuncture and sensory thresholds. *The American Journal of Chinese Medicine, 17*, 99–110.

Lundeberg, T., Kjartansson, J., & Samuelsson, U. (1988). Effect of electrical nerve stimulation on healing of ischaemic skin flaps. *Lancet, 2*, 712–714.

Lundeberg, T., & Lund, I. (2008). Acupuncture for preconditioning of expectancy and/or Pavlovian extinction. *Acupuncture in Medicine, 26*, 234–238.

Macdiarmid, S. A., Peters, K. M., Shobeiri, S. A., et al. (2010). Long-term durability of percutaneous tibial nerve stimulation for the treatment of overactive bladder. *The Journal of Urology, 183*, 234–240.

MacLachlan, J. (1999). *Galileo Galilei: first physicist*. Oxford: Oxford University Press.

MacPherson, H., Thomas, K., Walters, S., & Fitter, M. (2001a). A prospective survey of adverse events and treatment reactions following 34,000 consultations with professional acupuncturists. *Acupuncture in Medicine, 19*, 93–102.

MacPherson, H., Thomas, K., Walters, S., & Fitter, M. (2001b). The York acupuncture safety study: prospective survey of 34 000 treatments by traditional acupuncturists. *BMJ, 323*, 486–487.

Manheimer, E., Cheng, K., Linde, K., et al. (2010). Acupuncture for peripheral joint osteoarthritis. *Cochrane Database of Systematic Reviews*, CD001977.

Manheimer, E., Linde, K., Lao, L., Bouter, L. M., & Berman, B. M. (2007). Meta-analysis: acupuncture for osteoarthritis of the knee. *Annals of Internal Medicine, 146*, 868–877.

Manheimer, E., White, A., Berman, B., Forys, K., & Ernst, E. (2005). Meta-analysis: acupuncture for low back pain. *Annals of Internal Medicine, 142*, 651–663.

Mann, F. (1998). A new system of acupuncture. In J. Filshie & A. White (Eds.), *Medical acupuncture — a Western scientific approach* (1st ed., pp. 61–66). Edinburgh: Churchill Livingstone.

Mann, F. (2000). *Reinventing acupuncture: a new concept of ancient medicine* (2nd ed.). Oxford: Butterworth Heinemann.

Martin, G. (2000). Was Hippocrates a beginner at trepanning and where did he learn? *Journal of Clinical Neuroscience, 7*, 500–502.

Meissner, K., Fässler, M., Rücker, G., et al. (2013). Differential effectiveness of placebo treatments: a systematic review of migraine prophylaxis. *JAMA Internal Medicine, 173*, 1941–1951.

Melchart, D., Linde, K., Fischer, P., et al. (2001). Acupuncture for idiopathic headache. *Cochrane Database of Systematic Reviews*, CD001218.

Melzack, R., Stillwell, D. M., & Fox, E. J. (1977). Trigger points and acupuncture points for pain: correlations and implications. *Pain, 3*, 3–23.

Molsberger, A. F., Schneider, T., Gotthardt, H., & Drabik, A. (2010). German randomized acupuncture trial for chronic shoulder pain (GRASP) — a pragmatic, controlled, patient-blinded, multi-centre trial in an outpatient care environment. *Pain, 151*, 146–154.

Moré, A. O., Cidral-Filho, F. J., Mazzardo-Martins, L., et al. (2013). Caffeine at moderate doses can inhibit acupuncture-induced analgesia in a mouse model of postoperative pain. *Journal of Caffeine Research, 3*, 143–148. https://doi.org/10.1089/jcr.2013.0014.

NICE (2009). Guideline on low back pain: early management of persistent non-specific low back pain. http://guidance.nice.org.uk/CG88 accessed on 13/5/2009.

NICE (2012). Guideline on headaches: diagnosis and management of headaches in young people and adults. http://guidance.nice.org.uk/CG150.

NICE (2014). Guideline update on osteoarthritis: the care and management of osteoarthritis in adults. http://guidance.nice.org.uk/CG177.

NICE (2016). Guideline on low back pain and sciatica in over 16s: assessment and management. https://www.nice.org.uk/guidance/ng59.

Park, J., White, A., Stevinson, C., Ernst, E., & James, M. (2002). Validating a new non-penetrating sham acupuncture device: two randomised controlled trials. *Acupuncture in Medicine, 20*, 168–174.

Parry, T. W. (1936). A case of primitive surgical holing of the cranium practised in Great Britain in mediaeval times, with a note on the introduction of trepanning instruments. *Proceedings of the Royal Society of Medicine, 29*, 898–902.

Peters, K. M., Carrico, D. J., Perez-Marrero, R. A., et al. (2010). Randomized trial of percutaneous tibial nerve stimulation versus sham efficacy in the treatment of overactive bladder syndrome: results from the SUmiT trial. *The Journal of Urology, 183*, 1438–1443.

Rampes, H., & Peuker, E. (1999). Adverse effects of acupuncture. In E. Ernst & A. White (Eds.), *Acupuncture — a scientific appraisal* (pp. 128–152). Oxford: Butterworth Heinemann.

Rous, P., & Gilding, H. P. (1930). Is the local vasodilatation after different tissue injuries referable to a single cause? *The Journal of Experimental Medicine, 51*, 27–39.

Sandberg, M., Larsson, B., Lindberg, L. G., & Gerdle, B. (2005). Different patterns of blood flow response in the trapezius muscle following needle stimulation (acupuncture) between healthy subjects and patients with fibromyalgia and work-related trapezius myalgia. *European Journal of Pain, 9*, 497–510.

Sandberg, M., Lindberg, L. G., & Gerdle, B. (2004). Peripheral effects of needle stimulation (acupuncture) on skin and muscle blood flow in fibromyalgia. *European Journal of Pain, 8*, 163–171.

Sandberg, M., Lundeberg, T., Lindberg, L. G., & Gerdle, B. (2003). Effects of acupuncture on skin and muscle blood flow in healthy subjects. *European Journal of Applied Physiology, 90*, 114–119.

Sato, A., Sato, Y., Shimura, M., & Uchida, S. (2000). Calcitonin gene-related peptide produces skeletal muscle vasodilation following antidromic stimulation of unmyelinated afferents in the dorsal root in rats. *Neuroscience Letters, 283*, 137–140.

Sato, A., Sato, Y., Suzuki, A., & Uchida, S. (1993). Neural mechanisms of the reflex inhibition and excitation of gastric motility elicited by acupuncture-like stimulation in anesthetized rats. *Neuroscience Research, 18*, 53–62.

Shinbara, H., Okubo, M., Sumiya, E., et al. (2008). Effects of manual acupuncture with sparrow pecking on muscle blood flow of normal and denervated hindlimb in rats. *Acupuncture in Medicine, 26*, 149–159.

Simons, D. G., Travell, J. G., & Simons, P. T. (1999). *Travell & Simons' myofascial pain & dysfunction. The trigger point manual. Volume 1. Upper half of body* (2nd ed.). Baltimore: Williams & Wilkins.

Skootsky, S. A., Jaeger, B., & Oye, R. K. (1989). Prevalence of myofascial pain in general internal medicine practice. *The Western Journal of Medicine, 151*, 157–160.

Stener-Victorin, E., Fujisawa, S., & Kurosawa, M. (2006). Ovarian blood flow responses to electroacupuncture stimulation depend on estrous cycle and on site and frequency of stimulation in anesthetized rats. *Journal of Applied Physiology, 101*, 84–91.

Stener-Victorin, E., Kobayashi, R., & Kurosawa, M. (2003). Ovarian blood flow responses to electro-acupuncture stimulation at different frequencies and intensities in anaesthetized rats. *Autonomic Neuroscience, 108*, 50–56.

Stener-Victorin, E., Kobayashi, R., Watanabe, O., Lundeberg, T., & Kurosawa, M. (2004). Effect of electro-acupuncture stimulation of different frequencies and intensities on ovarian blood flow in anaesthetized rats with steroid-induced polycystic ovaries. *Reproductive Biology and Endocrinology, 2*, 16.

Stener-Victorin, E., Waldenstrom, U., Andersson, S. A., & Wikland, M. (1996). Reduction of blood flow impedance in the uterine arteries of infertile women with electroacupuncture. *Human Reproduction, 11*, 1314–1317.

Streitberger, K., & Kleinhenz, J. (1998). Introducing a placebo needle into acupuncture research. *Lancet, 352*, 364–365.

Takakura, N., & Yajima, H. (2007). A double-blind placebo needle for acupuncture research. *BMC Complementary and Alternative Medicine, 7*, 31.

Takakura, N., & Yajima, H. (2008). A placebo acupuncture needle with potential for double blinding — a validation study. *Acupuncture in Medicine, 26*, 224–230.

Thoren, P., Floras, J. S., Hoffmann, P., & Seals, D. R. (1990). Endorphins and exercise: physiological mechanisms and clinical implications. *Medicine and Science in Sports and Exercise, 22*, 417–428.

Torres-Rosas, R., Yehia, G., Peña, G., et al. (2014). Dopamine mediates vagal modulation of the immune system by electroacupuncture. *Nature Medicine, 20*, 291–295. https://doi.org/10.1038/nm.3479.

Tough, E. A., White, A. R., Cummings, T. M., Richards, S. H., & Campbell, J. L. (2009). Acupuncture and dry needling in the management of myofascial trigger point pain: a systematic review and meta-analysis of randomised controlled trials. *European Journal of Pain, 13*, 3–10.

Uchida, S., & Hotta, H. (2008). Acupuncture affects regional blood flow in various organs. *Evidence-based Complementary and Alternative Medicine, 5*, 145–151.

van Balken, M. R., Vandoninck, V., Gisolf, K. W., et al. (2001). Posterior tibial nerve stimulation as neuromodulative treatment of lower urinary tract dysfunction. *The Journal of Urology, 166*, 914–918.

van Balken, M. R., Vandoninck, V., Messelink, B. J., et al. (2003). Percutaneous tibial nerve stimulation as neuromodulative treatment of chronic pelvic pain. *European Urology, 43*, 158–163.

Vas, J., Ortega, C., Olmo, V., et al. (2008). Single-point acupuncture and physiotherapy for the treatment of painful shoulder: a multicentre randomized controlled trial. *Rheumatology (Oxford), 47*, 887–893.

Veith, I. (1972). *The Yellow Emperor's classic of internal medicine*. Berkeley: University of California Press.

Vickers, A. J. (1996). Can acupuncture have specific effects on health? A systematic review of acupuncture antiemesis trials. *Journal of the Royal Society of Medicine, 89*, 303–311.

Vickers, A. J., Cronin, A. M., Maschino, A. C., et al. (2012). Acupuncture for chronic pain: individual patient data meta-analysis. *Archives of Internal Medicine, 172*, 1444–1453.

White, A. (1999). Neurophysiology of acupuncture analgesia. In E. Ernst & A. White (Eds.), *Acupuncture — a scientific appraisal* (pp. 60–92). Oxford: Butterworth Heinemann.

White, A. (2004). A cumulative review of the range and incidence of significant adverse events associated with acupuncture. *Acupuncture in Medicine, 22*, 122–133.

White, A. (2009). Western medical acupuncture: a definition. *Acupuncture in Medicine, 27*, 33–35.

White, A., & Cummings, M. (2009). Does acupuncture relieve pain? *BMJ, 338,* a2760.

White, A., & Cummings, M. (2012). Inconsistent placebo effects in NICE's network analysis. *Acupuncture in Medicine, 30,* 364–365.

White, A., Cummings, M., Barlas, P., et al. (2008a). Defining an adequate dose of acupuncture using a neurophysiological approach—a narrative review of the literature. *Acupuncture in Medicine, 26,* 111–120.

White, A., Cummings, M., & Filshie, J. (2008b). *An introduction to Western medical acupuncture.* London: Churchill Livingstone.

White, A., Foster, N. E., Cummings, M., & Barlas, P. (2007). Acupuncture treatment for chronic knee pain: a systematic review. *Rheumatology (Oxford, England).*

White, A., Hayhoe, S., Hart, A., & Ernst, E. (2001a). Adverse events following acupuncture: prospective survey of 32 000 consultations with doctors and physiotherapists. *BMJ, 323,* 485–486.

White, A. R., Filshie, J., & Cummings, T. M. (2001b). Clinical trials of acupuncture: consensus recommendations for optimal treatment, sham controls and blinding. *Complementary Therapies in Medicine, 9,* 237–245.

Witt, C. M., Pach, D., Brinkhaus, B., et al. (2009). Safety of acupuncture: results of a prospective observational study with 229,230 patients and introduction of a medical information and consent form. *Forschende Komplementärmedizin, 16,* 91–97.

Zhao, Z. Q. (2008). Neural mechanism underlying acupuncture analgesia. *Progress in Neurobiology, 85,* 355–375.

CHAPTER 15

Intramuscular Stimulation

STEVEN R. GOODMAN • CORY B. CHOMA

INTRODUCTION

Gunn intramuscular stimulation (Gunn-IMS) is a technique for the treatment of patients with myofascial pain syndrome (MPS) based on a comprehensive diagnostic and therapeutic model that identifies the aetiology of myofascial pain as neuropathic (i.e., due to disease or dysfunction in the nervous system). Further, it identifies the nerve root as the locus of the pathology, and thus it is a radiculoneuropathic model. It was developed in the 1970s by Dr. C.C. Gunn when treating injured workers and evolved from his clinical observations distinguishing those workers who succeeded in returning to work from those who failed to do so (Gunn & Milbrandt, 1976a).

Gunn's model is a derived clinical model. What grew out of the desire to understand his patients' persistent pain and offer them treatment ended in a completely new way to see and treat this most universal of all human afflictions: pain. He was the first physician to recognise the subtle physical examination signs of neuropathy and to describe the pathophysiology of neuropathic pain (Gunn & Milbrandt, 1978; Gunn et al., 1980).

Gunn's work reflects not only the great tradition of empirical science, but is also built upon the work of great scientists before him. In an example par excellence of the often quoted homage of scientific progress to the work of all who precede one in the history of science and medicine, 'dwarfs standing on the shoulders of giants', Gunn realised the pathophysiological explanation for what he observed clinically in the work of Walter Cannon, the distinguished early 20th century physiologist. Cannon's research on 'The Supersensitivity of Denervated Structures, a Law of Denervation' is an important law of neuropathophysiology that has been previously underrecognised by the medical community (Cannon, 1939; Cannon & Rosenblueth, 1949). Although an entire field of basic and animal neuromuscular physiology research has grown out of this work known as 'Cannon's Law' (CL), it had remained a purely academic and nonclinical pursuit limited to the laboratory until Gunn: Gunn built a bridge from the research laboratory to the medical clinic and rescued CL from experimental obscurity to practical posterity.

The prevailing medical–surgical management of persistent spinal and regional musculoskeletal pain is based on what could be called the 'spondylosis-nociception-inflammation' model. This model attributes pain to nociceptive and inflammatory aetiologies due to altered structure in a normal peripheral nervous system. Typical diagnoses in this model include 'disc rupture, degeneration, and inflammation', 'nerve root impingement', 'facet joint arthropathy', 'rotator cuff tear', 'extensor elbow/Achilles tendonitis', 'hip bursitis', 'patella-femoral dysfunction', and 'plantar fasciitis', to name a few. Diagnosis and treatment decisions in this model are based largely on the structural findings of imaging studies (plain x-ray, CT/MRI, nuclear medicine) or the presumption of inflammation, and myofascial pain syndrome is not thought of as bearing any relationship to these entities. This model, however, cannot account for many clinically 'inconvenient' facts, including the lack of correlation between anatomic findings and pain (Savage et al., 1997; Borenstein et al., 2001) or the absence of examination findings or histological evidence of inflammation (Khan et al., 1999; Alfredson & Lorentzon, 2002).

Connecting the dots between radiculopathy, neuropathy, and myofascial pain, one could say that Gunn discovered the 'missing link' between three entities previously thought of as separate, even disparate. Gunn's radiculo-neuropathic-myofascial pain (RNMP) model explains many of the failures and paradoxes of the traditional model and accounts for many of the facts that a nociceptive and inflammatory model alone cannot. These include the common clinical observations of painless nerve impingement, why pain may resolve despite imaging evidence of persistent nerve impingement or electrodiagnostic evidence of ongoing acute denervation, or why pain may persist even after surgical nerve root decompression or in the absence of detectable inflammation. Understanding persistent spinal and regional musculoskeletal syndromes as manifestations of RNMP and not inflammatory in aetiology explains the common failure of antiinflammatory therapy for these conditions. It also explains why strengthening exercise, which normally produces muscle shortening, often fails to relieve pain, and not infrequently worsens it as it aggravates the already present muscle shortening seen in RNMP syndromes. Alternatively, it explains why such therapies as osteopathic manipulation, myofascial release, stretching, transcutaneous electrical nerve stimulation (TENS), diathermy, acupuncture, trigger point injection, and spinal cord stimulation may be effective. It would predict that muscle relaxant as well as antineuropathic medications such as gabapentin might be effective (Audette et al., 2005).

Gunn's identification of myofascial pain as essentially a neuropathic condition leads to additional insights. As a treatment for MPS, Gunn-IMS is hardly different from the other techniques of superficial and deep dry needling described in this textbook, and not only predicts but readily recognises the efficacy of these approaches. Yet although Gunn-IMS does not differ from dry needling (DN) in much of its technique, or the 'how', it does differ substantially from other DN techniques in its understanding of the 'what', 'where', 'why', and 'when' of MPS. It differs in explaining 'what' causes MPS and trigger points and so how to examine the patient and thus 'what' for and 'where' to look on physical examination. This leads to a rationale for 'where' to treat the patient (i.e., in a segmental or radiculoneuropathic pattern of myotomal involvement). In its recognition of MPS as a fundamentally neuropathic condition, it proposes an explanation of 'why' Gunn-IMS and many other forms of counterirritation reflex stimulation are effective in reversing neuropathic supersensitivity. Understanding the time frame for experimental reversal of neuropathic supersensitivity (Lomo & Rosenthal, 1972; Lomo & Westgaard, 1975), it also provides a 'when'—that is, a rationale for the expected length and course of treatment based on the severity of the physical examination findings. These and not the technique per se are what differentiate Gunn-IMS from DN.

Gunn's model recognises the 'myofascial trigger point' (TrP), but it recognises the TrP as just one of many clinical manifestations of RNMP. Because it is a radiculopathic model, it predicts the presence of TrPs in a myotomal distribution, including the posterior ramus, and recognises the importance of treating such points. Yet despite these differences Gunn-IMS practitioners share in common with all practitioners who treat MPS the recognition of both the prevalence of MPS and the success in treating it early and properly.

Indeed the most important aspect of Gunn's contribution is not even necessarily the technique of Gunn-IMS (although important), but that it will hopefully lead to wider recognition by the medical community of the significant incidence and prevalence of MPS in the general population. Epidemiological studies suggest that MPS is an important source of morbidity in the community (Cummings & White, 2001), yet it is commonly overlooked in the clinic (Skootsky et al., 1989). This is corroborated by the fact that it is found in 85% of patients seen in chronic pain clinics (Fishbain et al., 1989). MPS is the most common cause of chronic pain, and so 'it is essential to authenticate that chronic refractory myofascial pain is...a ubiquitous neuromusculoskeletal disease resulting from spondylotic radiculopathies induced partial denervation with denervation supersensitivity' and to recognise it as a 'global public health disease' (Chu et al., 2016). Despite all of the rich resources we have thrown at this problem by pursuing the standard paradigm of 'spondylosis-nociception-inflammation'—strengthening exercise programs, imaging studies, spinal injections, surgery, multidisciplinary pain clinics, opioids, spinal cord stimulators, and pumps—we have ended up with increasing suffering, impairment, opioid dependence, disability, and unsustainable costs (Deyo et al., 2009). The only things we have not done is recognise and treat myofascial pain early and properly. By placing myofascial pain squarely within the pathophysiological schema and thus diagnostic algorithm of spondylotic pain, myofascial pain can be properly seen as the prevalent condition that it is. Clinical presentations of myofascial pain are protean in their manifestations: pain referral, although adhering to general patterns, is individually variable, inconsistent, and sometimes enigmatic, and it can be overshadowed by the nonspecific nature of the nonpain complaints referable to autonomic mediation that suggest primary visceral pathology (Fricton et al., 1985). All of these features make it difficult to standardise case definition, thus making diagnosis elusive. Gunn's model accounts for this variability and provides an objective approach to the evaluation and treatment of these patients. Rather than a possible afterthought when the existing model fails, MPS will hopefully be moved to the forefront of the algorithmic evaluation of pain that persists for more than 3 to 6 months. With greater recognition and proper early treatment there is hope of stemming the global epidemic tide of chronic pain that is overwhelming Western medical systems.

Yet, although Gunn-IMS is a treatment for myofascial pain, the RNMP model that it is employed within represents more than simply a technique for treating TrPs. It represents an entirely new way to understand, examine, and effectively treat patients with persistent pain. As such, his work represents a true paradigm shift. Gunn's RNMP model provides a unified model of peripheral neuromusculoskeletal pain that points the way to improved treatment for these costly clinical and societal problems.

Although Gunn has exploited CL in the service of treating pain primarily, the implications of this law and Gunn's therapeutic model go beyond the treatment of neuromusculoskeletal pain. Although beyond the scope of this chapter, taken to its logical and inevitable conclusion, Gunn's model proposes a rational basis for the treatment of syndromes caused by the autonomically mediated visceral epiphenomena of segmental radiculoneuropathy, including such varied complaints as vertigo, tinnitus, irritable bowel syndrome, and infertility, to name but a few. Current research interest in the role of the nervous system in chronic, or 'parainflammation', suggests even broader and significant implications of Gunn's model (Tracey, 2002).

Gunn-IMS is a procedure that can carry significant risks, especially when treating deeper paraspinal muscle contractures or anywhere overlying the lungs or near vascular structures. Despite these risks, properly qualified healthcare providers, both primary care and specialist, can be taught to apply it safely and readily to many of the most commonly encountered clinical problems. In addition, Gunn-IMS, similar to all DN techniques, is 'low tech', inexpensive, and easily employed in clinics worldwide. Yet although any practitioner can easily be taught to stick a pin into a muscle, as mentioned previously it is the understanding of 'what' may cause the TrP, 'where' and 'how' to treat the patient, 'what' responses are sought by needling, 'why' needling is likely effective, and 'when', or how often and for how long to treat the patient that constitute the proper application of Gunn-IMS.

NEUROPHYSIOLOGICAL MECHANISM OF GUNN INTRAMUSCULAR STIMULATION

In seeking to understand his clinical findings, Gunn found an explanation in Cannon and Rosenblueth's 'The Supersensitivity of Denervated Structures, a Law of Denervation'. After the identification of segmental myalgic hyperalgesia ('tenderness at motor points') as a correlate of radiculopathy (Gunn & Milbrandt, 1976a), subsequent observations included the heretofore unrecognised neuropathic findings in these patients: increased muscle tone, neurogenic oedema, vasomotor disturbances with hypothermia, exaggerated pilomotor and sudomotor reflexes, and dermatomal hair loss (Gunn & Milbrandt, 1978).

Cannon is credited with originating the concept of the 'fight or flight' response, introducing the term 'homoeostasis', and popularising the use of barium to visualise the gastrointestinal tract. He and Arturo Rosenblueth, former head of the department of physiology and pharmacology at University of Mexico, also performed animal research demonstrating the effects of motor nerve denervation. CL quantified experimentally the pathophysiological responses to somatic and autonomic motor denervation in a variety of target end organ tissues, including skeletal and smooth muscle, spinal neurons, sympathetic ganglia, adrenal glands, sweat glands, and brain cells. These reactions can all be described as forms of supersensitivity (i.e., abnormal tissue responses to stimuli) and although Cannon investigated the effects of motor denervation (techniques to study sensory receptors did not exist then), the phenomena of neuropathic supersensitivity first described by him is the same as that which we recognise clinically in peripheral sensory neuropathies (e.g., diabetic, alcoholic) as dysesthesia, allodynia, and hyperalgesia. In other words, stimuli that normally should not trigger a response now do: it is not the stimuli that are abnormal but the system that senses them.

Cannon & Rosenblueth's Law is summarised as: 'When a unit is destroyed in a series of efferent neurons, an increased irritability to chemical agents develops in the isolated structure or structures, the effect being maximal in the part directly denervated'. Gunn, as a practicing physician, first recognised the clinical manifestations of CL: 'This law is seldom cited to explain neuropathic pain; it deserves to be better known. It points out that the normal physiology and integrity of all innervated structures are dependent on the arrival of nerve impulses via the intact nerve to provide a regulatory or trophic effect. When this flow, which is probably a combination of axoplasmic flow and electrical input, is blocked, innervated structures are deprived of the trophic factor, which is vital for the control and maintenance of cellular function… A-trophic structures become highly irritable and develop abnormal sensitivity or supersensitivity' (Loeser et al., 2001).

All of the tissues studied by Cannon and Rosenblueth (skeletal and smooth muscle, spinal neurons, sympathetic ganglia, adrenal glands, sweat glands, and brain cells) develop denervation supersensitivity.

Their research quantified this phenomena as: (1) increased susceptibility: lessened stimuli, which do not have to exceed a threshold, can produce responses of normal amplitude; (2) hyperexcitability: the threshold of the stimulating agent is lower than normal; (3) superreactivity: the capacity of the muscle to respond is augmented; and (4) superduration of response: the amplitude of response is unchanged but its time course is prolonged. Numerous animal experiments have confirmed that denervation supersensitivity is indeed a general phenomenon.

In the muscle, the previous responses are demonstrated by a lowered threshold to acetylcholine (ACh) inducing a contraction. It has also been shown in both striated and smooth muscle that the surface area of the muscle fibre that is sensitive to ACh increases. That is to say 'extrajunctional' areas on the surface away from the zone of innervation, normally the only area receptive to ACh stimulation, now respond to ACh. This phenomenon is detectable 4 to 5 days after denervation and reaches a maximum within about a week, at which time the entire surface of the muscle fibre is as sensitive to ACh as the neuromuscular junction (Axelsson & Thesleff, 1959).

Another manifestation of denervation supersensitivity in the muscle fibre is the development of spontaneous electrical activity called fibrillation. In contrast to an action potential in the muscle fibre occurring only in response to the release of neurotransmitter, action potentials now occur spontaneously due to changes in membrane potentials and conductivity. In electromyography, spontaneous depolarisations are called 'denervation potentials' and reflect loss of motor innervation; they are seen in diseases of the anterior horn cells, nerve roots, plexus, peripheral nerve, and muscle (Chu-Andrews & Johnson, 1986). They are manifestations of CL, reflecting the abnormally elevated sensitivity and reactivity of the muscle membrane to both ACh and the mechanical stimuli of the electromyography needle as it provokes depolarisation, a result of the disinhibiting effect of denervation. Significantly, in addition to the spontaneous depolarisations that produce action potentials, ACh slowly depolarises the supersensitive muscle membrane, inducing electromechanical coupling in which tension develops slowly without generating action potentials (Eyzaguirre & Fidone, 1975).

Cannon and Rosenblueth's original work was based on complete loss of motor innervation for supersensitivity to develop. Subsequently it became recognised that actual physical interruption and total denervation are not necessary: any injury or illness that impedes the flow of motor impulses for a period of time can rob the target organ of its excitatory input and cause supersensitivity in that structure and, significantly, in associated spinal reflexes (Loeser et al., 2001; Cangiano et al., 1977; Gilliatt et al., 1978). Supersensitive skeletal muscle fibres overreact to a wide variety of chemical and physical inputs, including stretch and pressure.

This process of nerve dysfunction with impaired or interrupted neural impulses (neurapraxia with partial or complete conduction block from dysmyelination/demyelination) and at times associated with partial denervation (incomplete axon loss from axonostenosis, axonocachexia, axonotmesis, Wallerian degeneration) is not uncommon in adults and is known as 'neuropathy', or 'nerve-sickness', literally. It is important to recognise that such nerves can still conduct nerve impulses, can synthesise and release transmitted substances, and, in the case of motor nerves, can evoke both muscle action potentials and muscle contraction. The causes of neuropathy are legion and include congenital, neoplasms, inflammatory, traumatic, vascular, toxic, metabolic, infectious, degenerative, and idiopathic aetiologies. Commonly recognised neuropathies include the peripheral sensory neuropathies associated with diabetes, nutritional deficiencies, chemotherapeutic agents, alcoholism, and postherpetic; however, the far more common cause of nerve dysfunction is injury, especially that due to spinal strain and trauma, including acute, subacute, and chronic. Sciatica, a type of spondylotic traumatic compressive neuropathy, accounts for the highest incidence of all causes of neuropathy, five times that of the second most common cause, diabetic neuropathy (Bridges et al., 2001). Spondylosis is defined as the subacute or chronic (gradual, insidious) structural disintegration and morphological alterations in the intervertebral disc and pathoanatomic changes in surrounding structures that leads to damage of the nerve roots and spinal nerves (Wilkinson, 1971). In addition to disc degeneration and bulging, osteophyte and spur formation, ligamentous hypertrophy, spondylolisthesis, decreased disc height, and facet joint arthropathy all combine to cause narrowing of the spinal canal and intervertebral foramina leading to radiculopathy and myelopathy in some patients. Evidence of spondylosis on imaging studies is common: it is found in more than 50% of those over 40 and 85% of those over 60 years old, yet as many as 75% to 90% of asymptomatic 60- to 65-year-olds show significant disc degeneration at one or more levels, confirming the poor correlation between structural abnormality and symptoms (Kelly et al., 2012).

The spinal nerve roots and spinal nerves are especially vulnerable to injury as result of anatomic features specific to these structures, especially the absence of the protective perineurium and epineurium around the roots; experimental research has documented the significantly lower compressive forces that the nerve roots are able to withstand compared with peripheral nerves before developing electrical conduction block (Sharpless, 1975). Axonal transport is blocked experimentally at pressures as low as 30 mm Hg, and the spinal nerves are limited to 15% elongation beyond their original length by stretching before developing intraneural blood flow and electrical conduction block (Rydevik et al., 1985); tethering by the dura, the intertransverse and mamilloaccessory as well as accessory ligaments further limit their mobility, with the mamilloaccessory a common source of entrapment neuropathy in patients with chronic low back and/or leg pain (Sihvonen, 1992). As little as 9 degrees of axial rotation will produce a myelographic filling defect at L5-S1 in normal subjects, with the angulation of the nerve over the edge of the vertebral body producing beyond normal physiological stretching of the nerve and potential neural deficit (Farfan, 1984). Spondylosis is thus associated with repetitive and cumulative compression, angulation, traction, and torsional injuries to the spinal nerves and roots, some leading to transient impaired intraneural blood flow, axonal transport, and electrical conduction block, and contributing to the development of neuropathic supersensitivity (Lorkovic, 1975; Gilliatt et al., 1978; Rydevik et al., 1985). Yet extrinsic neural compression may be absent, and the patient may have only partial denervation with intraneural fibrosis, with no evidence of a 'pinched nerve' on MRI and no evidence of acute denervation on EMG (Murphy, 1977; Sihvonen, 1992). Many of these cumulative injuries to the spinal nerves associated with reversible electrical conduction block may produce no or only transient symptoms (e.g., the 'stinger' in football) before the patient returns to an asymptomatic state, although subclinical neuropathic morbidity persists. When considered in its totality, spondylosis accounts for the most common form of neuropathy seen clinically: radiculoneuropathy, representing a far larger group of patients than those with radiculopathy, in which there are reflex and sensorimotor deficits on physical examination, a herniated disc seen compressing a nerve on MRI, and/or an abnormal EMG revealing acute denervation.

Because the nerve roots and spinal nerves contain motor, sensory, and autonomic fibres, it follows that the clinical manifestations of injury to them reflect the effects of neuropathy that develop to varying degrees in each of these three components. Ochoa and colleagues have demonstrated experimentally that tourniquet compression selectively demyelinates larger diameter fibres, sparing the smaller diameter myelinated and unmyelinated fibres (Ochoa et al., 1972). Because the largest diameter myelinated fibres in the spinal nerve and roots consist of the alpha motor neuron efferents and proprioceptive muscle spindle afferents, these are typically the earliest fibres damaged by the spondylotic process due to compression, either transient or prolonged.

As noted earlier, in neuropathic skeletal muscle ACh slowly depolarises the supersensitive muscle membrane, inducing electromechanical coupling of actin and myosin in which tension develops slowly without generating action potentials. Due to the extended time frame over which this occurs, no action potentials are seen on electromyography, and this shortening is called contracture rather than contraction (Eyzagguire & Fidone, 1975). In addition, Gunn has proposed that radiculoneuropathic involvement of muscle spindle afferent fibres leads to hyperexcitability of the muscle spindle mechanism, potentiating the length-regulating feedback mechanism of the gamma loop and contributing to the development of these contractures (Gunn & Milbrandt, 1977). This mechanism may be amplified even further by sympathetic supersensitivity activating intrafusal fibres of the muscle spindle (Chu, 1995). Dysfunction of this mechanism is sometimes referred to as the 'facilitated segment', 'somatic dysfunction', or the 'osteopathic lesion' (Korr, 1975).

Consistent with the experimental evidence showing the earliest involvement of nonnociceptive large diameter myelinated fibres (alpha motor neuron and proprioceptive muscle spindle afferents), it is noteworthy that muscle contracture and hyperexcitability of the muscle spindle produce the earliest symptoms the patient often reports: these are typically not the pain we associate with nociception (i.e., sharp, or even dull and aching). Early symptoms associated with MPS are often described as stiffness or tightness and have a peculiar cramplike sensation. This is the same phenomena seen in significant numbers of patients diagnosed with irritable bowel syndrome (IBS), who experience sensitivity to abdominal distension that is perceived as pain: hypersensitivity of the mechanoreceptors for stretch and contractile tension are implicated in this entity, although involving smooth muscle rather than striated muscle (Johnson, 2012). So, just as 'all that glitters is not gold', 'all that 'pains' is not nociception'. Muscle spindle dysfunction also results in impaired proprioceptive and neuromuscular function, producing impaired standing balance or cursive handwriting; these symptoms even often preceding the onset of 'painful' symptoms.

On physical examination these muscle contractures are palpable in the more superficial muscles and are commonly referred to as 'taut bands', 'ropy bands', or 'contraction knots' (Baldry, 2001). Deeper, nonpalpable contractures are what Gunn terms 'the silent lesion' (Gunn, 1996). Over time, when enough regions of the muscle develop contractures, the muscle's overall resting length shortens, at which point the patient may become aware of decreased flexibility, noting, for example, the need to turn their upper body to check automotive traffic behind them, as the active range of motion in the cervical spine is diminished. As the process of spondylosis advances with additional acute injuries superimposed on preexisting subclinical neuropathy, the model postulates that small diameter nerve fibres eventually develop supersensitivity leading to myalgic allodynia (tenderness to light touch/palpation that is normally nonpainful) and hyperalgesia (elevated levels of pain to light touch/palpation that is normally painful). The patient may still not complain of pain but may report impaired balance, stiffness, and decreased flexibility; the patient is often surprised by the pain elicited by palpation of these tender contractures, or 'latent TrPs' (Sola et al., 1955; Baldry, 2001). It is this morbid but generally pain-free phase that Gunn terms 'prespondylosis' (Gunn et al., 1980).

With progressive sensitisation of small diameter nociceptor fibres and muscle shortening compressing the intramuscular type III and IV nociceptors, the patient develops 'active TrPs' and complains of pain at rest, in the absence of either external nociceptive stimuli or tissue inflammation. Lactic acidosis and other biochemical changes in the local milieu of the trigger point (Shah et al., 2008) chemically sensitise the nociceptive fibres further, contributing to the pain.

When radiculoneuropathy involves the autonomic division of the spinal nerve, vascular, smooth muscle, pilomotor, sudomotor, and trophic responses are exaggerated. Although one of the clinical hallmarks of inflammation is warmth/heat, neuropathy results in vasoconstriction and relative coolness of affected segments. Because Cannon's Law applies to smooth muscle fibres as well as striated skeletal muscle, they respond similarly to denervation and neuropathy by developing shortening contractures. The architecture of smooth muscle is distinct, however, from the arrangement of skeletal muscle fibres, which lay parallel to each other. The smooth muscle cells lining vascular,

lymphatic, and visceral organs are arranged adjacent to each other, in sheets or layers; when they develop shortening contractures, the potential space between adjacent cells ('cell gap') increases, and intraluminal fluids leak out, creating neurogenic oedema (recognised as 'cellulite' when located in the hip girdle and thighs).

Neuropathy induced smooth muscle contractures also result in impairment of efficient synchronous muscular contractile function, which can produce symptoms that can be mistaken for primary visceral pathology. Depending on the spinal segments involved, otolaryngological, cardiorespiratory, gastrointestinal, and genitourinary signs and symptoms may occur, including dizziness, bronchospasm with neurogenic oedema/ARDS, 'irritable' bowel, urinary frequency-urgency, and even infertility due to fallopian tube smooth muscle dysfunction precluding passage of the ova.

The quality of collagen in soft and skeletal tissues is degraded in neuropathy with replacement collagen weaker due to fewer crosslinks. With muscle contractures creating increased mechanical tension on these weaker ligaments, tendons, cartilage, and bones, neuropathy expedites degenerative wear and tear, especially in activity-stressed parts of the body, causing 'spondylosis', 'discogenic' disease, and 'osteoarthritis'. Although these entities continue to be regarded as primary diseases, they are the 'down-stream' cumulative effects of RNMP. Enthesopathy, thickening of the musculotendinous junction, is also seen as a result of and possibly compensation for the factors mentioned previously.

Autonomic neuropathy also leads to exaggerated sudomotor and pilomotor responses, producing hyperhidrosis and 'goose bumps/flesh'. The presence of dermatomal rather than stocking distribution hair loss (as seen in peripheral neuropathy) is another common finding, attributable to trophic changes. Gunn refers to the constellation of these autonomically mediated signs and symptoms as the 'epiphenomena' of spondylotic neuropathy.

The combined motor, sensory, and autonomic effects of RNMP manifest as all manner of subjective complaints, including coolness, paresthesias (including tingling, buzzing, vibration, pressure), dysesthesias (including 'pins and needles'), neuralgic pain (shooting-stabbing-lancinating-paroxysmal), and itching (Stellon, 2002). Complaints of unsteadiness, dizziness, stiffness, weakness, fatigue, and swelling are attributable to muscle shortening, muscle spindle dysfunction, and neurogenic oedema. Physical findings may include impaired single leg standing balance, decreased range of motion, coolness to touch, hyperhidrosis, goose-flesh, dermatomal hair loss, myalgic hyperalgesia with generation of referred pain, and either spontaneous or elicited local fasciculation, known as the 'local twitch response' (LTR). There may be cutaneous hypoesthesia and allodynia, rather than anaesthesia which is present in denervation.

Over time RNMP leads to both localised intramuscular contractures and shortening of the resting length of the muscle, as well as the persistent increased mechanical tension on the musculotendinous attachments to bone leads to what previously was labelled tendonitis, implying an inflammatory aetiology, now preferably called tendinopathy or tendinosis (Khan et al., 1999). These include most of the subacute and chronic tendonitis and bursitis syndromes (Achilles, extensor forearm, bicipital, rotator cuff, DeQuervain's tenosynovitis, patella, gluteal) as well as such entities as iliotibial band syndrome, chondromalacia patellae, muscle tension headache, pyriformis syndrome, plantar fasciitis, and temporomandibular joint. Many of these are thus seen as the effects of muscle shortening that, due to increased tension at the periosteum, create pain as well as bone spurs according to Wolff's Law, which describes the process of bone deposition in response to mechanical tensile forces. Thus extensor elbow tendinosis, or 'tennis elbow', is seen not as a local pathology but the 'downstream' effect of subacute and chronic C6-C7 radiculoneuropathic–myofascial pain that can sometimes be treated successfully by treatment to the cervical spine alone (Gunn & Milbrandt, 1976b).

The constellation of symptoms and signs noted previously collectively constitute a picture and definition of what is called MPS, myofascial pain being a term popularised by Dr. Janet Travell, who also 'popularised the use of the term TrP (Baldry, 2001). The pathognomonic feature of MPS is the TrP, the hallmark of which is hyperalgesia with referred pain, and which is 'structurally…made up of a collection of dysfunctional motor endplates, juxtapositional contraction knots and neurovascular bundles with each containing blood vessels and contiguous sympathetic fibres; a motor axon and its nerve terminals; and sensory afferents attached to proprioceptors and nociceptors' (Baldry, 2001).

Whereas Gunn's model recognises TrPs as most often found beneath motor points and the importance of directing treatment to these points (Gunn et al., 1980), the TrP is seen as just one of the many diverse manifestations of radiculoneuropathic–myofascial pain syndromes. It recognises that needling can 'occasionally actuate muscle to fasciculation: this is usually accompanied by near-instantaneous muscle relaxation' (LTR). It also recognises that, due to supersensitivity, the entire surface of the neuropathic muscle may respond to needling. Penetration into almost any part of the muscle can lead to relaxation, but the most rewarding sites are at tender and painful points in muscle bands (Gunn, 1989).

Gunn's finding of a correlation between tender motor points and electromyographic (EMG) evidence of partial denervation radiculopathy has been corroborated by Chu using a semiquantitative motor unit action potential (MUAP) EMG technique (Chu, 1995). Although EMG abnormalities were found in a myotomal distribution correlating with clinical findings of MPS, Chu suggested that single-fibre EMG (SFEMG) may be more useful than conventional EMG in establishing the cause of abnormalities as 'neurogenic, myogenic, or otherwise'. The presence and severity of motor neuroaxonal degeneration correlating with TrPs and disease duration using SFEMG technique has been established by Chang, who has also found evidence of spinal accessory neuropathy in cervical MPS (Chang et al., 2008, 2011). Clinical studies (Letchuman et al., 2005; Sari et al., 2012) have also confirmed the association between (cervical) radiculopathy and myofascial tender points as originally demonstrated by Gunn (Gunn & Milbrandt, 1976a).

Cannon originally experimentally documented neuropathic supersensitivity from motor denervation in both the peripheral (skeletal muscle/neuromuscular junction, autonomic ganglia) (Cannon & Rosenblueth, 1936) and central (brain, spinal neurons) (Cannon & Haimovici, 1939) nervous systems, defining it quantitatively using the neurotransmitter acetylcholine. Since then the phenomena of central sensitisation that develops in response to peripheral nociception and/or nerve damage has been further elaborated experimentally, with evidence of biomarker, neurotransmitter and neuroplastic changes in the dorsal horn, cingulate nucleus, hippocampus and other regions of the CNS leading to amplified and sustained pain in the absence of ongoing peripheral nociception; it has been precisely defined as an 'amplification of neural signaling within the CNS that elicits pain hypersensitivity' (Woolf, 2011). Partial deafferentation of the CNS (as in radiculoneuropathy) can result in both chronic 'central' pain (Loeser, 2012) and peripheral findings of supersensitivity. Gunn's localisation of the pathology to the spinal nerve therefore accounts for both retrograde proximal–central and anterograde distal–peripheral neuropathic abnormalities. Clinically, however, the central and peripheral nervous systems function simultaneously and seamlessly as an integrated system and cannot be separated—research has confirmed the presence of peripheral sensitisation manifesting as trigger points in many syndromes associated with central sensitisation, contributing to the cluster of signs and symptoms seen in these patients (Dommerholt, 2011).

What then is the evidence that Gunn-IMS can reverse RNMP? Evidence that neuropathic supersensitivity can be reversed was demonstrated experimentally by Lomo, who showed that ACh supersensitivity in denervated animal skeletal muscle could be abolished by graded electrical stimuli (Lomo & Rosenthal, 1972; Lomo & Westgaard, 1975; Thesleff, 1976). Fig. 15.1 shows how experimental denervation affects the sensitivity of a muscle membrane to ACh (bold line). Additionally, Fig. 15.1 shows how this hypersensitivity returns toward normal after electrical stimulation and does so more quickly with continuously applied stimuli. Gunn has proposed that the 'current of injury' (the measureable electrical microcurrent associated with damage to a cell wall membrane) created by the minor muscle fibre trauma of needling provides an intrinsic source of electrical stimulation that facilitates reversal of neuropathic supersensitivity similar to that provided exogenously by Lomo (Gunn, 1978).

Supporting evidence for Gunn's claim that DN can reverse neuropathic supersensitivity is found in animal studies which have shown that the spontaneous endplate activity (SEA) associated with TrPs (and predicted by a neuropathic model of MPS) can be diminished by DN (Chen et al., 2000). Chu studied the electromyographic effects of DN in humans and stated 'that the presence of discharges of sustained or grouped endplate potentials and twitch responses are gradations of the same phenomena of achieving focal muscle contraction of varying forces at a physiological level. Stretching occurs at the myofibrillar level, with breaking of the actin–myosin bonds responsible for sarcomere shortening and stiffness' (Chu, 1995, 1997).

CLINICAL APPLICATION OF GUNN INTRAMUSCULAR STIMULATION
Introduction
The proper practice of Gunn-IMS requires that the clinician remains mindful of the radiculopathic model and the effects of partial denervation supersensitivity. In doing so, the practitioner will easily be able to collect signs and symptoms that focus attention on the appropriate spinal levels. Treatment directed at the affected spinal levels is mandatory in Gunn-IMS (Gunn & Milbrandt, 1976b) and, along with the corresponding segmentally innervated muscles exhibiting positive findings, will provide the best outcomes (Gunn & Milbrandt, 1976b; Ga et al., 2007b). Neuropathic signs and symptoms will often improve, along with an increase in limited range of motion and restoration of normal movement patterns. Without ensuring that the radiculopathic model is the basis of all decisions, client outcomes and therapist satisfaction with this technique may suffer. Kim and colleagues (2003) documented a study in which neuropathic signs and symptoms helped to identify the true cause of pain in patients for which surgery had failed. In this study, failed back surgery syndrome patients were assessed with a simple and general Gunn-IMS clinical examination and treatment. All patients showed improvement in their symptoms, leaving doctors to consider Gunn-IMS as an alternative effective treatment modality for failed back surgery syndrome patients.

One of the most notable and consistent comments offered by newly certified Gunn-IMS practitioners

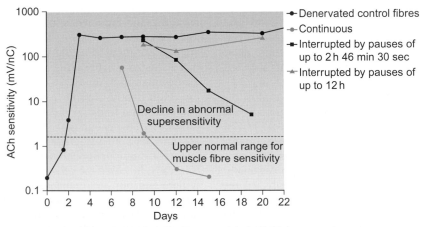

FIG. 15.1 Experimental reversal of denervation supersensitivity.

is how its use immediately translates into better outcomes in clinical practice. Many conditions that have been resistant to standard therapies will improve dramatically when the neuropathic component is treated using Gunn-IMS. Therapy that adheres to the tenets of Gunn-IMS will identify neuropathy, where present, and treat the myotomal level(s) affected. When a myotomal pattern is present, both proximally in the paraspinal and distally in the distribution of the anterior ramus, radiculopathy is confirmed (Gunn, 1996). The ensuing treatment must target both the erector spinae and distal myotomally linked muscles.

The information that follows is sufficient to understand how the clinical examination is used to determine the presence of neuropathy and provide basic information regarding what is required of a therapist to treat using Gunn-IMS. In order to become a safe, competent, and certified Gunn-IMS practitioner, instruction from a certified Gunn-IMS instructor is required. Gunn's textbook, 'The Gunn approach to the treatment of chronic pain—Intramuscular stimulation for myofascial pain of radiculopathic origin' (Gunn, 1996) has been translated into several languages and is the standard reference text and bedside manual used at international Gunn-IMS courses.

Patient History and Past Treatment

Gunn-IMS is the most appropriate treatment technique when the patient presents with clear signs of neuropathy. For patients in which inflammation is the dominant presentation, a strategy specific for the control and resolution of an inflammatory process must be followed. The determination of pain type is simplified by reviewing the characteristics of each class of pain. Nociception produces immediate pain in the presence of noxious stimuli associated with the threat of tissue damage and precipitates the 'fight-or-flight' behavioural response. Inflammation can produce acute pain by damage to tissue that releases chemicals that activate nociceptors, and behaviourally precipitates care, concern, and anxiety. When due to direct trauma, inflammation is a self-limited process that responds to supportive measures. Strains and sprains should typically heal within weeks. Chronic pain, by definition pain lasting more than 3 months, may occur in the presence of ongoing nociception, psychological factors, or alterations in the central or peripheral nervous system and behaviourally can lead to depression (Gunn, 1996). A review of the injury mechanism, current presentation, and overall duration will help in determining which of the classes fit the patients' pain characteristics. Current and recent use of medication is a valuable tool in understanding the class of pain. In radiculopathic patients, antiinflammatories are often of limited use, and muscle relaxants may help in the short term, both being discontinued if the side effects outweigh the usefulness of the drug. More recently, a tour through the different (anti) neuropathic medications is often attempted with varying levels of effectiveness. In these cases, the patient often presents with a desire to further decrease their pain while decreasing their use of medications.

The patients' history will often be characterised by pain with no obvious cause. If a history of an injury is present, it may seem trivial compared with the severity and consequence of the patient's pain. The insidious nature of neuropathy is often the result of spondylosis, the most common cause of radiculopathy (Gunn et al., 1980). Multiple diagnostic tests (x-ray, MRI, CT, and EMG/nerve conduction tests) may have been ordered but offer little to correlate with the presentation of pain. There must be no obvious signs of complete denervation (e.g., severe atrophy, absent reflex, complete anaesthesia) as the radiculopathic model is specific to partial denervation supersensitivity. Partial denervation, or neuropathy, causes any tissue supplied by an affected nerve to become abnormally sensitive to a variety of normally nonnoxious stimuli. From the perspective of patient complaints, the most common and significant tissue that develops supersensitivity is skeletal muscle (Gunn, 1996). This supersensitivity causes the 'shortened muscle syndrome', creating long standing tension throughout the muscle and its tendon(s). The muscles and tendons may respond to this pull by chronically thickening (enthesopathy). The patient may have been told incorrectly that this is a tendonitis, even though the only clinical feature is tenderness and there is a lack of inflammatory signs. When the muscle exerts force on or over a bursa the popular diagnosis may be bursitis, even though repeated treatments and local injection prove unsuccessful. Past treatment, which has been directed locally, may have decreased the pain; however, the response is often short lived or minimal. The local treatments that may have proven partially effective often include massage, physical therapy, and finally TrP injections. The radiculopathic model explains why these treatments may be only partially effective for this subgroup of patients. All physical methods of treatment that provide some relief in neuropathic pain are ultimately forms of energy which stimulate specific receptors, and, as such, they may help to decrease the supersensitivity of a neuropathic region (Gunn, 1984). When the patient demonstrates a history of partial success with short-acting stimulation type treatments such as massage, TENS, exercise, or manipulation,

Gunn-IMS may serve as the necessary additional supply of a more specific, localised, higher intensity, and prolonged stimulation through the current of injury. In the case of stubborn pain when simple methods prove ineffective, Gunn-IMS is indicated (Gunn, 1996). There is no need to waste time and money on expensive tests and long wait lists for specialist referrals.

Physical Assessment

It is reasonable to expect that the clinical examination be straightforward, focused, and easy to carry out. Gunn-IMS is based on the recognition that neuropathy most often occurs at the level of the spinal nerve root (radiculopathy) with its three divisions (motor, sensory, autonomic). For ease of presentation the physical signs that follow are organised according to these three divisions. When radiculopathy is present and pain is a presenting symptom, it is often accompanied by muscle shortening, tender focal areas in muscle (TrPs), and autonomic and trophic manifestations (Gunn, 1996).

Sensory findings

Peripheral nerve supersensitivity affecting sensory fibres may present as altered pain reports. Allodynia and hyperalgesia refer to complaints of excessive muscle tenderness to typically nonnoxious or mildly noxious stimuli (e.g., tenderness using flat palpation or gentle squeezing). Hyperpathia refers to client reports of prolonged duration of pain from nociceptive stimuli, reflecting the phenomenon of superduration as described originally by Cannon. Testing for hyperpathia is typically performed using a pinwheel over suspected dermatomes. The presence of these signs may be indicative of peripheral sensitisation secondary to peripheral nerve dysfunction, neuropathy.

Motor Findings

Observation

The observation and assessment of motor involvement are perhaps the most familiar and recognisable components of the neuropathy–radiculopathy assessment. They are important in that muscle shortening is an early feature of radiculopathy and may occur in the absence of pain (Gunn et al., 1980). Therefore identification of shortened muscles allows for early intervention before the perception of pain. Observations such as scoliosis, nonanatomical leg length discrepancies, elevated shoulders, or skin creasing will draw the therapist's attention to muscle shortening without the use of expensive imaging tests. The innervation of each indicated muscle directs the clinician to specific spinal levels where further testing may support or refute the observational findings.

Range of motion

The shortening of muscle at rest is easily measured as decreased range of motion. The use of a simple and inexpensive goniometer or tape measurement is the only equipment required to accurately quantify current status and future improvements in most cases.

Palpable Bands

Tenderness at motor points was the first clinical feature commented on by Gunn and Milbrandt (1976a). They postulated that partial denervation supersensitivity may lead to increased irritability of muscle and contribute to the muscle shortening seen in neuropathy (Gunn & Milbrandt, 1978). On examination, muscle contractures ('taut' or 'ropy bands', 'contraction knots') with exaggerated tenderness (myalgic hyperalgesia) are identified by utilising a snapping palpation directed perpendicular to the muscle, the presence of which must be notated with attention to the corresponding level of motor innervation.

Autonomic Findings

The autonomic portion of peripheral nerves is responsible for controlling many visceral functions. The effects are often not noted or overlooked as they are thought to be unrelated to the report of pain. Because autonomic patterns of innervation do not always strictly follow dermatomal, myotomal, or sclerotomal distributions, their clinical manifestations are less segmentally localising. Yet attention to this division of the spinal nerve root rounds out the evidence for radiculopathy and was first commented on by Gunn and Milbrandt (1976b). As with the sensory and motor signs, the approximated affected segmental level must be noted for each autonomic sign observed.

Vasomotor Disturbances

Vasoconstrictor disturbance secondary to smooth muscle contracture may be observed as mottling of the skin. Additionally, affected areas will be perceptively cooler to palpation, as tested with the back of the examiner's hand. In recent times thermographic scans have become more popular, although are unnecessary for the purpose of this assessment.

Sudomotor Reflex

The pattern of sweating and tendency to sweat is noted. In partial nerve palsies there is an increased sweat response, and hyperhidrosis may be noted in affected areas in a characteristic nerve root pattern (Gunn & Milbrandt, 1978). This may manifest as a 'wet' hand-shake or perspiration footprints seen on a laminate floor.

Pilomotor Reflex

The pilomotor reflex ('gooseflesh' or 'goose-bumps') may be observed when the affected area is undraped for examination. This reflex may also be elicited when palpating or needling muscles of the affected segmental level.

Trophic Changes

When the nutritional supply to a tissue is decreased, proper growth may be delayed or absent. A change in nutrition may be observed as alterations in skin, nails, subcutaneous tissues, muscles, bones, and joints (Gunn & Milbrandt, 1978). The pattern of hair loss is a common indicator for altered nutritional status. Fig. 15.2 shows loss of hair at the L2-L3 nerve root level in a hirsute male. Figs 15.3 and 15.4 show additional similar patterns of hair loss at other dermatomal levels (L5, C5). Essential in the Gunn-IMS assessment is the identification and consideration of clinical signs that have often gone unnoticed or were not considered relevant.

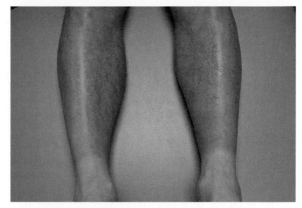

FIG. 15.3 L5 dermatomal hair loss due to trophic disturbance.

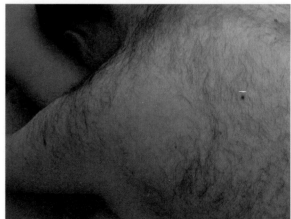

FIG. 15.4 C5 dermatomal hair loss due to trophic disturbance.

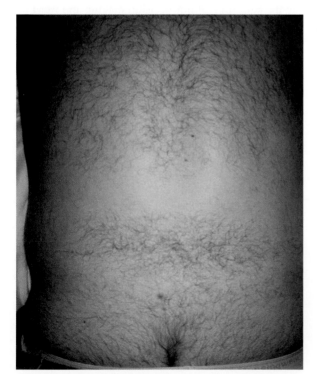

FIG. 15.2 L2-L3 dermatomal hair loss due to trophic disturbance.

Neuropathy may also lead to decreased collagen quality and fewer crosslinks with subsequent compromise of the integrity and strength of ligaments, cartilage, and bone, thus contributing to a variety of degenerative conditions in weight-bearing and activity-stressed structures. 'These secondary conditions...are probably only the ultimate sequelae of neuropathy. Degenerative disc disease itself may not be a primary condition' (Gunn et al., 1980). Findings may include ligamentous and capsular joint laxity, subluxation, or instability.

Trophic Oedema

When efferent impulses in an autonomic peripheral nerve are partially interrupted, smooth muscle contracture ensues, and trophic oedema occurs (Haymaker & Woodhall, 1953). The presence of neurogenic oedema can be easily identified by specific examination techniques, but it is clinically distinct from the 'pitting' oedema due to cardio–renal pathologies and cannot be elicited by digital depression in the pretibial pedal region. The matchstick test is another example of the high degree of specificity afforded with this assessment without the need for expensive procedures or imaging (Fig. 15.5). Although the matchstick has been replaced by the blunt end of a swab, the test remains the same. The blunt end is firmly pressed into the skin throughout the tested area. A positive test is indicated when the indentation appears deeper, has defined edges and does not resolve for some time (Gunn, 1996).

The presence of a peau d'orange effect may also be used to identify trophic changes. Fig. 15.6 shows a

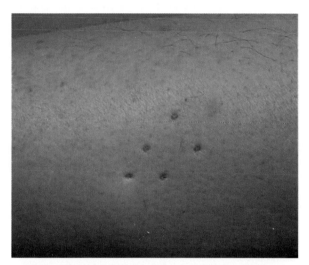

FIG. 15.5 Matchstick test for neurogenic oedema.

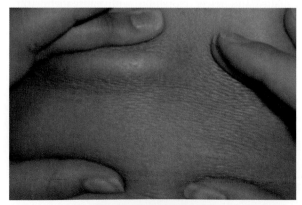

FIG. 15.6 Peau d'orange ('orange peel') appearance of skin and subcutaneous tissue by skin rolling technique.

clinician performing this test by bunching up a section of skin to see if it appears similar in appearance to an orange peel—the 'skin rolling technique'. Neurogenic oedema can also manifest as the variable and intermittent swelling around joints, often mistakenly attributed to inflammation despite the absence of evidence of tissue damage. Enthesopathy can often be palpated along the base of the occiput, at the mastoid process, over the common extensor origin/lateral epicondyle of elbow, and along the Achilles tendon and segmental origins of the erector spinae.

These sensory, motor and autonomic signs may identify both the presence of neuropathy and the affected spinal segment(s). Treatment should be directed to the segment indicated with retesting performed in each future session.

TREATMENT

Evidence-based medicine requires clinical practice to rely on the therapist's individual clinical expertise and the best available scientific evidence. Clinical expertise increases with our experience and practice, whereas evidence increases with advances in the basic sciences and patient-centered clinical research. These two aspects are the backbone of our decision making and must be combined with the patient's predicaments, rights, and preferences (Sackett et al., 1996).

When planning Gunn-IMS treatments, clinicians must keep in mind the history and pathophysiology that supports the radiculopathic model as the science is both growing and unbiased in its support. We must also keep in mind the evidence for the use of Gunn-IMS in this group of clients as accessibility and treatment results often favour Gunn-IMS techniques for RNMP. Clinical research continues to expand our understanding of treatments for neuropathy. By using a needle, the clinician makes use of an ancient technique for stimulating the body. The ancient practice of acupuncture is credited with the discovery of the effects of stimulation on the body, and modern techniques have updated the practice with modern needles. Gunn spoke of the use of needles for treatment in terms of stimulation of motor points in 1976. Lewitt directly compared an injection technique to noninjection stating: 'in reviewing techniques for therapeutic local anaesthesia of pain spots, it appeared that the common denominator was puncture by the needle and not the anaesthetic employed' (Lewit, 1979).

The current use of Gunn-IMS follows this rich history of nonpharmaceutical treatment and updates it with modern science and physiology. In clinical practice the treatment must be combined with patient rights and preferences, assisting in the growth of clinical experience. Karakurum and colleagues (2001) published a paper titled 'The 'dry-needle technique': intramuscular stimulation in tension-type headache.' They compared treatment with intramuscular stimulation (IMS) with a placebo group that utilised shallow needle insertions. The insertion points used in each group were consistent, differing only in depth of penetration. The study concluded that the treatment (IMS) group was more effective in reducing the tenderness score and increasing neck range of motion. Studies by Ga and colleagues (2007a, 2007b, 2007c) directly compared different needling techniques for their effect in treating TrPs in myofascial pain. In the first study, acupuncture was compared with lidocaine injection (Ga et al., 2007a). Both groups demonstrated improvement in pain reports and range of motion but were not found to be significantly different. In another study intramuscular and nerve root stimulation was compared with lidocaine injection (Ga et al., 2007b). The intramuscular stimulation technique was found to be superior in reducing pain, increasing range, and decreasing depression. The DN technique used was described as modified TrP needling as described by Simons with nerve root stimulation as described by Gunn. A final study directly compared DN of TrPs with and without paraspinal needling (Ga et al., 2007c). The results were similar to the previously mentioned study, with the authors stating, 'TrP and paraspinal DN is suggested to be a better method than TrP DN only for treating in elderly patients.'

A well-designed, placebo-sham control study that included only patients with a neuropathic component on the Neuropathic Pain Diagnostic Questionnaire (DN4) demonstrated greater efficacy of multiple trigger point deep DN combined with paraspinal deep intramuscular stimulation in the spinal segment where hyperalgesia was identified, compared with lidocaine trigger point injection (Couto et al., 2014). All outcome measures including the visual analogue scale (VAS), algometric pressure point threshold (PPT), visual analogue sleep quality scale (VASQS), health-related quality of life (SF-12 Physical and Mental Health Summary Scales), and—perhaps the 'gold standard' of objective outcome measurements—analgaesic medication usage, all significantly improved with the DN intervention compared with injection of lidocaine. This 'combined' technique is identical to Gunn-IMS, and the authors

conclude that their results are supported by Gunn's theory that myofascial pain syndrome is due to 'disordered function in the peripheral nerve'. Additional clinical research is currently looking at the efficacy of IMS in comparison with sham placebo needling, trigger point injection, and neural prolotherapy in chronic whiplash associated disorder and chronic midportion Achilles tendinopathy.

Chu has developed an electrotherapeutic device called 'eToims' (electrical twitch obtaining intramuscular stimulation) that can objectively identify, grade, and treat myofascial trigger points associated with partial denervation and supersensitivity due to spondylotic neuropathy (Chu et al., 2016, 2017). Although this is not a needling therapy, it quantifies and effectively reverses motorpoint neuropathic sensitivity through afferent stimulation and elicitation of graded LTRs as described by Gunn; stimulation is surface–electrical rather than needle–intramuscular–mechanical as in IMS, but otherwise applied within and consistent with Gunn's RNMP model. Using a single case study design sequentially over time (which can produce superior statistical results compared with random controlled trials (RCTs)), use of the eToims device demonstrated significant reduction in pain and increased function in a patient with chronic refractory myofascial pain.

As mentioned earlier, clinically the peripheral and central nervous systems function in a simultaneous and integrated manner and cannot be separated; so even though the objective findings of peripheral sensitisation are more readily clinically diagnosable, they likely are accompanied by some degree of central sensitisation, even if the clinical diagnosis of 'central sensitisation syndrome' is still elusive (Dommerholt, 2011; Srebly et al., 2016). The LTR is mediated by CNS spinal reflexes (Hong, 1994), and DN has been shown to have both local and remote effects, supporting that its mechanism of action occurs at the spinal cord segmentally as well as suprasegmentally in the CNS. In addition to reversing peripheral sensitisation, by stimulating spinal reflexes IMS also likely modulates central sensitisation through its antinociceptive, segmental and suprasegmental CNS effects (Srebly et al., 2010; Dommerholt, 2011; Woolf, 2011).

With sufficiently supportive scientific clinical evidence (Gunn et al., 1980; Chu, 1995, 1997, 1999; Karakurum et al., 2001; Ga et al., 2007a, 2007b, 2007c; Couto et al., 2014), the clinician can be confident that treating paraspinal muscle segments as well as corresponding distal muscles will provide optimal results in this group of patients. With this in mind, the number of treatments, duration of each session and style of needle insertion will be explained.

Number of Treatments

It is common for treatment of a noncomplex condition to be completed in 6 to 8 sessions, although more severe cases require a more prolonged course of intervention. Treatments occur once per week, on consecutive weeks. Gunn and colleagues (1980) found the average number of treatments/condition to be 7.9 sessions in injured workers with chronic low back pain. Other studies reporting successful outcomes with the Gunn-IMS model have used as few as three (Ga et al., 2007b, 2007c) or four treatments (Karakurum et al., 2001) and as many as 36 or more for patients with long duration symptoms associated with lumbar spinal stenosis, postlaminectomy, and fibromyalgia (Chu, 1999). These studies did not attempt to identify the number of treatments required for optimal results and, as such, should not be considered for this purpose. The resolution of supersensitivity and reversal of neuropathic signs must be the most important factors used to determine the length of a course of treatments. A detailed reevaluation after six treatments will establish a baseline of initial response and allow for a prognosis for the likely frequency and length of additional treatment.

Duration of Session

It is advised that assessment and treatment be scheduled for 45 to 60 minutes. A typical treatment time recommended for Gunn-IMS is 30 minutes. This allows time for updating the patient's report of interval responses to treatment, proper testing, explanation, thorough treatment, and retesting with final explanations and advice. The invasive nature of the treatment must also be considered. Permitting sufficient time for the treatment allows the patient to remain calm. If the client feels rushed and nervous, strong autonomic response may accompany treatment and precipitate treatment limiting vasovagal responses.

Needle Insertion

Gunn-IMS treatment requires needle stimulation of skeletal muscle. With the choice of muscle being driven by the assessment findings, how does one choose the site of needle insertion? Gunn's initial observation was the tender motor point. Today, palpation of tight bands combined with allodynia and hyperalgesia are the typical findings that finely focus needling practice. The motor point is the locus on the surface of the body that corresponds to an underlying neuromuscular

endplate zone and where electrical conductivity is normally lower than the surrounding tissues (Shultz et al., 2007). Contractures leading to trigger points initially develop and are most often found in these endplate zones. The use of a handheld device commonly called a 'point finder' that measures electrical skin resistance/conductivity can be useful to more precisely localise the sites likely to provoke the strongest responses, but it is not routinely necessary.

The amount of stimulation administered is dependent first on the patient needs and tolerances and then by the goals of treatment. In the first treatment the number of points and stimulation administered is considerably less than in later treatments. This number will often fall within 12 treatment points, including treatment of up to four spinal segments. The number of points used is considerably less important than the patient's comfort with treatment and the amount of supersensitivity present. Highly supersensitive patients will usually respond favourably to fewer points than those who are moderately or minimally supersensitive. Even patients with a history of prior Gunn-IMS treatment that appear to tolerate points well should only receive a minimal number of points on their initial visit. In later sessions the number of needle insertions may increase as supersensitivity decreases. Audette and colleagues (2004) demonstrated that 'in subjects with active TrPs, bilateral motor unit activation could be obtained with unilateral needle stimulation of the TrP', suggesting that treatment in the presence of active TrPs and bilateral symptoms does not necessarily require bilateral treatment. The decision regarding the number of points to needle in each session is made using clinical evidence but requires clinician experience. If a smaller number of points are used initially, an increase in points may subsequently be required and tolerated by the patient.

Needle-Grasp

Gunn and Milbrandt stated in 1977 that 'when needle agitation occurs in a partially denervated or neuropathic muscle, the intense local muscular contraction causes the needle-grasp and in extreme cases bending of the needle.' They expand on this phenomenon stating that the exaggerated discharge on needle insertion 'may cause the muscle to fasciculate and relax'. Fasciculation, also called the 'local twitch response', is the term for clinically observable twitching of a group of muscle fibres belonging to a single motor unit. This muscular reaction assists in the identification of muscles that both require treatment and will respond best to Gunn-IMS. The needle-grasp is characterised by resistance to needle removal, reflecting increased reflex muscle contracture-shortening, whereas a LTR is characterised by a brief contraction.

There appears to be current interest in discerning the difference between these graded manifestations of response to the needle. In the Gunn-IMS model this is of interest but not of fundamental importance. The act of properly targeted stimulation is the goal, and not all spots elicit a LTR or a needle-grasp. In particular, the paraspinal muscles appear to twitch less frequently but are often found to harbour many contractured muscles that are important to treat with needle penetration. The use of snapping palpation is useful in identifying TrPs in distal and more superficial muscles but may be less relevant for identifying deep paraspinal muscles in need of treatment. Systematic examination and treatment of the paraspinal muscles, especially the deeper multifidi, is thus required to probe and feel a tightened band, fibrosis, or even a deep needle-grasp, the 'silent lesion'. As previously discussed, this will often elicit subclinical fasciculations that are therapeutic (Chu, 1997).

Treatment with needle stimulation is a function of the number of points, the duration of stimulation per point, and the style of needle manipulation used. It is not possible to provide a clear single formula to quantify stimulation during treatment, as this has not been adequately tested. The field of treatment using DN is still growing and future testing will help to quantify and qualify answers to these questions. Perhaps most importantly, the clinician should consider the effect of stimulation on the patient. If the patient is too sensitive to handle the current application, it must be changed to accommodate both the patient's tolerance and the therapeutic need for stimulation. For example, a quick insertion that elicits a LTR may be enough stimulation in a highly sensitive shortened muscle. In this case the LTR can occur immediately, even with a short duration of stimulation. In the event that an LTR has not occurred, the clinician may wish to explore the muscle further. Within a short period of time, an LTR may be found, or in the absence of a twitch or deep ache, the clinician may deem the tissue normal and not in need of treatment. For those muscles in which needle-grasp is intense and more sustained than with the LTR, leaving the needle in place for some time allows for more gradual release of contractures and improved patient tolerance. Attempting to prematurely remove the needle leads to the potential of the patient moving or 'jumping', and introduces unnecessary risk. It is therefore advisable to treat additional areas only after the release of muscle contracture and removal of the needle. These examples illustrate that stimulation parameters are often varied for both patient comfort and desired treatment affect. As this field grows, it is expected that more guiding principles on treatment parameters will be developed. In the meantime, we must make use of the experience of the founders of DN techniques. According to Gunn, 'failure to induce needle-grasp signifies that muscle shortening is not the cause of pain and that the condition would probably not respond to this type of treatment. Penetration into almost any part of the muscle can lead to relaxation, but the most rewarding sites are at tender and painful points in muscle bands. These points (which often correspond to traditional acupuncture points) are generally situated beneath muscle motor points, and at musculotendinous junctions' (Gunn, 1996).

Considering these possibilities, one can see that providing the optimal amount of stimulation requires experience. If the therapist elicits an LTR by gently penetrating the area, multiple insertions may be tolerated. Alternatively, overly forceful insertions provoking a strong needle grasp and accompanied by premature attempts at needle removal may often result in decreased client tolerance and may unnecessarily risk an adverse reaction such as fainting or noncompliance due to discomfort. When acquiring experience it is advised to remain on the light side of stimulation. By doing so, the shortened muscle and supersensitivity will respond favourably to treatment while respecting patient comfort and tolerance.

Concurrent Treatments

From the perspective of treatment goals, it must be remembered that all treatments are forms of stimulation, and in supersensitive patients, excessive stimulation can result in poor outcomes. Treatments occurring concurrently should therefore be discouraged by the therapist to avoid potentially negative additive effects. From a safety perspective therefore it is contraindicated to have joint manipulation immediately after Gunn-IMS. The decrease in protective muscle spasm leaves weakened ligaments and vessels at risk. If Gunn-IMS is being spaced out by 5 to 7 days and needle insertion is adding the correct amount of stimulation, concurrent treatments could introduce the risk of overstimulating the patient. Thus by having the patient receive Gunn-IMS alone, the results of treatment can be more accurately evaluated. For similar reasons patients are encouraged to avoid undue physical stress or activity in the days after treatment.

On the second visit, the clinician will assess the efficacy of care and the client's response to treatment. The patient is encouraged to perform gentle functional activities that allow the neuromuscular unit a period of normalised action posttreatment. Gunn-IMS must be seen as a method to encourage normal function within the neuromuscular unit rather than a tool that loosens a muscle in order to allow for other mechanical treatments such as manipulation. The effectiveness of this treatment demonstrates that the condition is an electrical problem for which mechanical treatment alone will be insufficient to fully address the signs and symptoms.

Reassessment

The response to treatment can often be surprisingly quick and deserves reassessment each session. The start of each treatment session includes questioning the patient to determine the effects of care. A miniassessment should also be used to retest appropriate critical assessment findings for evidence of change that correlate to the patient's subjective reports. Choosing outcomes that are a possible consequence and measure of radiculopathy is an important requirement. Their use will remind the therapist of the need for tracking of motor, autonomic, and trophic signs that affect both anterior and posterior primary rami of the affected nerve root.

The Tools of Gunn Intramuscular Stimulation

Although the Gunn-IMS plunger used to hold the needle is often seen as the distinguishing tool of the Gunn-IMS technique, it is given far too much emphasis. The most important tools are the clinical examination and the interpretation of findings. Without these, a needle or plunger will not provide consistently positive outcomes. Having adequately discussed the examination and interpretation of results, the remaining tools to present are the needles, plungers, and required sterilisation equipment.

Needle/Sizes

Gunn-IMS uses standard solid filament needles. The most common lengths used vary between 10 mm and 50 mm, the choice of which is entirely dictated by safety and depth required. It is common when treating the cervical paraspinals to limit the needle size to 25 mm. Treatment in the gluteal muscle may often need lengths of 50 mm or 60 mm. Although traditional acupuncture needles are used, needles that are compatible with plungers are also common. These needles do not have the characteristic coiled wire end. Instead they have a small blunt end that fits easily into the locking mechanism of a plunger.

Plunger

The Gunn-IMS plunger is made up of two stainless steel or plated alloy pieces, an outer tube and an inner shaft.

The needle handle fits into a locking mechanism on the tip of the shaft. This shaft and needle are inserted into the hollow tube and secured by a tightening screw. The loaded plunger will allow for easy insertion while preventing contamination of the needle from contact with nonsterile or unclean items during treatment. A disposable version of this reusable medical device has recently become available (Fig. 15.7). The disposable plunger is packaged with a needle and guide tube as is typical of any acupuncture style needle (Fig. 15.8). An additional shorter guide tube is fit snugly overtop of the standard tube. Upon needle insertion, the longer guide tube is then removed, leaving the short tube available for securing the insertion site and preventing over bending of longer needles. This novel device is a useful advance, allowing for easy manipulation of the needle once inserted. It is, however, relatively cumbersome compared with the Gunn-IMS plunger because resheathing the needle and resetting the shorter guide tube requires more time and focus to avoid a needle-stick injury while introducing a risk of contamination resulting from the needle touching nonsterile surfaces.

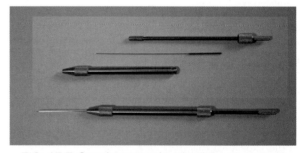

FIG. 15.7 Gunn intramuscular stimulation plunger with needle.

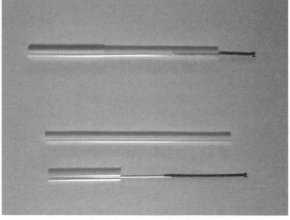

FIG. 15.8 Disposable plunger.

Cleaning and Sterilisation

Use of a standard plunger requires specialised equipment and thorough cleaning and sterilisation procedures. The policies that dictate these procedures are dependent on the local governing bodies for healthcare, as well as the clinician's professional licensing body. Typical requirements include a mechanical cleaning followed by sterilisation that utilises steam under intermittent pressure (autoclaving). Clinic policy and procedures should allow for tracking of the use and effectiveness of properly validated sterilisation techniques and equipment. It is imperative that national, regional and local requirements be consulted and implemented.

CASE STUDY EXAMPLE

Newly certified Gunn-IMS practitioners may find consistent success by treating a classic case of pseudosciatica due to a gluteus medius TrP. The term 'classic' is intended to exclude significant disc injury or nerve root compression. There must be low back dysfunction with radiating leg pain and neuropathic findings indicating a lumbar source. Treatment should be directed at the spinal levels indicated by the assessment as well as to other muscles supplied by the affected nerve root. In this case you may wish to track pain reports (amount, duration, intensity), medicine usage, sleep disturbance, and range of motion for the affected joints. Treat the patient once per week for the duration of symptoms using 30 minute appointments. The only additional treatment suggested is the typical client education one would expect for low back care. Avoid the use of other treatments such as mobilisation, manipulation, and bracing, as long as it is safe and pertinent to do so. In this way you will be able to compare your typical results with that of Gunn-IMS using outcome measures that are of significance to the patient's quality and enjoyment of life. In this patient case, needling of shortened paraspinals as well as distal muscles innervated by the affected myotome distinguishes Gunn-IMS from other DN techniques.

REFERENCES

Alfredson, H., & Lorentzon, R. (2002). Chronic tendon pain: no signs of inflammation but high concentrations of the neurotransmitter glutamate. Implications for treatment? *Current Drug Targets, 3,* 43–54.

Audette, J. F., Eminike, E., & Meleger, A. (2005). Neuropathic low back pain. *Current Pain and Headache Reports, 9,* 168–177.

Audette, J. F., Wang, F., & Smith, H. (2004). Bilateral activation of motor unit potentials with unilateral needle stimulation of active myofascial trigger points. *American Journal of Physical Medicine & Rehabilitation. 83,* 368–374.

Axelsson, J., & Thesleff, S. (1959). A study of supersensitivity in denervated mammalian skeletal muscle. *The Journal of Physiology, 147,* 178–193.

Baldry, P. E. (2001). *Myofascial pain and fibromyalgia syndromes: a clinical guide to diagnosis and management* (p. 62). Edinburgh: Churchill Livingstone.

Borenstein, D. G., O'Mara, J. W., Boden, S. D., et al. (2001). The value of magnetic resonance imaging of the lumbar spine to predict low-back pain in asymptomatic subjects: a seven-year follow-up study. *Journal of Bone and Joint Surgery [American], 83,* 1306–1311.

Bridges, D., Thompson, S. W. N., & Rice, A. S. C. (2001). Mechanisms of neuropathic pain. *British Journal of Anaesthesia, 87,* 12–26.

Cangiano, L., Lutzemberger, M., & Nicotra, L. (1977). Non-equivalence of impulse blockade and denervation in the production of membrane changes in rat skeletal muscle. *The Journal of Physiology, 273,* 691–706.

Cannon, W. B. (1939). A law of denervation. *American Journal of the Medical Sciences, 198,* 737–750.

Cannon, W. B., & Haimovici, H. (1939). The sensitization of motor neurons by partial "denervation". *American Journal of Physiology, 126,* 731–740.

Cannon, W. B., & Rosenblueth, A. (1936). The sensitization of a sympathetic ganglion by preganglionic denervation. *American Journal of Physiology, 116,* 408–413.

Cannon, W. B., & Rosenblueth, A. (1949). *The supersensitivity of denervated structures: a law of denervation.* New York: Macmillan Co.

Chang, C. W., Chang, K. Y., Chen, Y. R., & Kuo, P. L. (2011). Electrophysiological evidence of spinal accessory neuropathy in patients with cervical myofascial pain syndrome. *Archives of Physical Medicine and Rehabilitation, 92,* 935–940.

Chang, C. W., Chen, Y. R., & Chang, K. F. (2008). Evidence of neuroaxonal degeneration in MFPS. *European Journal of Pain, 12,* 1026–1030.

Chen, J. T., Chung, K. C., Hou, C. R., et al. (2000). Inhibitory effect of dry needling on the spontaneous electrical activity recorded from myofascial trigger spots of rabbit skeletal muscle. *American Journal of Physical Medicine & Rehabilitation, 80,* 729–734.

Chu, J. (1995). Dry needling (intramuscular stimulation) in myofascial pain related to lumbosacral radiculopathy. *European Journal of Physical and Rehabilitation Medicine, 5,* 106–121.

Chu, J. (1997). Does EMG (dry needling) reduce myofascial pain symptoms due to cervical nerve root irritation? *Electromyography and Clinical Neurophysiology, 37,* 259–272.

Chu, J. (1999). Twitch-obtaining intramuscular stimulation: observations in the management of radiculopathic chronic low back pain. *Journal of Musculoskeletal Pain, 7,* 131–146.

Chu, J., Bruyninckx, F., & Neuhauser, D. V. (2016). Chronic refractory myofascial pain and denervation supersensitivity as global public health disease. *BMJ Case Reports*, https://doi.org/10.1136/bcr-2015-211816.

Chu, J., McNally, S., Bruyninckx, F., & Neuhauser, D. (2017). American football and other sports injuries may cause migraine/persistent pain decades later and can be treated successfully with electrical twitch-obtaining intramuscular stimulation (ETOIMS). *BMJ Innovations*, https://doi.org/10.1136/bmjinnov-2016-000151x. Published online: March 24, 2017.

Chu-Andrews, J., & Johnson, R. (1986). *Electrodiagnosis: an anatomical and clinical approach* (p. 211). Philadelphia: Lippincott.

Couto, C., de Souza, I. C. C., Torres, I. L. S., Fregni, F., & Caumo, W. (2014). Paraspinal stimulation combined with trigger point needling and needle rotation for the treatment of myofascial pain: a randomized sham-controlled clinical trial. *Clinical Journal of Pain*, 30, 214–223.

Cummings, T., & White, A. R. (2001). Needling therapies in the management of myofascial trigger point pain: a systematic review. *Archives of Physical Medicine and Rehabilitation*, 82, 986–992.

Deyo, R. A., Mirza, S. K., Turner, J. A., & Martin, B. I. (2009). Over treating chronic back pain: time to back off? *Journal of the American Board of Family Medicine*, 22, 62–68.

Dommerholt, J. (2011). Dry needling — peripheral and central considerations. *Journal of Manual/Manipulative therapy*, 19(4), 223–237.

Eyzaguirre, C., & Fidone, S. J. (1975). *Physiology of the nervous system*. Chicago: Year Book Medical Publishers.

Farfan, H. F. (1984). The torsional injury of the lumbar spine. *Spine*, 9, 53.

Fishbain, D. A., Goldberg, M., Steele, R., & Rosomoff, H. (1989). DSM-III diagnoses of patients with myofascial pain syndrome (fibrositis). *Archives of Physical Medicine and Rehabilitation*, 70, 433–438.

Fricton, J. R., Kroening, R., Haley, D., & Siegert, R. (1985). Myofascial pain syndrome of the head and neck: a review of clinical characteristics of 164 patients. *Oral Surgery, Oral Medicine, and Oral Pathology*, 60, 615–623.

Ga, H., Choi, J. H., Park, C. H., & Yoon, H. J. (2007a). Acupuncture needling versus lidocaine injection of trigger points in myofascial pain syndrome in elderly patients: a randomised trial. *Acupuncture in Medicine*, 25, 130–136.

Ga, H., Choi, J. H., Park, C. H., & Yoon, H. J. (2007b). Dry needling of trigger points with and without paraspinal needling in myofascial pain syndromes in elderly patients. *Journal of Alternative and Complementary Medicine*, 13, 617–624.

Ga, H., Koh, H. J., Choi, J. H., & Kim, C. H. (2007c). Intramuscular and nerve root stimulation vs lidocaine injection of trigger points in myofascial pain syndrome. *Journal of Rehabilitation Medicine*, 39, 374–378.

Gilliatt, R. W., Westgaard, R. H., & Williams, I. R. (1978). Extrajunctional acetylcholine sensitivity of inactive muscle fibers in the baboon during prolonged nerve pressure block. *The Journal of Physiology*, 280, 499–514.

Gunn, C. C. (1976). Trans-cutaneous neural stimulation, needle acupuncture & 'Teh Ch'i' phenomenon. *American Journal of Acupuncture*, 4, 317–322.

Gunn, C. C. (1978). Trans-cutaneous neural stimulation, acupuncture and the current of injury. *American Journal of Acupuncture*, 6, 191–196.

Gunn, C. C. (1984). *Pain and misperceptions in neuropathways*. I.F.O.M.T Proceedings.

Gunn, C. C. (1989). *Treating myofascial pain: intramuscular stimulation (IMS) for myofascial pain syndromes of neuropathic origin* (p. 16). University of Washington, Seattle: Health Sciences Center for Educational Resources.

Gunn, C. C. (1996). *The Gunn approach to the treatment of chronic pain — intramuscular stimulation for myofascial pain of radiculopathic origin*. London: Churchill Livingstone.

Gunn, C. C., & Milbrandt, W. E. (1976a). Tenderness at motor points. A diagnostic and prognostic aid for low-back injury. *Journal of Bone and Joint Surgery [American]*, 58, 815–825.

Gunn, C. C., & Milbrandt, W. E. (1976b). Tennis elbow and the cervical spine. *Canadian Medical Association Journal*, 114, 803–809.

Gunn, C. C., & Milbrandt, W. E. (1977). The neurological mechanism of needle-grasp in acupuncture. *American Journal of Acupuncture*, 5, 115–120.

Gunn, C. C., & Milbrandt, W. E. (1978). Early and subtle signs in low-back sprain. *Spine*, 3, 267–281.

Gunn, C. C., Milbrandt, W. E., Little, A. S., & Mason, K. E. (1980). Dry needling of muscle motor points for chronic low-back pain. A randomized clinical trial with long-term follow-up. *Spine*, 5, 279–291.

Haymaker, W., & Woodhall, B. (1953). *Peripheral nerve injuries; principles of diagnosis* (pp. 145–151). Philadelphia: WB Saunders Company.

Hong, C. Z. (1994). Persistence of local twitch response with loss of conduction to and from spinal cord. *Archives of Physical Medicine and Rehabilitation*, 75, 12–16.

Johnson, L. (Ed.), (2012). *Physiology of the gastrointestinal tract* (5th ed., p. 636). London: Elsevier.

Karakurum, B., Karaalin, O., Coskun, O., et al. (2001). The 'dry-needle technique': intramuscular stimulation in tension-type headache. *Cephalalgia*, 21, 813–817.

Kelly, J. C., Groarke, P. J., Butler, J. S., Poynton, A. R., & O'Byrne, J. M. (2012). The natural history and clinical syndromes of degenerative cervical spondylosis. *Advances in Orthopedics*, 1–5. Article ID 393642.

Khan, K. M., Cook, J. L., Bonar, F., et al. (1999). Histopathology of common tendonopathies. Update and implications for clinical management. *Sports Medicine*, 27, 393–408.

Kim, J. K., Lim, K. J., Kim, C., & Kim, H. S. (2003). Intramuscular stimulation therapy in failed back surgery syndrome patients. *Journal of the Korean Pain Society*, 16, 60–67.

Korr, I. M. (1975). Proprioceptors and somatic dysfunction. *The Journal of the American Osteopathic Association*, 74, 638–650.

Letchuman, R., Gay, R. E., Shelerud, R. A., & VanOstrand, L. A. (2005). Are tender points associated with cervical radiculopathy? *Archives of Physical Medicine and Rehabilitation*, 86, 1333–1337.

Lewit, K. (1979). The needle effect in the relief of myofascial pain. *Pain*, 6, 83–90.

Loeser, J. D. (2012). Chronic pain is more than a peripheral event. *Journal of Pain*, 13(10), 930–931.

Loeser, J. D., Butler, S. H., Chapman, C. R., & Turk, D. C. (2001). Bonica's management of pain. In C. C. Gunn (Ed.), *Neuropathic myofascial pain syndromes* (3rd ed., pp. 518–525). Hagerstown: Lippincott Williams & Wilkins.

Lomo, T., & Rosenthal, J. (1972). Control of ACh sensitivity by muscle activity in the rat. *The Journal of Physiology*, 221, 493–513.

Lomo, T., & Westgaard, R. H. (1975). Further studies on the control of ACh sensitivity by muscle activity in the rat. *The Journal of Physiology*, 252, 603–626.

Lorkovic, H. (1975). Supersensitivity to ACh in muscles after prolonged nerve block. *Archives of International Physiology and Biochemistry*, 83, 771–781.

Murphy, R. W. (1977). Nerve roots and spinal nerves in degenerative disc disease. *Clinical Orthopaedics and Related Research*, 129, 46–60.

Ochoa, J., Fowler, T. J., & Gilliatt, R. W. (1972). Anatomical changes in peripheral nerves compressed by a pneumatic tourniquet. *Journal of Anatomy*, 113, 433–455.

Rydevik, B., Brown, M. D., & Lundborg, G. (1985). Pathoanatomy and pathophysiology of nerve root compression. *Spine*, 9, 7–15.

Sackett, D. L., Rosenberg, W. M. C., Muir Gray, J. A., Haynes, R. B., & Richardson, W. S. (1996). Evidence based medicine: what it is and what it isn't. *British Medical Journal*, 312, 71–72.

Sari, H., Akarirmak, U., & Uludag, M. (2012). Active myofascial trigger points might be more frequent in patients with cervical radiculopathy. *European Journal of Physical and Rehabilitation Medicine*, 48(2), 237–244.

Savage, R. A., Whitehouse, G. H., & Roberts, N. (1997). The relationship between the magnetic resonance imaging appearance of the lumbar spine and low back pain, age and occupation in males. *European Spine Journal*, 6, 106–114.

Shah, J. P., Danoff, J. V., Desai, M. J., Parikh, S., Nakamura, L. Y., Phillips, T. M., et al. (2008). Biochemicals associated with pain and inflammation are elevated in sites near to and remote from active myofascial trigger points. *Archives of Physical Medicine and Rehabilitation*, 89(1), 16–23.

Sharpless, S. K. (1975). Suceptibility of spinal roots to compression block. In *NINCDS Monograph #15, Goldstein M ed. NIH Workshop* (pp. 155–161).

Shultz, S. P., Driban, J. B., & Swank, C. B. (2007). The Evaluation of electrodermal properties in the identification of myofascial trigger points. *Archives of Physical Medicine and Rehabilitation*, 88, 780–784.

Sihvonen, T. (1992). The segmental dorsal ramus as a common cause of chronic & recurrent LBP. *Electromyography and Clinical Neurophysiology*, 32(10-11), 507–510.

Skootsky, S. A., Jaeger, B., & Oye, R. K. (1989). Prevalence of myofascial pain in general internal medicine practice. *The Western Journal of Medicine*, 151, 157–160.

Sola, A. E., Rodenberger, M. L., & Gettys, B. B. (1955). Incidence of hypersensitive areas in posterior shoulder muscles; a survey of two hundred young adults. *American Journal of Physical Medicine & Rehabilitation*, 34(6), 585–590.

Srbely, J. Z., Dickey, J. P., Lee, D., & Lowerison, M. (2010). Dry needle stimulation of myofascial trigger points evokes segmental anti-nociceptive effects. *Journal of Rehabilitation Medicine*, 42, 463–468.

Srbely, J., Vadasz, B., Shah, J., Gerber, N. L., Sikdar, S., & Kumbhare, D. (2016). Central sensitization: a clinical conundrum. *The Clinical Journal of Pain*, 32(11), 1011–1013.

Stellon, A. (2002). Neurogenic pruritis: an unrecognized problem? A retrospective case series of treatment by acupuncture. *Acupuncture in Medicine*, 20, 186–190.

Thesleff, S. (1976). *Motor innervation of muscle*. New York: Academic Press.

Tracey, K. J. (2002). The inflammatory reflex. *Nature*, 420, 853–859.

Wilkinson, J. (1971). *Cervical spondylosis: early diagnosis and treatment*. Philadelphia: WB Sanders.

Woolf, C. J. (2011). Central sensitization: implications for the diagnosis and treatment of pain. *Pain*, 152, S2–S15.

CHAPTER 16

Fu's Subcutaneous Needling

ZHONGHUA FU • LI-WEI CHOU

Concept and Terminology

Myofascial trigger points (TrPs) are discrete, focal, hyperirritable spots located in skeletal muscles. They produce pain and often accompany chronic musculoskeletal disorders. A TrP is a key concept for musculoskeletal pain problems. We have used the theory of TrPs for several years in our clinical practice; however, we have found that the concept of TrPs is not always suitable to our practice, which is why in 2014 we developed a new concept, referred to as 'tightened muscle (TM)'.

TM (in Chinese: 患肌) refers to the condition in which a normal muscle remains semicontracted for a prolonged period of time. This condition results in a tight, hard band felt in a part of the muscle or throughout the entire muscle, but most commonly in the area of the muscle belly. TrPs are in embedded in TM. Fu developed the term 'TM' in 2014 with collaboration by other practitioners of Fu's subcutaneous needling (FSN) in China. In one of his Chinese FSN books, he translated '患肌' into 'pathological tight muscle', but after the recommendation by Dr. Jidong Wu in Cambridge, UK, Dr. Fu agreed to the term 'tightened muscle' instead (Fu, 2016).

Before answering the question why the term TM is preferred over TrP, an introduction to the FSN technique is indicated. FSN is a therapeutic approach for musculoskeletal painful disorders and some chronic benign visceral disorders, which originated from traditional acupuncture. This procedure is performed by inserting a solid needle, usually a special trocar needle, into the subcutaneous layer around a TM to achieve a desired effect (Fig. 16.1). Different from traditional acupuncture, FSN has no special insertion point. The FSN needle is inserted anywhere in the vicinity of a TM with the needle tip pointing towards the TM. Apart from not having fixed insertion points, other aspects of FSN also contributed to the need to replace the more traditional TrP construct and terminology.

1. The term 'myofascial' is an adjective referring to skeletal muscle and its fascia. Fascia has been described in detail in Chapter 3. Myofascial refers not only to muscle tissue. The perception with palpation is that TM is mostly muscle tissue, especially in the muscle belly. Fascia does not have the same TM quality with palpation.

2. The word 'trigger', as used in TrP, is more or less meaningless in the practice of FSN. The trigger reaction is felt when a needle touches muscle fibres. In FSN, needles do not touch the muscles as the technique is strictly used subdermally.

3. The word 'point', as used in TrP, is also not suitable in the practice of FSN because FSN targets what is perceived as a slice or band.

The name FSN, or *Fu Zhen* (浮针, in simplified Chinese; 浮針, in Traditional Chinese), has some profound implications. 'Fu Zhen' is the Chinese pronunciation for FSN. Fu is the surname of the inventor, who is also the first author of this chapter. In Chinese, 'Fu, 浮' means floating, and it could also mean superficial. 'Zhen' means acupuncture or needling. Therefore in some English-language papers, FSN is also called 'floating acupuncture' (Huang et al., 1998), Fu's acupuncture (Zhang, 2004), Fu needling (Xia & Huang, 2004), and floating needling (Fu & Huang, 1999). However, neither *floating* nor *superficial* are precise translations; the word 'subcutaneous' is a better substitute in terms of demonstrating the manipulation features of FSN.

Although FSN originated from classic acupuncture, FSN's manipulation and theory have nothing to do with the concepts of traditional acupuncture such as meridians, acupoints, Yin-Yang, and Qi. Therefore FSN is not some variety of acupuncture and should not be referred to as acupuncture. Fig. 16.2 shows the FSN needle in a subcutaneous layer of a human cadaver. Another approach, called intradermal needle therapy, is easily confused with FSN. The intradermal needle (Fig. 16.3) is a type of short needle made of stainless steel wire, especially used for embedding in the skin rather than in the subcutaneous layer (Cheng, 1987).

The term 'Fu's subcutaneous needling' was first mentioned in a 2005 article by Fu and Xu, in which

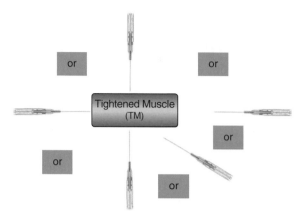

FIG. 16.1 A graphical map of Fu's subcutaneous needling.

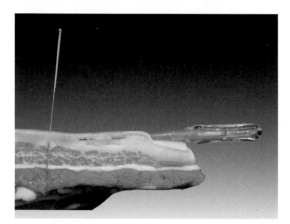

FIG. 16.2 Fu's subcutaneous needling needle located in the subcutaneous layer of a human cadaver.

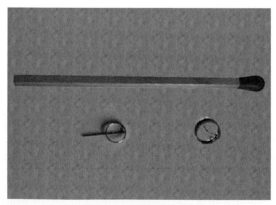

FIG. 16.3 The intradermal needle.

they described the treatment method (Fu & Xu, 2005), followed by several other research papers (Fu et al., 2006, 2007). FSN should be clearly distinguished from dry needling (DN), which involves the insertion of a fine single-use sterile needle into a TrP for the treatment of myofascial pain. DN has been in use since the 1970s and differs from the use of needling from an Oriental paradigm (Baldry, 1995, 2000, 2002; Hsieh et al., 2007; Hong, 2000, 2002, 2004, 2006; Simons, 2004, 2008). TrP DN is based on a Western anatomical and neurophysiological paradigm and has been increasingly utilised in the Western world, especially in the US, UK, The Netherlands, Canada, Belgium, Norway, Australia, Switzerland, Ireland, Brazil, South Africa, and Spain, among others (Dommerholt et al., 2006). Unlike traditional acupuncture, DN does not consider ancient Chinese philosophy and traditional ideas. Traditional acupuncture is based on prescientific ideas such as meridians, Qi (a kind of invisible energy), and Yin–Yang (Ellis & Wiseman, 1991; White & Ernst, 2001; Kim, 2004), whereas DN is entirely based on the recent understanding of scientific neurophysiology, anatomy, and pain sciences (Ghia et al., 1976; Melzack et al., 1977; Melzack, 1981). The manipulation method used in acupuncture differs from that used in DN and is based on different theoretical foundations and principles.

Contemporary research and the emergence of DN have reduced the sense of mystique surrounding non-injection therapies for pain (Amaro, 2008). Although acupuncture and DN have different theoretical bases, they are similar in some aspects.

1. Nothing is injected into the body.
2. Needles may target the same points known as either a trigger point in DN or an Ah-shi point in Chinese medicine.
3. Many of the pain indications overlap.

Further, in TrP DN the importance of the local twitch response is emphasised, which is a reaction during needling with some resemblance to the 'De-Qi' effect in acupuncture (Hong, 1994). Chou and associates (2008, 2009, 2011, 2014) have modified the technique used in acupuncture into a procedure similar to Hong's DN technique. Therefore in a 'broad sense' acupuncture can be considered as one type of DN.

FSN borrowed some ideas from traditional acupuncture, but the essential features are different from those of traditional acupuncture. Acupuncture and FSN are based on different theories and techniques and manipulations are employed with entirely different kinds of needles. Traditional acupuncture theory is mystical, even to Chinese doctors. FSN is a much easier approach, which does not consider the traditional theories. Compared with the current practice of DN, FSN has several unique features. There are at least two differences between FSN and DN. FSN needles are inserted into nondiseased areas and FSN is confined to subcutaneous layers, whereas DN inserts the needles into TrPs and often deep into the muscles. FSN is considered a particular type of DN. FSN shares the same scientific neurophysiological and anatomical foundation as TrP DN.

ORIGIN OF FU'S SUBCUTANEOUS NEEDLING

The following three sources led to FSN's evolution from traditional acupuncture.

Contemplation of De-Qi

De-Qi or Qi is an acupuncture phenomenon that occurs during needle manipulation, experienced by the patient as a particular sensation (e.g., soreness, aching, numbness, or 'needle grasp') or by the acupuncturist as a pulling sensation (Cheng, 1987; Lin, 1997; Langevin et al., 2006; White et al., 2008). Traditionally, De-Qi must be achieved in the process of acupuncture regardless of the manipulation used; otherwise, the therapeutic results are poor (Cheng, 1987). In every textbook on acupuncture in Chinese, the importance of De-Qi is always emphasised and reiterated and acupuncturists repeatedly highlight De-Qi. As a result, most Chinese patients believe in the adage, 'no De-Qi, no effect.' Sometimes patients will be disappointed in the acupuncturist if they fail to acquire De-Qi, even though it may cause discomfort to the patient.

Acupuncturists and patients are not the only ones who consider De-Qi to be pivotal. Some scientists also believe that De-Qi plays an important role in acupuncture analgesia (Cao, 2002; Park et al., 2005). Acupuncture needling may activate afferent fibres of peripheral nerves to elicit De-Qi, the signal that ascends to the brain, activates the antinociceptive system, including certain brain nuclei, modulators (opioid peptides) and neurotransmitters, and through the descending inhibitory pathway, which results in analgesia (Cao, 2002).

However, occasionally acupuncture does work without De-Qi and could fail even when the patients achieve strong De-Qi. Furthermore, many acupuncture substitutes, such as cupping, moxibustion, transcutaneous electrical nerve stimulation (TENS), and so on, do not elicit De-Qi, but they appear to be effective nevertheless (Chen & Yu, 2003).

Therefore De-Qi may be not as relevant as traditionally is often suggested. To prove the insignificance of De-Qi, the best method is to stimulate the tissue without obvious direction and then observe what will happen. The elicitation of De-Qi is related to the needling depth (Lin, 1997). There are few free nerve endings and proprioceptive receptors in the subcutaneous layer, whereas free nerve endings are abundant in the epidermis and dermis. Proprioceptive receptors do exist in the muscular layer (Tortora, 1989). Therefore there should be no occurrence of De-Qi even if the subcutaneous layer is stimulated. Under such a condition, does the needling effect still exist? For an acupuncturist, it is easy to verify the existence of the needling effect, and this simple trial was one of several factors resulting in the discovery and development of FSN. One example of a form of acupuncture where achieving De-Qi has been shown to not be critical is wrist–ankle acupuncture.

Clinical Application of Wrist–Ankle Acupuncture

Wrist–ankle acupuncture (WAA) (Jiang et al., 2006) is also called wrist–ankle needling (Song & Wang, 1985). Dr Xinshu Zhang, a neurologist who has worked at the Second Military Medical University in Shanghai, developed WAA in 1972. WAA divides the whole body into 12 longitudinal regions, six for each half of the body (Fig. 16.4). There are six points 2 *cun* (about 50 mm) above the wrist joint corresponding to the six regions above the diaphragm, and there are six points 3 *cun* (about 75 mm) above the ankle joint corresponding to the other six regions (Fig. 16.5). A *cun* is a measure of distance relative to a person's body dimensions that is commonly used in traditional Chinese medicine. If a disorder occurs in one of the regions, the corresponding point should be chosen. Unlike conventional acupuncture, WAA inserts an acupuncture needle only superficially in the subcutaneous layer; some authors claim that WAA is effective in the treatment of pain with various origins (Zhu & Wang, 1998). Needling superficially in WAA wrist or ankle points to treat distant disorders often has a good effect (Song & Wang, 1985; Chu & Bai, 1997), leading to the idea that needling close to the afflicted area could be at least as effective as needling in an area remote from that which is afflicted, and that needling closer may be preferable. These thoughts motivated the principle author to seek answers through clinical trials.

Ancient Techniques

The Medical Classic of the Yellow Emperor (also known as *The Yellow Emperor's Canon on Internal Medicine* or *The Yellow Emperor's Inner Classic*), written thousands of

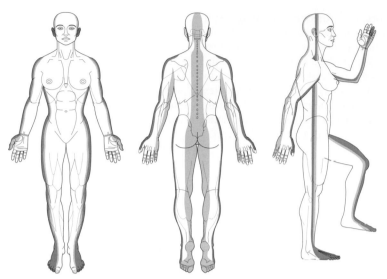

FIG. 16.4 Twelve longitudinal regions according to wrist–ankle acupuncture.

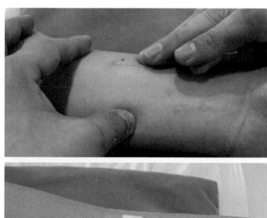

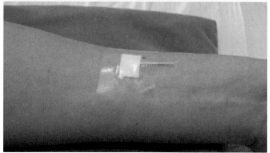

FIG. 16.5 The insertion style of wrist–ankle acupuncture.

years ago, is a fundamental book of traditional Chinese medicine. The book states that needling superficially and needling nearby are two characteristics of the ancient techniques for the treatment of painful problems. The principle author of this chapter learned from and was inspired by these techniques in the process of developing FSN. In *The Medical Classic of the Yellow Emperor*, there is a chapter entitled 'Guanzhen,' which records 26 special techniques. The 26 techniques are classified into three groups: a 9-technique group, a 12-technique group, and a 5-technique group.

The characteristic of superficial needling refers to quite a few techniques such as *MAO Ci* in the 9-technique group, *Zhizhen Ci* and *FU Ci* in the 12-technique group, and *Ban Ci* in the 5-technique group. Among them, especially *Zhizhen Ci* resembles FSN: hold up the skin with the thumb and index fingers of the left hand; insert the filiform needle into the skin; and then go forward toward the painful spot obliquely. *Zhizhen Ci* can be said to be a precursor to FSN without FSN needling and its swaying movement.

Needling nearby is often seen in the 26 techniques such as *Fen Ci* in the 9-technique group; *Hui Ci, Qi Ci, Yang Ci, Duan Ci,* and *Pangzhen Ci* in the 12-technique group; and *Baowen Ci, Guan Ci,* and *Hegu Ci* in the 5-technique group.

Aside from the practicable techniques mentioned previously, *The Medical Classic of the Yellow Emperor* also describes many systemic theories such as meridians, acupoints, and Yin–Yang. Nevertheless, from then on, most ancient acupuncture texts adopted meridians, acupoints and other theories instead of practicable techniques as their main interests. The long-term neglect of more practicable techniques resulted in today's acupuncturists having little knowledge about this valuable ancient technique, which really is a precursor to FSN.

Based on these ideas and thoughts, Fu devoted himself to seeking a new and effective treatment strategy and finally developed FSN in 1996, when he worked at the First Military Medical University in Guangzhou, China. The university ran a TCM Clinic in Zengcheng, a city near Guangzhou. In the clinic, patients who were in significant pain were more numerous than the author could deal with, which encouraged him to find ways to relieve the painful problems much more efficiently and quicker.

Fu attempted to treat a patient with tennis elbow, or lateral epicondylitis, by needling the patient near the painful spot, which caused a positive response, and as such became the first successful case of FSN. From then on, a series of clinical trials were completed, and positive results were commonly achieved. In the same year, Fu wrote a brief introduction to FSN, which was published in a Chinese health newspaper (Fu, 1996). The next year Fu published his first research paper in Chinese in the *Journal of Clinical Acupuncture and Moxibustion* (Fu, 1997).

DEVELOPMENT OF FU'S SUBCUTANEOUS NEEDLING

Fu continued using FSN in his clinics and accumulated more and more evidence, which improved the technique and clinical efficacy of FSN. The initial focus was on developing the FSN needle and on increasing the indications of FSN.

Innovation of the Fu's Subcutaneous Needling Needle

In physics, scientific theories usually precede technologies. However, in traditional medicine, technologies or therapies often precede theories. Without any past experience to draw from or previous theories to follow, Fu had to develop FSN by trial and error. During FSN's early months, he used a filiform acupuncture needle, but over time several factors changed his thinking:

- When the range of the lesion was large or deep, FSN did not work well with filiform needles even when using many needles simultaneously.
- FSN needs a period of retention, and the patients could not stay in any settled position for extended periods of time. The patients should be able to move their bodies and limbs during needle retention. With a stainless-steel filiform needle patients easily can get hurt.
- In spite of the absence of discomfort or pain, patients often worried about the steel needle.
- FSN requires the needle to sway from side to side. The filiform needle is too elastic to allow for the swaying movement.

Fu realised that certain changes had to be made to the FSN needle; however, the challenge he faced was how to determine what kind of needle would go through the skin quickly and stay beneath the skin safely.

Initially, a physical method was developed: a needle was invented using a new material. The material was solid at low temperatures and became soft at high temperature. When not in use, the needle was stored in a refrigerator to keep it solid. When FSN was used, the needle would become soft after insertion due to the patient's body temperature. The concept was acceptable, but the material used for the needle and the refrigerators were too expensive for most acupuncturists.

Next, a chemical method was considered. Fu tried to produce a biological hard needle made of a high-polymer material such as absorbable catgut, which would dissolve subsequently by tissue fluids. A large amount of time and energy was devoted to finding such a material, but none was found. Finally, Fu invented a trocar needle, which is still used at this time. The FSN needle consists of two parts: a solid stainless steel needle and its soft casing tube. The former is hard enough to break through the skin quickly and to ensure that the FSN needle can be easily controlled; the latter is soft enough to remain beneath the skin without continuously sticking the patient. A patent application for the FSN needle was filed in December 1997. A Chinese invention patent was granted in August 2002.

Increase of Fu's Subcutaneous Needling Indications

To determine whether a particular disorder would be a suitable indication for FSN, an immediate effect would need to occur with FSN, which was later referred to as 'the golden criterion'. Disorders or symptoms for which FSN did not get immediate results were not included in the indications for FSN. After the first successful case, Fu continued searching for other FSN indications, a process which occurred in roughly four stages.

Stage 1: Fu's subcutaneous needling was mainly used to treat patients with soft tissue injuries of the extremities

In the early months, FSN was used mainly for the treatment of patients with painful problems in the extremities, such as epicondylitis, stenosing tenosynovitis of the styloid process of the radius, snapping finger, osteoarthritis of the knee, sprain and strain of ankle, among others. Due to limited experience with FSN in those early days, the success rate of the treatment of painful problems of the extremities was only about 40%. Therefore FSN was not considered for the treatment of complex diseases or diagnoses of the trunk.

Stage 2: Fu's subcutaneous needling was used to treat patients with nonvisceral diseases in the trunk

In the autumn of 1998, the primary author saw a patient who was suffering from severe neck pain and who had been treated unsuccessfully in the university hospital for nearly 1 month. A friend of the author requested his assistance and pleaded whether something could be done for the patient, who happened to be her father-in-law, before leaving in a couple of days. The author had no better option for treatment than FSN. Surprisingly, the neck pain was immediately relieved, after which the author started using FSN to treat patients with nonvisceral painful diseases in the trunk such as low back pain with or without sciatica, cervical syndrome, and mild ankylosing spondylitis.

Stage 3: Fu's subcutaneous needling was used to treat patients with benign painful visceral problems

FSN is performed superficially; hence superficial illnesses such as soft tissue injuries were regarded as primary FSN indications. FSN was never expected to be used for the treatment of persons with visceral diseases, until an 80-year-old Chinese acupuncturist wrote the author that he had treated a patient with appendicitis using FSN. Although FSN may not always be suitable for the treatment of appendicitis for a variety of reasons, the letter implied that FSN may in fact be used in the treatment of persons with visceral diseases. From then on, FSN was used to treat individual with acute and chronic gastritis, cholecystitis, pain due to urinary calculus and painful menstruation, among others.

Stage 4: Fu's subcutaneous needling was used to handle painful problems in the head and face and nonpainful diseases

After the successful treatments of patients with visceral diseases, more confidence in FSN was gained. The primary author moved on to treat patients with painful head and face problems. The experiences convincingly showed that FSN is effective for the treatment of localised headaches and for painful problems of the face caused by temporomandibular pain and dysfunction and accessory sinusitis. FSN was mainly used to deal with painful problems for which an immediate response could always be achieved. The question was raised whether FSN could effectively manage nonpainful diseases. After many years of practice, it was found that FSN can also deal with nonpainful problems. At present, several nonpainful indications have been treated successfully, including chronic cough without sputum, onset of chronic asthma, and localised numbness.

FU'S SUBCUTANEOUS NEEDLING MANIPULATIONS

Although FSN originated from traditional acupuncture, the technique of FSN is quite different, especially in the way the needle is manipulated.

Structure of the Fu's Subcutaneous Needling Needle

FSN needles, individually packaged and presterilised with ethylene oxide gas, are designed for single use. The FSN needle is made up of three parts (Fig. 16.6): a solid steel needle core (bottom), a soft casing tube (middle), and a protecting sheath (top).

The needle core consists of a needle and the needle core handle. The needle is made of stainless steel with a beveled tip. When the needle enters the skin, the bevel of the tip should face upward. The handle is made of plastic and square-shaped, and one of the four sides has 10 protuberances. The protuberances are on the same side as the bevel of the tip. If the protuberances face upward, the bevel will also face upward. The needle core allows the FSN needle to have sufficient rigidity to quickly go through the skin, go forward along the superficial layer, and smoothly sway from side to side. A soft casing tube encases the FSN needle.

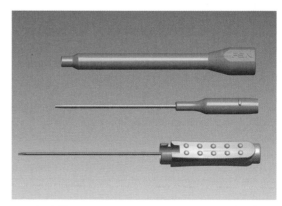

FIG. 16.6 Three parts of a Fu's subcutaneous needling needle.

The soft casing tube consists of two parts, namely a fluoroplastic body and the tube's hub, which is made of regular plastic. The two parts are connected to each other by a metal wedge. The tip of the casing tube is about 3 mm beyond the tip of the needle core when the needle core is embedded inside the casing tube. The casing tube has two functions. It covers the tip of the needle until the needle is pulled back by 3 mm; thus the tip of needle stick will not damage surrounding organs or tissues during the swaying movement. The casing tube can substitute for the steel needle core beneath the skin and reduce the patient's pain during retention.

The protective sheath covers the needle core and the casing tube and keeps the FSN needle sterile.

Preparation Before Treatment

Select a treatment posture

The FSN needle is thicker than an acupuncture needle, and the FSN manipulation lasts longer than an acupuncture or DN treatment. Therefore selecting a suitable treatment posture is crucial for FSN manipulation. The following postures are commonly used with FSN:

- *Sitting position:* Appropriate for manipulating locations in the head, face, neck, shoulder, upper back, and upper extremities.
- *Supine position:* Appropriate for manipulating in the abdomen.
- *Prone or sidelying:* An appropriate posture when treating diseases of the back and the posterior side of the lower extremities.

The treatment postures may need to be modified dependent on the patient's condition. More accurately, we should change the patient's postures, especially when there is no immediate effect after several minutes of the FSN swaying movement. For example, although the sitting posture is the first choice for the treatment of neck and upper back pain, if there is no relief of symptoms, changing to the prone position may be a better option. When a particular posture causes too much pain, a different treatment posture would be indicated. For example, if back pain is felt only during standing, the FSN needle could be inserted while the patient is in the prone position (Fig. 16.7). Before performing the swaying movement, the patient would be asked to stand up (Fig. 16.8).

Palpate the tightened muscles

In most cases, TMs are the cause of painful musculoskeletal problems and are also the main targets of the FSN needle. To locate the clinically relevant TM, follow these steps.

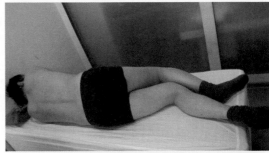
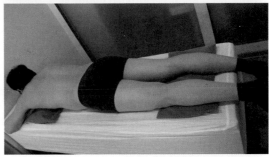

FIG. 16.7 Prone or sidelying position.

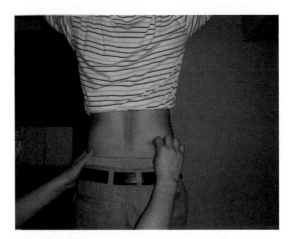

FIG. 16.8 Swaying movement during standing position.

1. Identify the suspected TMs—suspected TMs are those muscles with at least a partial anatomical relationship to the painful area.
2. Exclude irrelevant TMs—exclude TMs whose function is irrelevant to the movement limitation.
3. Confirm the TMs—palpate the TMs with the thumb or middle three fingers with medium strength. TM feels hard, tight, stiff, and sometime slippery. When in doubt, palpate the contralateral muscle for comparison.

Locate the insertion area

Unlike traditional acupuncture, FSN does not require the insertion of needles into acupoints or Ah-shi points. The needles are inserted into the area surrounding TMs. After identifying clinically relevant TMs, the needles can be inserted anywhere within the direct vicinity of the TMs. Several principles are employed to select the proximity of the needle insertion to the TMs:

- *Principle A:* For a single small nodule, the insertion area should be close to the TM. For a large-sized taut band or for nodules clustered in one area, the insertion points should be farther removed. For example, the insertion points should be close to the TM with a tennis elbow and farther away with more generalised upper extremity pain. The farther the tip, the less the intensity of FSN, although its coverage area may be enlarged. This phenomenon is called the *flashlight effect* (Fig. 16.9). The illumination of a flashlight becomes weaker, but covers a wider area when the light is used from a greater distance.
- *Principle B:* The FSN needle should not be inserted into scars or into hollow or prominent regions, such as the tip of the elbow, patella, styloid processes of the radius and ulna, malleolus lateralis, or malleolus medialis between the treated TM and the FSN needle insertion point.
- *Principle C:* For different types of diseases, the FSN needle insertion site should follow the guidelines listed in Table 16.1 if the needle insertion area would be far from the lesion site.
- *Principle D:* To reduce pain during needle insertion, surface blood vessels, most of which are veins, should be avoided.

TABLE 16.1
Insertion Areas Corresponding to the Dysfunctional Regions

Dysfunctional Region	Insertion Area
Head, face, upper back	Thumb side of forearm, outside of upper arm
Chest, epigastric zone	Inner side of forearm and upper arm
Lower abdomen	Middle part of inner side of leg, anteromedial part of thigh
Lower back	Rear or outside part of leg, outside of thigh
Genital organ, anus	Middle part of inner side of lower limb

Sterilise

Disinfection is necessary and essential before insertion of the needle. All persons administering FSN treatments should be aware of current methods of infection prevention, subject to their local skin-penetration regulations (see Chapter 5). To protect both clinicians and patients from needlestick injuries and contamination from bloodborne infections, the skin at the insertion point and the practitioner's fingers should be disinfected and sharps disposed of in appropriate biohazard containers.

Needling Method

In this section, the needling procedure for FSN is described, including needle insertion, needle swaying, needle direction, and needle retention.

Needle insertion

The posture of the patient should be adjusted to ensure that the skin on the inserting point is neither tight nor loose. If the skin is too tight, relevant blood vessels dilate, and the FSN needle is more prone to inducing pricking; on the other hand, if the skin is too loose, it is harder to penetrate. During the whole process, the needle tip should always be directed toward the TM.

First, the protective sheath of FSN needle is removed. Next, place fixes the FSN needle into the groove of the FSN device (Fig. 16.10) and lock the needle. Hold the device as shown in Fig. 16.11, then push and press the device to the area of intended insertion to form an indentation in the skin (Fig. 16.12). Press the control button with your index finger to eject the needle (Fig. 16.13). Use your other hand to take the

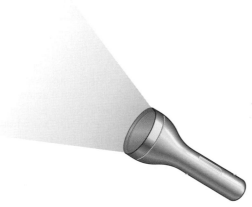

FIG. 16.9 Flashlight effect.

FSN needle out from the fixing groove, and remove the device with your hand.

Next, the needle should be laid flat and carefully pushed into the skin until fully inserted. When being pushed forward, the needle tip should be slightly

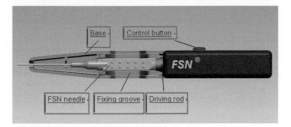

FIG. 16.10 A Fu's subcutaneous needling (FSN) inserting device with an FSN needle (Fu, Z., & Shepherd, R. (2013). Fu's subcutaneous needling, a modern style of ancient acupuncture? In L. L. Chen & T. O. Cheng (Ed.), *Acupuncture in modern medicine*. London: IntechOpen.)

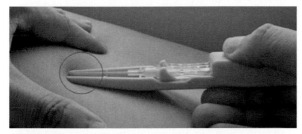

FIG. 16.11 The method of holding the inserting device.

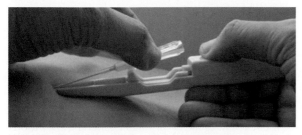

FIG. 16.12 Before ejecting, the device should be pushed to the direction of the area of intended insertion.

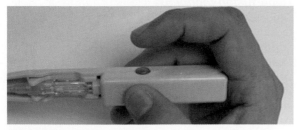

FIG. 16.13 Demonstrating the method to separate the needle from the device after the insertion of the needle.

elevated in order to observe if the skin hunch is moving along with the needle tip. At this point, the clinician's hand should feel loose with no resistance, while the patient feels something moving under the skin, but there is no feeling of De-Qi.

After the casing tube is totally embedded beneath the skin, the needle core handle should be withdrawn by about 3 mm and turned 90 degrees to the left; this way, an embossment in the tube goes into a groove in the needle core handle. The swaying movement can be done. Once the swaying movement is finished, the needle core handle is turned right by 90 degrees out of the groove, and then the steel needle core is withdrawn. The steel needle core is placed into the protective sheath for safety and to meet hygiene requirements. The casing tube is then embedded beneath the skin using an adhesive tape waterproof dressing. After 1 to 2 hours of retention, the adhesive tape is removed and the tube is pulled out. At the same time, the insertion point should be pressed using a sterilised cotton ball for at least 1 minute to prevent bleeding.

It is highly recommended to use a special designed device to insert the FSN needle. But if the clinician does not have access to the device, FSN can still be performed. First, remove the protective sheath. For a right-handed clinician, the FSN needle should be held using the right thumb, index, and middle fingers (Fig. 16.14). Care should be taken to avoid touching the casing tube in any way with the fingers.

Next, using the force of the wrist joint (not the elbow joint or shoulder joint), the skin is obliquely penetrated as quickly as possible with the tip of the needle at an angle of about 15 degrees to 25 degrees until the

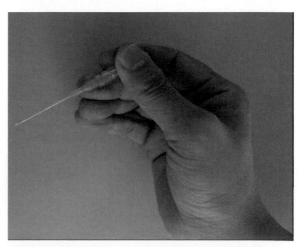

FIG. 16.14 Holding position of a Fu's subcutaneous needling needle.

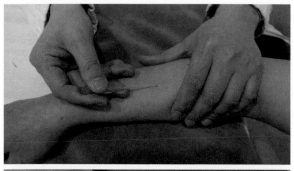

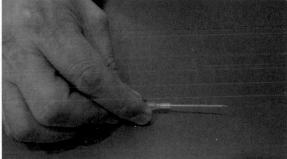

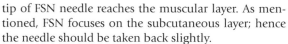

FIG. 16.15 Adjusting the method of holding the needle before taking back.

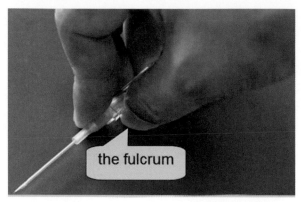

FIG. 16.16 The fulcrum of the swaying movement.

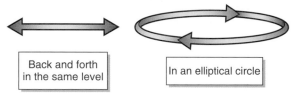

Back and forth in the same level

In an elliptical circle

FIG. 16.17 Two different types of swaying movement.

tip of FSN needle reaches the muscular layer. As mentioned, FSN focuses on the subcutaneous layer; hence the needle should be taken back slightly.

Before taking the FSN needle back, the method of holding the needle should be adjusted: the needle should be loosened first and grasped upward (Fig. 16.15). While slowly moving the needle backwards, the clinician will feel a sudden loosening, which indicates that the needle tip has entered the subcutaneous layer, and at the same time, a skin hunch appears at the insertion point.

Swaying movement

The swaying movement, a key procedure for FSN, is a smooth, soft, fan-style waggle using the thumb as its fulcrum. The index, middle, and ring fingers stay in a line. The middle finger and thumb affix the needle in a face-to-face way, while the index finger and ring finger alternately move back and forth (Fig. 16.16).

The frequency of the swaying movement is about 100 times a minute. The duration of the swaying movement for one insertion point is often less than 2 minutes. After 50 repetitions of the swaying movement (about half a minute), the clinician can palpate the TM or ask the patient about the condition of the problems. If the TM has been deactivated or the patient says the problem has resolved, the swaying movement can be

stopped; otherwise, it should be continued. If the problem persists, the entire needle should be pulled out and the insertion point should be adjusted. In addition, during the swaying movement, the needle tip could be moved back and forth in a line or moved in an elliptical circle (Fig. 16.17).

Together with the work of the right hand, the clinician's left hand or leg should keep on rocking to relax the relevant muscles or joints. Fig. 16.18A through C shows successive photos taken while manipulating the needle in a patient with forearm pain. Note the movement of the sleeve by the practitioner's left hand and the movement of the practitioner's left thigh. Rocking of the relevant muscles or joints is one of the methods referred to as the reperfusion technique.

Reperfusion technique

Chinese acupuncturists often use a particular kind of technique for the treatment of acute painful problems, which is implemented by patients. The patients move their afflicted body part while acupuncturists insert the needles in an area other than the afflicted region. For example, when Chinese acupuncturists treat an acute sprain in a patient with low back pain, they will ask the patient to stand up and rock his back during needling at the acupoint *Renzhong* (DU26). Although widely used, this practical rocking technique has seldom been

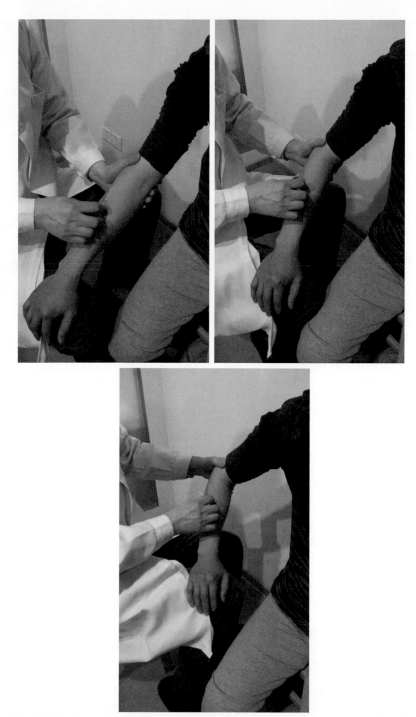

FIG. 16.18 Successive photos when manipulating an arm with upper extremity pain.

introduced in textbooks. At present, this technique has no specific name; sometimes, it is called *Yundong needling* (kinetic needling; Liu et al., 2010), other times, *Dong-Qi* (meaning moving the energy) therapy and movement therapy (Luo & Han, 2010). In the Western world, there are also some similar techniques such as stretching (Edwards & Knowles, 2003).

Inspired by these techniques, Fu applied them to the practice of FSN. To his surprise and delight, these techniques immediately enhanced FSN in many patients, especially those with persistent pain. To say that these techniques are a much better fit for FSN than acupuncture is no exaggeration. The insertion point of acupuncture should be far from the afflicted area when these techniques are applied, but there is no such restriction in FSN because FSN needles are not inserted deep into the muscles. Thus these techniques could be done easily during FSN manipulation, regardless of whether the FSN insertion point is far from or near the afflicted area.

Fu wondered about the mechanism of these techniques, and his search for relevant studies was disappointing as there are only a few studies on these techniques both in Chinese and English. The limited number of studies can probably be blamed on the shortage of appropriate techniques, such as ischaemic compressions, that can be done while exercising. These techniques are known to increase the effectiveness of FSN. Why do they work this way?

In the energy crisis theory (Hong 2002, 2006), the contraction of a muscle segment creates a demand for energy and may restrict the local circulation. Thus improving the local circulation is crucial. FSN can relieve contractures and then improve the local circulation, but this consumes both time and the practitioner's energy. FSN can be better utilised with the help of other methods that can improve the circulation. Can these reperfusion techniques help in improving the circulation? The answer can be illustrated using the change in the hand's skin colour when a fist is clenched and loosened alternately. Fig. 16.19 shows that as soon as the clenched fist loosens, the palm colour resembles a rising tide. After a few minutes, the tide ebbs. This state of flux and reflux is useful for improving circulation.

Fu named the series of techniques the *Reperfusion Approach* (RA). RA refers to the mechanical methods that can cause recirculation in noninflamed ischaemic tissues and includes the repetitive actions applied to relevant soft tissues. Reperfusion is a word found in the phrase 'reperfusion injury', which refers to tissue damage caused when blood supply returns to the tissue after a period of ischaemia. Reperfusion injury is often involved in cerebral vascular accidents, brain trauma, and some-

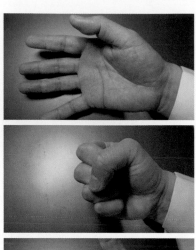
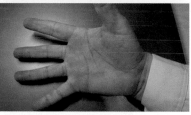

FIG. 16.19 This state of flux and reflux when the fist is clenched and loosened.

times in muscular trauma. Could RA lead to reperfusion injury in ischaemic tissues? This is very unlikely because: (1) ischaemia is a chronic state; and (2) the approach calls for the performance of actions in a successive and repetitive way, which can only improve the circulation.

Fu distinguishes active and passive RA. Active RA means that the actions are carried out by the patient's involved joints or organs. Passive RA means that the actions are implemented by the practitioner or the patient's healthy limbs. The application range of active RA is broader than that of passive RA. Active RA can be used in most instances. Passive RA is more applicable in the following conditions: (1) the patient does not know how to perform the RA; (2) the patient has no idea how to control the amplitude and frequency; and (3) the TM is located in a body part that the patient finds hard to move such as the scalp.

Active RA and passive RA could be used alternatively. Passive RA in small joints can often be implemented by the practitioner, whereas passive RA in large joints can be carried out by either the practitioner or the patient. For different body parts afflicted with musculoskeletal disease, practitioners should use different methods of RA during FSN. The following illustrates some common RAs.

Reperfusion approach for the neck area. In the neck area, passive RAs are applied more commonly than active RAs because the latter easily cause dizziness in nervous or anxious patients. The RAs for the neck should be conducted gently. When the patient is seated, passive RAs can be conducted using several methods. Fig. 16.20 shows the most common types of passive RAs for the neck. When the patient feels uncomfortable with moving the head from side to side, the practitioner could move the patient's head from side to side during FSN. Active RAs for the neck can be performed in a similar way, but the speed should be slow.

Reperfusion approach for the shoulder. When using FSN treatment for painful shoulder problems, the patient is usually seated. RAs in the shoulder can be either passive or active, with the former being used more. Fig. 16.21 shows examples of both passive and

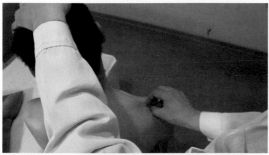
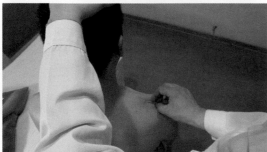
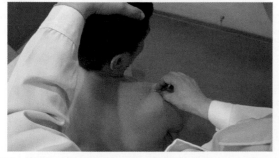

FIG. 16.20 Some reperfusion approaches for the neck area.

active RAs when the patient's upper limbs are difficult to stretch backwards and when patients feel pain while they are stretching their upper limbs. When patients have difficulty raising their arms or they experience pain when they raise the arms, both passive and active RAs are applicable (Fig. 16.22).

Usual reperfusion approach for back pain. For back pain, applicable RAs are summarised in Fig. 16.23. For stubborn painful problems, the patient should assume a kneeling position. In this position, active RAs in the back can often be performed as shown in Fig. 16.24.

Usual reperfusion approach for knee pain. For knee pain, the patient could assume either a sitting position (Fig. 16.25) or a decubitus position (Fig. 16.26).

Retention

After the swaying movement and RA, the solid steel needle core should be removed, while the soft casing tube is retained beneath the skin. Once the patient experiences relief of their symptoms, retention is necessary to maintain and prolong the immediate effects of the treatment. If a patient has no immediate relief another needle insertion point or a different posture should be used until relief is obtained.

The sterile adhesive dressing that is used for retention should be big enough to cover the tube hub and insertion point (Fig. 16.27). Sometimes, adhesive dressings can cause local itching and swelling due to allergy. In this case the rubberised dressing should be changed.

For how long should the retention be maintained? Based on clinical observations, the effect of 24-hour retention is a slightly better than that of 8-hour and 12-hour retention, whereas there are no differences between the effects of 24-, 48-, or 72-hour retention. Considering safety issues, retention time should be at least for 1 to 2 hours. In addition, during the retention the patient should be instructed: (1) not to wet the rubberised area of the fabric; (2) not to work or exercise too much and avoid contracting the muscles surrounding the needling site; (3) not to perspire too much as excessive perspiration may have a negative effect; (4) to pull out the casing tube immediately if the tube moves and causes a stabbing pain; and, (5) not to worry about bleeding when the tube is withdrawn. Simply press the insertion point and the area 2 cm around the insertion point with a sterilised cotton ball for 1 to 2 minutes, and cover with a small adhesive dressing.

In order to gain better effect and to be safer, some practitioners divide one session into two halves, with a retention break for 1 hour. During the break, the

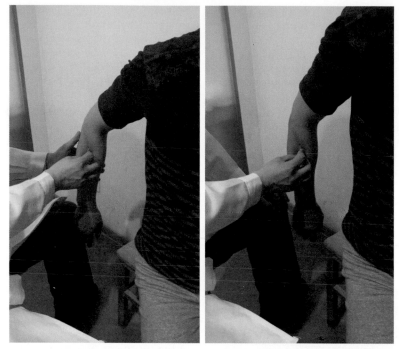

FIG. 16.21 Passive and active reperfusion approaches when it is difficult to stretch the patients' upper limbs backwards.

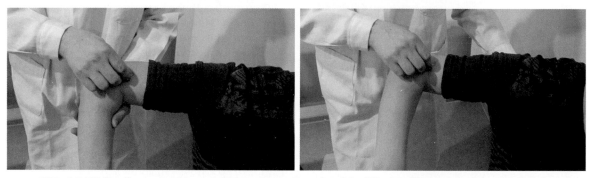

FIG. 16.22 Passive and active reperfusion approaches when it is difficult to lift the patients' upper limbs.

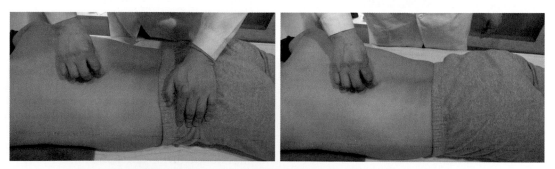

FIG. 16.23 Usual reperfusion approaches for back pain.

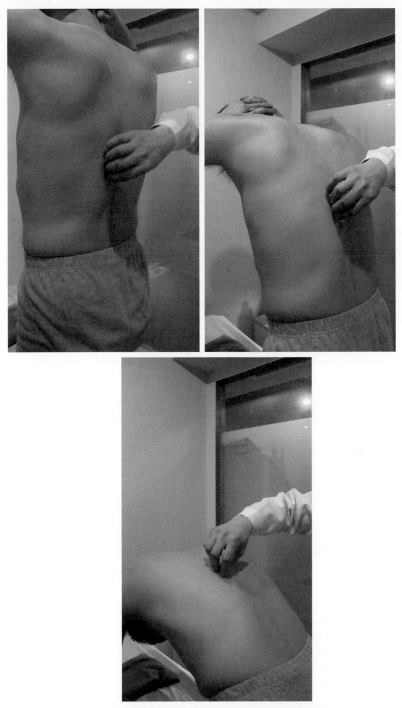

FIG. 16.24 Active reperfusion approach when in a kneeling position for back pain.

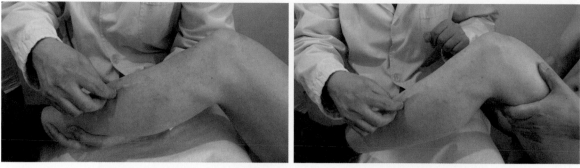

FIG. 16.25 Usual reperfusion approaches with a sitting position.

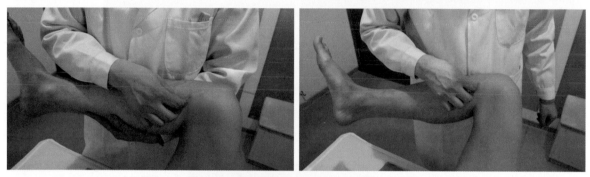

FIG. 16.26 Usual reperfusion approaches with a decubitus position.

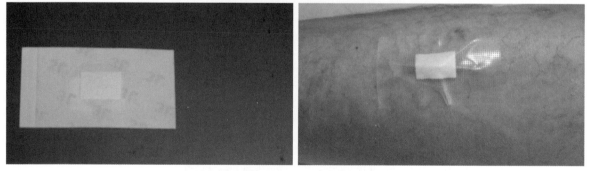

FIG. 16.27 Covering the casing tube.

patients walk around to see if the painful condition subsides. If the pain disappears completely, there is no need to continue the treatment. If the pain persists, the treatment continues. After completion of the second half of the treatment, the practitioner removes the FSN needle without follow-up retention.

PRECAUTIONS, CONTRAINDICATIONS, AND MANAGEMENT OF SIDE EFFECTS

Traditional acupuncture and DN have an extremely good safety record, but in theory, FSN is even safer as the needles are inserted only subcutaneously. However, no form of therapy is absolutely safe. When using FSN, close attention should be given to the following to gain satisfactory effects and to avoid causing patients discomfort.

- FSN treatment should be delayed for those patients who are famished or who have overeaten and also for patients who are intoxicated, overfatigued, or very weak, because these conditions can easily lead to fainting.
- The insertion of an FSN needle into the lower abdomen of pregnant women is contraindicated.

- During needling, blood vessels should be avoided to prevent bleeding, especially in the region of the superficial temporal artery, posterior auricular artery, and radial artery. When a patient suffers from spontaneous haemorrhage or is taking anticoagulant medications, FSN treatment are not indicated.
- FSN patients are more susceptible to infection compared with patients of traditional acupuncture due to the long duration of needle retention. The FSN needle can only be used once. For patients at increased risk of infection, such as patients with diabetes or HIV, more intensive sterilisation should be done.

When performed correctly, FSN is free from any adverse and addictive side effects. However, there are some temporary side effects.

- *Haematoma:* There are many small blood vessels, mostly veins, in the subcutaneous layer. During FSN manipulation, care should be taken to avoid the veins. However, some conditions make it impossible to avoid all blood vessels; hence bruising under the skin sometimes occurs. Bruises often feel tender or swollen in the first few days. If the congestion is severe and causes pain or affects local function, the casing tube should be removed immediately, and a cold compress applied to the local area.
- *Fainting:* Occasionally patients feel faint when undergoing FSN, especially at the start of the first treatment. When patients are faint, they may feel tired, dizzy, or nauseous, and their face may turn pale. Sometimes, patients exhibit autonomic signs such as profuse sweating, flushing, and coldness of the extremities, or even go into syncope or fall to the ground. The prevention of fainting is more important than its treatment. When a patient undergoes FSN treatment for the first time and feels nervous or is in a weak condition, the clinician should explain the FSN procedure and help the patient relax by selecting the most suitable posture. During manipulation, the patient's expressions should be observed; if any sign of faintness is seen, stop the FSN and let the patient lie down. In most cases, the patient will recover within 3 to 5 minutes. Drinking a glass of water may help.

FACTORS THAT INFLUENCE FU'S SUBCUTANEOUS NEEDLING EFFECTS

Many factors may influence the effects of FSN, but some of them such as smoking have not been proven. However, there is some clinical evidence for some of the factors.

Main Factors That Influence Short-Term Effects

- *Oedema:* Stopping FSN treatment is advisable when a patient is suffering from general oedema; that is, if a patient with lupus or rheumatoid arthritis and a painful problem received steroid treatments, FSN will have no effect on the painful problem.
- *Fever:* Regardless of the cause of fever, the effects of FSN are not as good, and FSN should be discontinued until the fever is controlled.
- *Other previous treatments:* Some previous treatments, such as local steroid injections, heavy cupping, herbal plaster medicine, local ointment medicine, and local application of the coupling medium for an ultrasound check, will influence the effects of FSN.
- *Poor manipulation:* If any step of FSN manipulation, especially the swaying movement, has not been performed well, the short-term effect will be negatively affected.
- *Wrong diagnosis:* FSN is good for nontraumatic soft tissue lesions, but not for traumatic lesions such as an acute ankle sprain or pain caused by a hairline fracture. If unsure, the patient should be evaluated further with an x-ray or sonography before proceeding.

Factors That Influence Long-Term Effects

- *Short-term effectiveness:* When there is a good short-term effect, it is likely that there will be a good long-term effect. If the short-term effect is not easily achieved, the long-term effect will probably not be as favourable.
- *Chronicity of the lesion:* When the nontraumatic soft tissue lesion has been present for a long time, the long-term effect will not be as good as when the lesion has only been present for a short time.
- *Completeness of FSN treatment for TMs:* Beginners of FSN can easily deactivate active TMs, but often ignore the palpation and the treatment of latent TMs, which frequently get activated, especially when patients are overfatigued or with changes in the weather.
- *Personal habit:* Some routine habits or customs diminish FSN's long-term effects. These routine habits include watching television in the bedroom, poor posture, repetitive movements at work or leisure activities, using an electric fan when sleeping, prolonged walking or standing, and sleep deprivation. For most chronic conditions, even if the painful problems have gone away after FSN treatment, the involved tissues need time and energy to recover. Under these situations, the effected tissues are over fatigued and the pain will often come back.

- *Health condition:* If the patient suffers from other concurrent diseases such as immunological diseases, chronic infections, hypothyroidism, diabetes, hyperuricemia, or malignancy, the treatment effects may be poor.

FU'S SUBCUTANEOUS NEEDLING FEATURES

As mentioned before, the way the needle is manipulated distinguishes FSN from traditional acupuncture and other needling approaches. In addition, the FSN is quicker and more effective than traditional acupuncture.

Manipulation Features

FSN differs from acupuncture in terms of manipulation of the needle in these aspects:

The selection of the Fu's subcutaneous needling insertion area is based on the nature of tightened muscles or other focal disorders

FSN abandoned traditional acupuncture theories such as meridians and acupoints. Where the FSN needles are inserted depends on where the TMs or other focal disorders are located. The insertion points are always in the vicinity of TMs and other focal disorders, although the distances between the insertion points and the local disorder are variable because of different characters of the disorders.

The Fu's subcutaneous needling needle is inserted into nondiseased areas

Common techniques used in traditional acupuncture include the application of medicated plaster, which is somewhat similar to the use of medicated patches in Western medicine (i.e., lidocaine or fentanyl patches). Another acupuncture technique is known as cupping, whereby local cutaneous suction is created to promote healing. These interventions are commonly applied directly to the afflicted or painful area. In other words, a medicated plaster or a cupping technique is applied where the patient complaints of pain. A solid filament needle used in DN is commonly inserted directly into a local TrP.

Based on the principles of traditional acupuncture, Tseng and colleagues (2008), Tsai and colleagues (2010), and Chou and colleagues (2009, 2011) have demonstrated an effective way to inactivate severely hyperirritable TrPs by needling other TrPs remote to these TrPs. Similarly, FSN acts on nonafflicted areas. The tip of the FSN needle usually does not reach the actual lesion. The FSN needle stimulates a nonafflicted area to

heal the afflicted area. If the patient has oedema, broken skin or swelling in the chosen insertion site, FSN needles should not be inserted and an alternative area must be used or the treatment should be suspended or cancelled. For example, if the surrounding area of the painful spot is swollen, the FSN needle should not be inserted into the swollen part.

The insertion of Fu's subcutaneous needling needle is restricted to the subcutaneous tissue

The needle used in DN goes through the skin, into the subcutaneous layer, and then enters deeply into muscles, whereas the FSN needle stops at the subcutaneous layer (Fig. 16.28).

De-Qi is not required during Fu's subcutaneous needling treatment

In traditional acupuncture, De-Qi is considered an indication of its curative effect (Park et al., 2005; White et al., 2008), which is why most acupuncturists try to induce De-Qi. However, FSN aims to avoid sensations of soreness, swelling, or numbness for the patient, while the clinician does not look for mild resistance or 'needle grasp'.

The Fu's subcutaneous needling needle is retained in the subcutaneous tissues for a prolonged period of time

Retention of needles is seldom mentioned in ancient acupuncture. In modern acupuncture, however, retention is widely used, and the retention often lasts for 15 or 20 minutes, but never goes over 60 minutes. FSN needs a longer retention time, often lasting more than 1 hour. The patient should be allowed to keep on moving even with the FSN needles retained in the subcutaneous region.

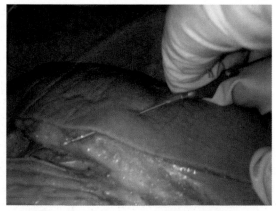

FIG. 16.28 Different layer of Fu's subcutaneous needling and traditional acupuncture.

The tip of Fu's subcutaneous needling needle is directed to the painful region

The acupuncture needle is often inserted perpendicularly or obliquely, whereas the FSN needle is inserted horizontally and directed toward the TM or other focal disorder.

The Fu's subcutaneous needling needle is swayed from side to side

The FSN applies a special technique referred to as 'the swaying movement'. The swaying movement is essential to FSN treatment and provides a curative effect, especially when dealing with chronic disorders. In most circumstances, FSN does not work well without the swaying movement.

The involved muscles and joints can move easily during Fu's subcutaneous needling treatment

Moving afflicted joints and muscles can effectively speed up the recovery from soft tissue injury. As mentioned, the FSN needle is manipulated above the muscular layer, which makes it easy for the medical staff or the patients themselves to move the afflicted joints or muscles even during FSN's swaying movement.

Characteristics of Effectiveness

After 20 years of clinical observations, the principle author defined these characteristics of FSN.

- FSN focuses on treating painful problems, although FSN can also have positive effects on some nonpainful disorders, such as numbness, chronic cough without sputum, and acute onset of asthma.
- FSN can provide relief under most conditions. After the swaying movement, the pain is reduced or completely absent.
- Retention of the FSN needle is usually necessary when symptoms recur frequently, although they are often suppressed after therapy.
- Generally, acupuncture has fewer side effects than many medications, but there are still several adverse effects such as haemorrhage, haematoma, dizziness, fainting, nausea, pneumothorax, prolonged De-Qi effect (paraesthesia), and increased pain (Ernst et al., 2003). However, FSN is safer than acupuncture because the needles do not penetrate deeply and fewer needles are required for each treatment. So far, there have been no cases of nausea, pneumothorax, or a prolonged De-Qi effect.
- FSN has short-term and long-term effectiveness in the treatment of a majority of nontraumatic soft tissue lesions if the afflicted joints and muscles can

have enough recovery time. However, for painful problems caused by malignant tumours, trigeminal neuralgia, and postherpetic neuralgia, FSN only has short-term effects.

- Empirically, FSN treatment appears to achieve an equal or better effect with fewer treatments compared with other manual techniques in current practice, saving time and resources. There is also a complete absence of 'post-treatment tissue soreness' often experienced by patients after other manual therapy interventions, including DN. In addition, because it can often relieve painful problems, such as lower back pain with sciatica, patients may avoid invasive surgical procedures.
- FSN provides immediate feedback, and occasionally FSN can modify the diagnosis based on whether the patient's symptoms are not relieved or reduced immediately. For example, FSN could be used in the neck region in an effort to treat dizziness without an obvious diagnosis. If there is immediate improvement, the diagnosis may be modified to a neck problem causing dizziness.

In the authors' experience, FSN is superior to traditional approaches, but there are also certain disadvantages. For example, FSN is more time-consuming and clinicians need to expend more energy on each patient. FSN can be easily misunderstood by patients and other healthcare providers, because the FSN rationale may be too unconventional. Chinese physicians often doubt the results and effects of FSN, probably because FSN does not obey the rules of traditional Chinese medicine. Furthermore, Chinese patients who are not familiar with FSN often think that their physicians have discreetly injected an anaesthetic or steroid. Future studies confirming the authors' clinical assumptions and experiences are imperative to further determine the effectiveness of FSN versus acupuncture.

ACKNOWLEDGEMENT

The authors thank Professor Chang-Zern Hong for his critical review of the manuscript.

REFERENCES

Amaro, J. (2008). When acupuncture becomes dry needling. *Dynamic Chiropractic, 26*, 1–2.

Baldry, P. (1995). Superficial dry needling at myofascial trigger point sites. *Journal of Musculoskeletal Pain, 3*, 117–126.

Baldry, P. (2000). Superficial dry needling. In L. Chaitow (Ed.), *Fibromyalgia syndrome: a practitioner's guide to treatment*. Edinburgh: Churchill Livingstone.

Baldry, P. (2002). Superficial versus deep dry needling. *Acupuncture in Medicine, 20*, 78–81.

Cao, X. (2002). Scientific bases of acupuncture analgesia. *Acupuncture Electro-Therapeutics Research, 27*, 1–14.

Chen, C. J., & Yu, H. S. (2003). Acupuncture, electro-stimulation, and reflex therapy in dermatology. *Dermatologic Therapy, 16*, 87–92.

Cheng, X. (1987). *Chinese acupuncture and moxibustion.* Beijing: Foreign Languages Press.

Chou, L. W., Hong, J. Y., & Hong, C. Z. (2008). A new technique for acupuncture therapy and its effectiveness in treating fibromyalgia syndrome: a case report. *Journal of Musculoskeletal Pain, 16*(3), 193–198.

Chou, L. W., Hsieh, Y. L., Chen, H. S., Hong, C. Z., Kao, M. J., & Han, T. I. (2011). Remote therapeutic effectiveness of acupuncture in treating myofascial trigger point of the upper trapezius muscle. *American Journal of Physical Medicine & Rehabilitation, 90*, 1036–1049.

Chou, L. W., Hsieh, Y. L., Kao, M. J., & Hong, C. Z. (2009). Remote influences of acupuncture on the pain intensity and the amplitude changes of endplate noise in the myofascial trigger point of the upper trapezius muscle. *Archives of Physical Medicine and Rehabilitation, 90*, 905–912.

Chou, L. W., Hsieh, Y. L., Kuan, T. S., & Hong, C. Z. (2014). Needling therapy for myofascial pain: recommended technique with multiple rapid needle insertion. *Biomedicine, 4*, 39–46.

Chu, J. (1997). Does EMG (dry needling) reduce myofascial pain symptoms due to cervical nerve root irritation? *Electromyography and Clinical Neurophysiology, 37*, 259–372.

Chu, Z., & Bai, D. (1997). Clinical observation of therapeutic effects of wrist-ankle acupuncture in 88 cases of sciatica. *Journal of Traditional Chinese Medicine, 17*, 280–281.

Dommerholt, J., Mayoral, O., & Gröbli, C. (2006). Trigger point dry needling. *The Journal of Manual & Manipulative Therapy, 14*, E70–E87.

Edwards, J., & Knowles, N. (2003). Superficial dry needling and active stretching in the treatment of myofascial pain: a randomised controlled trial. *Acupuncture in Medicine, 21*, 80–86.

Ellis, A., & Wiseman, N. (1991). *Fundamentals of chinese acupuncture.* Brookline, Massachusetts: Paradigm.

Ernst, G., Strzyz, H., & Hagmeister, H. (2003). Incidence of adverse effects during acupuncture therapy—a multicentre survey. *Complementary Therapies in Medicine, 11*, 93–97.

Fu, Z. (1996). Floating needling, a new approach to treat pain. *TCM.* Information 21 Dec, p. 4 (in Chinese).

Fu, Z. (1997). Some successful cases of Fu's acupuncture. *Journal of Clinical Acupuncture Moxibustion*, 24–25 [in Chinese].

Fu, Z. H. (2016). *The foundation of Fu's subcutaneous needling.* Beijing: People's Medical Publishing House Co. [in Chinese].

Fu, Z. H., Chen, X. Y., Lu, L. J., et al. (2006). Immediate effect of Fu's subcutaneous needling for low back pain. *Chinese Medical Journal, 119*, 953–956.

Fu, Z., & Huang, Y. (1999). Floating needling. *International Journal of Clinical Acupuncture, 10*, 51–52.

Fu, Z. H., Wang, J. H., Sun, J. H., Chen, X. Y., & Xu, J. G. (2007). Fu's subcutaneous needling: possible clinical evidence of the subcutaneous connective tissue in acupuncture. *Journal of Alternative and Complementary Medicine, 13*, 47–51.

Fu, Z., & Xu, J. (2005). A brief introduction to Fu's subcutaneous needling. *Pain Clinic, 17*, 343–348.

Ghia, J. N., Mao, W., Toomey, T. C., & Gregg, J. M. (1976). Acupuncture and chronic pain mechanisms. *Pain, 2*, 285–299.

Hong, C. Z. (1994). Lidocaine injection versus dry needling to myofascial trigger point. The importance of the local twitch response. *American Journal of Physical Medicine and Rehabilitation, 73*, 256–263.

Hong, C. Z. (2000). Myofascial trigger points: pathophysiology and correlation with acupuncture points. *Acupuncture in Medicine, 18*, 41–47.

Hong, C. Z. (2002). New trends in myofascial pain syndrome. *Chinese Medical Journal, 65*, 501–512.

Hong, C. Z. (2004). Myofascial pain therapy. *Journal of Musculoskeletal Pain, 12*(3-4), 37–43.

Hong, C. Z. (2006). Treatment of myofascial pain syndrome. *Current Pain and Headache Reports, 10*, 345–349.

Hsieh, Y. L., Kao, M. J., Kuan, T. S., et al. (2007). Dry needling to a key myofascial trigger point may reduce the irritability of satellite MTrPs. *American Journal of Physical Medicine & Rehabilitation, 86*, 397–404.

Huang, Y., Fu, Z. H., Xia, D. B., & Wu, R. K. (1998). Introduction to floating acupuncture: clinical study on the treatment of lateral epicondylitis. *American Journal of Acupuncture, 26*, 27–31.

Jiang, H., Shi, K., Xuemei, L., et al. (2006). Clinical study on the wrist–ankle acupuncture treatment for 30 cases of diabetic peripheral neuritis. *Journal of Traditional Chinese Medicine, 26*, 8–12.

Kim, D. H. (2004). Evolution of acupuncture for pain management. *Seminars in Integrative Medicine, 2*, 135–147.

Langevin, H. M., Bouffard, N. A., Badger, G. J., et al. (2006). Subcutaneous tissue fibroblast cytoskeletal remodeling induced by acupuncture: evidence for a mechanotransduction-based mechanism. *Journal of Cellular Physiology, 207*, 767–774.

Lin, J. G. (1997). Studies of needling depth in acupuncture treatment. *Chinese Medical Journal, 110*, 154–156.

Liu, W. A., Wu, Q. M., Lei, F., et al. (2010). Effect of kinetic needling combined with blood-letting puncturing and cupping on functions of upper limbs of patients with shoulder-hand syndrome after apoplexy. *World Journal of Acupuncture-Moxibustion, 1*, 24–27.

Luo, B. H., & Han, J. X. (2010). Cervical spondylosis treated by acupuncture at Ligou (LR 5) combined with movement therapy. *Journal of Traditional Chinese Medicine, 30*, 113–117.

Melzack, R. (1981). Myofascial trigger points: relation to acupuncture and mechanisms of pain. *Archives of Physical Medicine and Rehabilitation, 62*, 114–117.

Melzack, R., Stillwell, D. M., & Fox, E. J. (1977). Trigger points and acupuncture points for pain: correlations and implications. *Pain, 3*, 3–23.

Park, J., Park, H., Lee, H., et al. (2005). DeQi sensation between the acupuncture-experienced and the naive: a Korean study II. *The American Journal of Chinese Medicine, 33*, 329–337.

Simons, D. G. (2004). New aspects of myofascial trigger points: etiological and clinical. *Journal of Musculoskeletal Pain, 12*, 15–21.

Simons, D. G. (2008). New views of myofascial trigger points: etiology and diagnosis. *Archives of Physical Medicine and Rehabilitation, 89*, 157–159.

Song, B. Z., & Wang, X. Y. (1985). Short-term effect in 135 cases of enuresis treated by wrist–ankle needling. *Journal of Traditional Chinese Medicine, 5*, 27–28.

Tortora, G. J. (1989). *Principles of human anatomy* (5th ed.). London: Longman Higher Education.

Tsai, C. T., Hsieh, L. H., Kuan, T. S., et al. (2010). Remote effects of dry needling on the irritability of the myofascial trigger point in the upper trapezius muscle. *American Journal of Physical Medicine & Rehabilitation, 89*, 133–140.

Tseng, C. L., Kao, M. J., Chou, L. W., & Hong, C. Z. (2008). Injection of remote myofascial trigger points for pain control: a case report. *Taiwan Journal of Physical Medicine and Rehabilitation, 36*, 47–52.

White, P., Bishop, F., Hardy, H., et al. (2008). Southampton needle sensation questionnaire: development and validation of a measure to gauge acupuncture needle sensation. *Journal of Alternative and Complementary Medicine, 14*, 373–379.

White, A., & Ernst, E. (2001). Systematic reviews of acupuncture: is a more profitable discussion possible? *Clin. Acupuncture Oriental Med., 2*, 111–115.

Xia, D. B., & Huang, Y. (2004). Combination of Fu needling with electric acupuncture for tennis elbow. *Di Yi Jun Yi Da Xue Xue Bao, 24*, 1328–1329.

Zhang, C. (2004). An investigation on Fu's acupuncture treating lumbago. *Journal of Clinical Acupuncture Moxibustion, 20*, 2.

Zhu, Z., & Wang, X. (1998). Clinical observation on the therapeutic effects of wrist–ankle acupuncture in treatment of pain of various origins. *Journal of Traditional Chinese Medicine, 18*, 192–194.

Index

Note: Page numbers followed by *f* indicate figures, *t* indicate tables, and *b* indicate boxes.